Little, Brown's Paperback Book Series

Basic Medical Sciences

Boyd & Hoerl	Basic Medical Microbiology
Colton	Statistics in Medicine
Daube et al.	Medical Neurosciences
Friedman	Biochemistry
Kent	General Pathology: A Programmed Text
Levine	Pharmacology
Miller	Peery and Miller's Pathology
Reich	Hematology
Richardson	Basic Circulatory Physiology
Roland et al.	Atlas of Cell Biology
Selkurt	Physiology
Sidman & Sidman	Neuroanatomy: A Programmed Text
Siegel, Albers, et al.	Basic Neurochemistry
Snell	Clinical Anatomy for Medical Students
Snell	Clinical Embryology for Medical Students
Streilein & Hughes	Immunology: A Programmed Text
Valtin	Renal Dysfunction
Valtin	Renal Function
Watson	Basic Human Neuroanatomy

Clinical Medical Sciences

Clark & MacMahon	Preventive Medicine
Eckert	Emergency-Room Care
Grabb & Smith	Plastic Surgery
Green	Gynecology
Gregory & Smeltzer	Psychiatry
Judge & Zuidema	Methods of Clinical Examination
Nardi & Zuidema	Surgery
Niswander	Obstetrics
Thompson	Primer of Clinical Radiology
Wilkins & Levinsky	Medicine
Ziai	Pediatrics

Manuals and Handbooks

Alpert & Francis	Manual of Coronary Care
Arndt	Manual of Dermatologic Therapeutics
Berk et al.	Handbook of Critical Care
Bochner et al.	Handbook of Clinical Pharmacology
Children's Hospital Medical Center, Boston	Manual of Pediatric Therapeutics
Condon & Nyhus	Manual of Surgical Therapeutics
Friedman & Papper	Problem-Oriented Medical Diagnosis
Gardner & Provine	Manual of Acute Bacterial Infections
Iversen & Clawson	Manual of Orthopaedic Therapeutics
Klippel & Anderson	Manual on Techniques of Emergency and Outpatient Surgery
Massachusetts General Hospital	Clinical Anesthesia Procedures
Massachusetts General Hospital	Diet Manual
Massachusetts General Hospital	Manual of Nursing Procedures
Neelon & Ellis	A Syllabus of Problem-Oriented Patient Care
Papper	Manual of Medical Care of the Surgical Patient
Roberts	Manual of Clinical Problems in Pediatrics: Annotated with Key References
Samuels	Manual of Neurologic Therapeutics
Shader	Manual of Psychiatric Therapeutics
Snow	Manual of Anesthesia
Spivak & Barnes	Manual of Clinical Problems in Internal Medicine: Annotated with Key References
Wallach	Interpretation of Diagnostic Tests
Washington University Department of Medicine	Manual of Medical Therapeutics
Zimmerman	Techniques of Patient Care

Hematology : Physiopathologic Basis for Clinical Practice

Hematology:
Physiopathologic Basis
for Clinical Practice

Paul R. Reich, M.D.
Assistant Clinical Professor of Medicine,
Harvard Medical School; Department
of Medicine, Beth Israel Hospital, Boston

with a chapter on blood coagulation
by Daniel Deykin, M.D., Professor of Medicine,
Boston University and Tufts University
Schools of Medicine; Chief, Medical
Service, Veterans Administration Hospital,
Boston

Little, Brown and Company : Boston

Library of Congress Catalog Card No. 78-57424

ISBN 0-316-73860-3 (C)
ISBN 0-316-73861-1 (P)

Printed in the United States of America

To my wife, Dianne

Foreword
from the Series Editor

The goal of the Little, Brown Physiopathology Series is to provide textbooks that describe and illustrate the scientific foundations underlying the current practice of clinical medicine. The concept of this series developed from curricular changes that occurred in many medical schools during the early 1970s. These changes resulted in increased emphasis in the teaching of normal and abnormal human biology, usually to second-year medical students, as the bridge between the traditional basic science courses and the clinical clerkships. A need exists for textbooks in this "bridge" area.

Each book in this series will deal with a different medical subspecialty. Each book will aim to provide a clear and solid discussion of the basic scientific concepts and principles on which the clinical subspecialty is built. This discussion will include selected aspects of normal and abnormal physiology, biochemistry, morphology, cell biology, and so on, as appropriate. The discussion of the basic science material will usually be presented in the context of the approach to the study of clinical material. Major clinical phenomena and disease processes will, in turn, be analyzed in terms of normal and abnormal human biology. Thus, the books will try to show how the art of modern clinical medicine involves firm scientific knowledge and the scientific approach in order to be effective.

Although designed for second-year medical students, this series will, we hope, be useful as well to more advanced students and practitioners as a readable and up-to-date review of the scientific basis for clinical practice in a given area.

DeWitt S. Goodman, M.D.
Department of Medicine
Columbia University College
of Physicians and Surgeons

Preface

This textbook is designed for use by students in an introductory hematology course. Each chapter serves as a unit of study. First, basic physiology and pathology are reviewed with particular attention to defining a vocabulary of hematologic terms, understanding diagnostic tests, and learning normal and abnormal cellular morphology. Stained slides illustrating blood cell morphology should be studied along with the color illustrations bound into this book. Once basic physiopathology and morphology have been mastered, attention should be directed to the approaches outlined for the important problems encountered in medical practice. The case development problems at the end of each chapter serve as a final review that measures the student's fundamental knowledge of the concepts discussed in each chapter. Clinical material chosen to pique student interest is stressed in these problems. The chapter bibliographies are not annotated or complete, but rather direct students who desire to read more about a topic to readily available textbooks and review articles containing detailed discussions and references to original articles. Original articles are cited in areas of ongoing research or where controversies exist. A list of topics for theses, term papers, and seminars is supplied for each chapter. In many cases, particular topics have been selected because knowledge in these areas is growing, changing, and sometimes controversial.

Although primarily intended for medical students enrolled in a hematology course, this textbook should also be suitable for use by nursing and paramedical students, and by house officers and physicians who desire a concise, easily readable overview of common hematologic problems. It could not have been written without my ten-year exposure to students in the Harvard Medical School course in hematology. Nor would it have seen the light of day without the encouragement and patience of Dianne, my wife, and the expertise of Ms. Lin Richter and Ms. Jacqueline Cohen, my editors at Little, Brown.

P. R. R.

Contents

Hematology : Physiopathologic Basis for Clinical Practice

1 : Anemia

Anemia is usually defined as a condition in which the amount of hemoglobin in a patient's red blood cells is reduced. A physiologic definition stresses the inability of an anemic individual to maintain normal tissue oxygenation. This may result from decreased erythrocyte hemoglobin content or reduced red cell number, but it can also be the result of other abnormalities such as defective hemoglobin molecules that unload oxygen from hemoglobin poorly despite a low partial pressure of oxygen (PO_2). If oxygen-carrying capacity is reduced, then compensatory mechanisms come into play, such as increased pulse rate, stroke volume, and therefore cardiac output; increased erythropoietin production; decreased affinity of hemoglobin for oxygen; and diversion of blood from less vital to more vital organs, such as the brain.

These compensatory changes and the inability of blood to meet tissue oxygen requirements lead to signs and symptoms of anemia. These are listed on the next page more or less in order of their appearance in patients with increasingly severe anemia (p. 2). The rapidity of development of the anemia and the patient's physical activity greatly affect the development of these signs and symptoms.

The speed with which anemia develops determines which symptoms are prominent. In acute blood loss the decrease in blood volume, despite adequate cardiac output, leads to inability to maintain blood pressure. Shock, unconsciousness, and ultimately death follow. Once bleeding has stopped, plasma volume can be replenished from preformed stores of albumin, with restoration of blood volume in 24 to 72 hours. However, since there are no preformed stores of erythrocytes, red cell volume may not be replenished for days or weeks, depending on the magnitude of the bleeding. Thus patients recovering from blood loss may avoid the effects of low blood volume but may suffer the chronic symptoms of anemia until enough red cells are available for oxygen transport to meet tissue metabolic requirements.

Erythropoietin

As a result of decreased tissue oxygenation in the kidney, erythropoietin, a hormone that regulates red cell production, appears in increased quantities in the serum and urine. Erythropoietin is a glycoprotein with a molecular weight of 46,000. Although the

1

Symptoms of anemia (roughly in order of appearance in an increasingly anemic patient)

Pallor
Fatigue
Rapid pulse
Shortness of breath
Irritability, difficulty in concentrating
Headache
Dizziness
Nausea and decreased appetite
Menstrual irregularities
Loss of libido or potency
Heart murmurs
Angina pectoris (chest pain with exertion)
Heart failure
Coma

kidney is the chief site of its production or activation, erythropoietin has been difficult to extract from renal tissues. Two explanations have been proposed to explain this discrepancy. One suggests that a material called *renal erythropoietic factor* (REF) or *erythrogenin* is produced in the kidney and that this material acts on a substance manufactured by the liver to yield active erythropoietin. As REF is chemically and immunologically different from erythropoietin, it would not be detected by techniques aimed at extracting erythropoietin. An alternative hypothesis has been advanced by those who believe the kidney contains a lipid inhibitor of erythropoietin. Experimental addition of serum to an erythropoietin–lipid complex releases erythropoietin from the complex. Thus, the release or activation of renal lipid-bound erythropoietin may be moderated by a circulating serum factor. It is possible that both mechanisms are operative in controlling erythropoietin production.

Development of primitive cells into cells recognizable as belonging to the red cell or erythroid series is stimulated by erythropoietin. Cell physiologists found that marrow cells injected into lethally irradiated mice gave rise to homogenous colonies in the spleens of these mice. Using chromosomal markers, they showed that each colony was derived from a single hematopoietic colony-forming cell (CFC, also called colony-forming unit spleen, CFU_s). The CFC was thought to have the potential to develop into either an erythroid, a granulocytic, or a megakaryocytic cell precursor. The pluripotential cell (the CFUs) was called a *stem* cell; and the primitive but committed erythroid cell, which responded to erythropoietin by forming erythrocyte precursors, was designated an *erythropoietin-responsive* cell (ERC). Erythropoietin can act on the ERC to stimulate proliferation of more ERC and to develop ERC into recognizable early erythroid cells.

The effect of erythropoietin stimulation is recognizable in bone marrow and peripheral blood. Before discussing these changes we must review the normal maturation of red cell precursors in the bone marrow. The pluripotential stem cell and the committed erythropoietin-responsive cell have not been definitely identified, although some investigators believe they resemble lymphocytes.

With Wright stain the earliest recognizable erythroid cell is the *erythroblast* or *pronormoblast* (Plate 1), a large cell with blue cytoplasm. It contains a finely reticular and multinucleolated nucleus. When the nuclear chromatin becomes more clumped and nucleoli are lost, the cell is called a *basophilic normoblast* (Plate 2). Hemoglobin is first seen in the *polychromatic normoblast* (Plate 3) as pink material mixed with the blue cytoplasm.

Its nucleus is smaller and contains more clumped chromatin than the basophilic normoblast. This cell represents the last stage in which DNA synthesis and cell division can occur. The *orthochromatic normoblast* (Plate 4) has a pink or gray cytoplasm and a small pyknotic nucleus. With further maturation the nucleus is extruded, but some ribonuclear protein remains; with Wright stain the cytoplasm has a diffuse basophilic appearance. The overall cell size remains larger than the normal mature erythrocyte. This cell is called a *reticulocyte* (Plate 5), since the ribonuclear protein appears as a blue reticular network when stained supravitally with new methylene blue. The reticulocyte normally remains in the marrow for one day and then circulates in the bloodstream for another day before it becomes a normal adult red cell. If a nucleated erythroid precursor escapes into the peripheral blood, it is called a *nucleated red cell*. Ordinarily the complete maturation sequence from erythroblast to adult red cell takes 4 to 6 days. The normal life span of the adult erythrocyte is 120 days.

The erythropoietin-stimulated marrow has a greater than normal number of nucleated red cells. The peripheral blood contains macrocytic polychromatophils derived from early denucleation of basophilic and polychromatic normoblasts. These *stress reticulocytes* contain increased amounts of cytoplasmic ribonuclear proteins, which when stained supravitally show the blue reticular network characteristic of reticulocytes. Since they have been released early from the bone marrow, their maturation into normal erythrocytes takes approximately two days rather than one.

Biochemical studies have shown that erythropoietin acts first to increase production of several species of RNA and then to increase DNA and protein synthesis. New erythroid cell components are produced, and finally hemoglobin synthesis begins. It is not clear what is the primary biochemical event triggered by erythropoietin, nor how many of the effects attributed to erythropoietin are direct rather than a consequence of the initial inductive steps in the differentiation of the ERC.

Red Cell 2,3-Diphosphoglycerate (2,3-DPG)

Erythropoietin, by increasing the number of hemoglobin-containing erythrocytes in the peripheral blood, enhances blood oxygen-carrying capacity and thereby tissue oxygenation. Another mechanism by which tissue oxygenation is enhanced in the face of anemia involves the affinity of oxygen for hemoglobin. If oxygen is more easily released from hemoglobin, then less hemoglobin is required to maintain normal tissue oxygen supply. This is illustrated in Figure 1. In both normal and anemic individuals there is a blood oxygen dissociation curve, sigmoid in shape,

Fig. 1 : Oxygen dissociation curve of hemoglobin

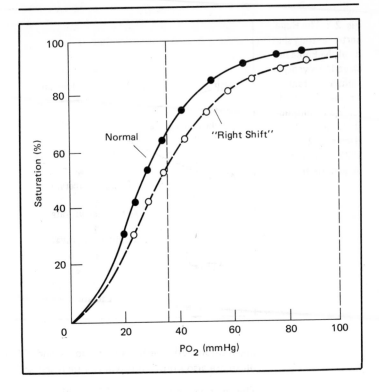

which describes the relationship between oxygen content (percentage of saturation), determined colorimetrically, and partial pressure of oxygen (PO_2), determined by special electrodes. At arterial PO_2 of 100 mm Hg a normal subject (upper curve in Figure 1) carries approximately 20 ml of oxygen per deciliter of whole blood, while at venous PO_2 of 40 mm Hg, the oxygen content is approximately 15 ml of oxygen per deciliter of whole blood. The 5.0 ml/dl of blood difference represents oxygen released to tissues. The sigmoid curve can be shifted to the right (decreased oxygen affinity) by a decrease in pH (Bohr effect), an increase in temperature, or hypoxic conditions such as altitude adaption or anemia. In an anemic patient, if arterial PO_2 is maintained, this rightward shift, or decrease in oxygen affinity, will lead to greater release of oxygen to hypoxic tissue.

The shift of the oxygen dissociation curve in anemic individuals is mediated by the phosphate ester 2,3,-diphosphoglycerate (2,3-DPG). It is produced from 1,3-diphosphoglycerate by the action of a mutase enzyme (Fig. 2). This enzyme is inhibited by free 2,3-DPG. Since 2,3-DPG binds readily with deoxygenated hemoglobin, hypoxia will release this product inhibition. Deoxygenated hemoglobin is more alkaline than oxygenated, and alkaline pH stimulates glycolysis, thereby increasing 2,3-DPG

Fig. 2 : The Rapoport-Luebering shuttle of the Embden Meyerhof glycolytic pathway. (From Grimes, A. J., Red cell 2,3-diphosphoglycerate. Br. J. Haematol. 25:555, 1973. Reproduced by permission.)

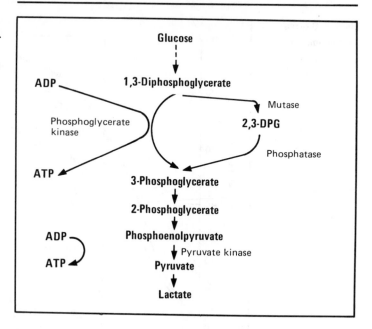

production. Other effects of hypoxia and pH on 2,3-DPG metabolism are also known but will not be discussed here.

The manner by which 2,3-DPG binding to deoxyhemoglobin affects oxygen affinity is complex. Basically the binding of the 2,3-DPG molecule to the central cavity between the β-chains of deoxyhemoglobin increases the affinity of the oxygen-binding site located near the heme irons, a so-called *heterotropic interaction*. These binding sites are also affected by their state of oxygenation, that is, oxygenation of one site on a hemoglobin molecule enhances affinity for oxygen at a different but chemically identical site. This *heme-heme* or *homotropic interaction* is expressed in the sigmoid shape of the hemoglobin oxygen dissociation curve. Certain characteristics of this curve — for example, P_{50}, the partial pressure at which 50 percent of hemoglobin is saturated — are used clinically to measure changes in hemoglobin oxygen affinity.

Quantitation and Characterization of Anemia

Hemoglobin concentration is determined by converting hemoglobin to methemoglobin (converting the elemental iron in heme from the ferrous to the ferric state) and then to cyanmethemoglobin. Cyanmethemoglobin absorbs light at 540 nanometers, and the concentration of hemoglobin varies logarithmically as a function of its light absorption at 540 nm. Sources of error include variations in patients' plasma volume and the relative insolubility of certain abnormal hemoglobins such as sickle cell hemoglobin, which clouds the solution and thereby falsely

Table 1-1 : Blood Counts in Normal Adults

Measurement	Males		Females	
	Mean	95% Range	Mean	95% Range
Hemoglobin (gm/dl)	16.0	14.0–18.0	14.0	12.0–16.0
Packed cell volume (PCV, L/L)	0.46	0.41–0.51	0.42	0.37–0.47
Erythrocyte ($\times 10^{12}$/L)	5.2	4.4–6.0	4.8	4.2–5.5

Adapted from Wintrobe, M. M., et al, *Clinical Hematology,* 7th ed., p. 1791. Philadelphia: Lea & Febiger, 1974.

elevates the hemoglobin concentration. All forms of hemoglobin (oxyhemoglobin and deoxyhemoglobin, carboxyhemoglobin, and methemoglobin) except sulfhemoglobin are converted to cyanmethemoglobin. Normal values for hemoglobin, packed cell volume (PCV), and erythrocyte number are shown in Table 1-1.

The packed cell volume (PCV) or *hematocrit* is determined by centrifugation of blood in a heparinized capillary tube. The volume of packed red cells relative to the total volume of blood, expressed as a decimal, is the PCV. Sources of error include changes in patient's plasma volume, inadequate mixing or centrifugation, and expression of relatively larger amounts of plasma than red cells when obtaining blood by fingerstick. This measurement is most frequently used in clinical practice, because it can be done quickly and accurately with minimal equipment.

The red cell count (RBC or RCC) was in the past performed with a hemocytometer or counting chamber. A suitably diluted specimen of blood was placed in a chamber of known volume and the red cells enumerated with the use of a microscope. This method was notoriously inaccurate because of a large dilution factor and the difficulty of evenly distributing the red cells in the counting chamber. The development of electronic particle counting meant a vast improvement in the accuracy of red cell counting and also allowed automated determination of the hematocrit.

The Coulter principle for cell counting is most widely used. A known volume of blood is mixed with a measured amount of isotonic electrolyte solution, and the mixture is passed through a small orifice between two electrodes. An electric current is applied to the electrodes. Since a red cell is a relative nonconductor and displaces a volume of conducting electrolyte solution it induces a change in the current flowing between the electrodes. This results in electric pulses whose number, when appropriately corrected for coincidence, represents the red cell count. By averaging the pulse heights and with proper standardization

Erythrocyte (Wintrobe) indices in normal adults*

MCV (mean corpuscular volume)

$$= \frac{\text{PCV (packed cell volume) (L/L)} \times 1000}{\text{red cell count } (\times 10^{12}/\text{L})}$$

Normal values: [†]82–101 femtoliters per cell

$$\text{MCH (mean corpuscular hemoglobin)} = \frac{\text{hemoglobin (gm/dl)} \times 10}{\text{red cell count } (\times 10^{12}/\text{L})}$$

Normal values: [†]27–34 picograms per cell

MCHC (mean corpuscular hemoglobin concentration)

$$= \frac{\text{hemoglobin (gm/dl)}}{\text{PCV (packed cell volume) (L/L)}}$$

Normal values: [†] 31.5–36.0 grams per deciliter

*Adapted from Wintrobe, M. M., et al, *Clinical Hematology,* 7th ed., pp. 117 and 1791. Philadelphia: Lea & Febiger, 1974.
[†]Using Coulter model S and 95 percent limits.

against particles of known volume, mean cell volume (MCV) is determined. Since packed cell volume is the product of mean cell volume and red cell number, a hematocrit value can be electronically calculated.

These electronic counters have the advantage of being able to count many cells and to disregard values distinctly different from the mean. Large numbers of white cells will affect the red cell count, but normal numbers are too small to be a problem. Another potential source of error is agglutination or sticking together of red cells. This results in falsely low red cell counts and hematocrit values. It is best to use blood obtained by venipuncture, since blood obtained by fingerstick may contain an unrepresentatively high concentration of plasma.

Other red cell indices (Wintrobe indices) can be calculated manually or by computer from the hemoglobin, hematocrit, and red blood cell count. The formulas for mean cell volume (MCV), mean cell hemoglobin content (MCH) and mean cell hemoglobin concentration (MCHC) are as shown here. Since these indices represent average values, their calculation does not replace a careful examination of the stained peripheral blood smear for abnormalities of size, shape, or color.

Reticulocyte Count and Reticulocyte Production Index

Bone marrow erythroid activity is usually reflected in the peripheral blood reticulocyte count. To obtain this count, one drop of whole blood is mixed with two drops of new methylene blue and, after incubation for 15 minutes, a blood smear is made. One thousand red cells are scanned with an oil immersion lens (2,000 cells give better statistical accuracy with reticulocyte counts of less than 5 percent), and the number of cells with dark blue strands or particles, usually appearing as a reticular network, are counted (see Plate 5). Normal values are 0.5-2.0 percent or, in "absolute" numbers (reticulocyte count as a decimal multiplied by RBC), $20-100 \times 10^9$ per liter.

In the presence of anemia the reticulocyte percentage does not accurately reflect reticulocyte production, since each reticulocyte released is being diluted into fewer adult red cells. A better measure of erythroid production is the *reticulocyte production index* (RPI). The reticulocyte percentage is first corrected to a normal hematocrit of 0.45. For example, a reticulocyte percentage of 10 percent in a patient with a hematocrit of 0.23 would be equivalent to a percentage of 5 percent in a patient with a hematocrit of 0.45. Another correction is made because erythropoietin production in response to anemia leads to premature release of newly formed reticulocytes, and these stress reticulocytes take two days rather than one to mature into adult erythrocytes. If many polychromatophils are seen, then a correction factor of 2.0 is divided into the corrected reticulocyte percentage, for example

$$RPI = \frac{10 \times 23/45 \text{ (hematocrit correction)}}{2.0 \quad \text{(maturation time correction)}} = 2.5$$

Maturation factors from 1.0 to 2.0 are used, the higher numbers if there is a great deal of polychromatophilia in the peripheral blood smear, and the lower numbers if there is little. A method of correction using only the hematocrit is also available (Fig. 3). The reticulocyte production index is an approximate measure of effective red cell production. A normal marrow has an index of 1. In hemolytic anemia, with excessive destruction of red cells in the peripheral blood and a functionally normal marrow, this index may be three to seven times higher than normal. When there is marrow damage, erythropoietin suppression, or a deficiency of iron, vitamin B_{12}, or folic acid, the index is less than expected from the degree of anemia — that is, 2 or less. Ineffective erythropoiesis, with intramedullary (marrow) destruction of erythroid precursors, can be deduced if the marrow contains many normoblasts but the reticulocyte production index is low.

Red Cell Mass

Since PCV and hemoglobin concentration are affected by abnormalities in plasma volume, a patient with a normal mass of erythrocytes will have a low PCV if his plasma volume is abnormally large. Similarly a high hemoglobin concentration can be due to salt depletion and dehydration with a resulting low plasma volume. To avoid these sources of error, red cell mass can be directly measured by a radioisotope dilution assay. An aliquot of the patient's blood is incubated with radioactive chromium 51, which attaches to the β-chains of hemoglobin within the erythrocyte, and then unbound chromium 51 is washed free. A known number of counts per minute of radiochromium in a known volume of blood (e.g., 5 ml) is injected back into the patient. After allowing time for mixing, another 5-ml blood sample is drawn and the counts per minute of radioactivity determined. A simple calculation

$$\frac{\text{counts per minute injected}}{\text{counts per minute sampled}} = \frac{\text{red cell mass (ml)}}{5 \text{ ml}}$$

yields the red cell mass (in milliliters) independent of plasma volume. The only major source of error is the potential for damaging red cells during the labeling procedure. If this occurs, the damaged radioactive red cells are removed from the circulation by the spleen, and a falsely high red cell mass is obtained.

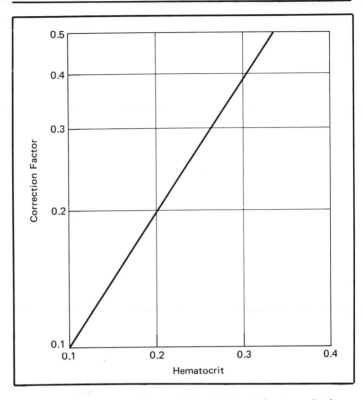

Fig. 3 : This graph is used for calculation of the reticulocyte production index from the patient's hematocrit (PVC) and percentage reticulocyte count. It corrects for the decreased number of adult erythrocytes in anemic patients and for the increased maturation time of reticulocytes, due to early release, in the peripheral blood of these patients. Maturation time lengthens progressively with increasing anemia. To calculate the reticulocyte production index, use the patient's hematocrit to determine the correction factor. Multiply the reticulocyte count, as a percentage, by the correction factor. For example, a patient with a 10% reticulocyte count and a PCV of 0.30 has a reticulocyte production index of 10 X 0.38 = 3.8. [Adapted from Hillman, R., and Finch, C., Red Cell Manual (4th ed.), p. 60. Philadelphia: F. A. Davis, 1974.]

Normal values for red cell mass are *25* to *30* ml per kilogram of body weight in the male and *22* to *28* ml per kilogram in the female. Red cell mass determinations are not used often in the clinical practice of hematology, since the PCV and hemoglobin concentration usually accurately reflect red cell mass.

APPROACH TO PATIENT WITH ANEMIA

Three steps are carried out in the diagnostic approach to an anemic patient (see pp. 12-13). First, the medical history is taken to obtain the patient's symptoms that provide clues to the cause of anemia (e.g., blood loss, drugs, and inherited diseases). Second, the physical examination is carried out to determine the effect of

Approach to patient with anemia

I. History
   A. Symptoms of anemia
      1. Chest pain on exertion (angina)
      2. Dizziness and syncope (fainting)
      3. Fatigue and weakness
      4. Rapidity of onset of symptoms
      5. Response of anemia to therapy
      6. Shortness of breath
   B. Blood loss
      1. Gastrointestinal — hematemesis (vomiting blood); melena (black stools); hemorrhoidal bleeding; hematochezia (red blood in stools)
      2. Bleeding at operation or delivery
      3. Respiratory — hemoptysis (coughing blood); epistaxis (nosebleed)
      4. Uterine — menorrhagia (excessive bleeding); metrorrhagia (irregular bleeding)
      5. Other — hematuria (blood in urine); purpura (black and blue marks)
   C. Bleeding tendency
      1. Bleeding after trauma, operations (circumcision, tonsillectomy), deliveries, and tooth extractions
      2. Bleeding into joints
      3. Menstrual bleeding
      4. Petechiae (capillary hemorrhages appearing as red splinters)
      5. Spontaneous purpura
   D. Iron deficiency anemia
      1. Blood loss (see B.)
      2. Glossitis (sore or inflamed tongue)
      3. Pregnancies and iron supplementation
   E. Megaloblastic anemia
      1. Foul-smelling diarrhea with greasy stools
      2. Glossitis
      3. Parasthesias (tingling toes or fingers); difficulty with gait
   F. Drugs and toxins
      1. Alcohol
      2. Occupational exposures
      3. Therapeutic medications
      4. Toxins
   G. Miscellaneous
      1. Bone pain
      2. Jaundice (yellow skin)
      3. Weight loss
   H. Family history
      1. Anemia
      2. Racial and geographic derivation
      3. Recurrent jaundice
      4. Splenomegaly
II. Physical examination
   A. Vital signs
      1. Blood pressure, pulse, temperature
      2. Orthostatic hypotension (lowered blood pressure, upon standing or sitting)
   B. Skin
      1. Leg ulcers
      2. Nail beds — koilonychia (spoon-shaped nails)
      3. Pallor (pale skin)
      4. Purpura, petechiae
      5. Spider angioma (spider-shaped capillaries) and other signs of chronic liver disease

C. Conjunctivae
   1. Jaundice
   2. Pallor
   3. Petechiae
D. Fundi
   1. Papilledema
   2. Petechiae, hemorrhage
E. Mouth
   1. Lips — cheilosis (split lips), angular stomatitis (sores at angles of lips)
   2. Mucus membranes — pallor, petechiae
   3. Tongue — redness, atrophy of papilla
   4. Uremic breath
F. Lymph nodes
   1. Enlargement in cervical (neck), axillary, inguinal (groin), epitrochlear (near elbow), or other areas
G. Bones
   1. Tenderness over sternum, ribs, or vertebrae
H. Cardiorespiratory system
   1. Cardiac gallop
   2. Heart murmurs
   3. Peripheral edema
   4. Pulmonary râles
I. Abdomen
   1. Hepatomegaly
   2. Splenomegaly
   3. Masses
   4. Ascites
J. Neurologic examination
   1. Loss of vibratory or position sense
   2. Positive Romberg sign (inability to stand upright with eyes closed)
   3. Peripheral neuritis
K. Pelvic and rectal examination
   1. Bleeding
   2. Tumors
III. Laboratory data
   A. Hematocrit and hemoglobin
   B. Wintrobe indices
   C. Reticulocyte count
   D. White cell count and differential
   E. Platelet estimation
   F. Peripheral blood smear
   G. Bone marrow aspirate or biopsy
   H. Special tests
      1. Schilling test for vitamin B_{12} absorption
      2. Serum iron and total iron-binding capacity
      3. Vitamin B_{12} and folic acid serum levels
      4. Others as determined by patient's problem

the anemia on vital functions and to help pinpoint its etiology (e.g., splenomegaly, tumors, bleeding). Important information obtainable from the history and physical examination is listed in the outline as are definitions of medical terms used for certain signs and symptoms. Finally, laboratory tests are performed to quantitate and characterize the anemia and the status of the other blood elements, white cells, and platelets. Most importantly, the peripheral blood smear is examined for clues to the etiology of the anemia. Often the bone marrow specimen must be examined before a definitive diagnosis can be made. Special tests (e.g., serum iron, vitamin B_{12}, and folate levels) are often done to confirm the diagnosis made from the history, physical examination, blood counts, and blood smear. The extensiveness of the laboratory testing depends on the nature of the hematologic problem, and the list of special tests is by no means complete. Subsequent chapters will explain how all this information is used to diagnose and treat anemia.

Since examination of the peripheral blood and bone marrow is central to the diagnostic workup, an approach to the interpretation of these specimens will be discussed here.

Peripheral Blood Smear

Blood obtained by venipuncture (anticoagulated with ethylene diaminetetraacetic acid [EDTA] or potassium oxylate) or by fingerstick is smeared on cover slips or glass slides and then stained with Wright stain. With the oil immersion objective (100X), the smear should first be examined for abnormalities in erythrocyte size or shape. Table 1-2 describes common morphologic abnormalities and the diseases associated with them. The white blood cells should be examined next, and a differential count performed. The platelet number can be estimated by counting how many of these small blue particles (Plate 6) are present in a high power field. Normally there is an average of 15-20 per high power field. The white cells and platelets are produced in the marrow, and any abnormality that produces anemia may affect these blood elements as well. White cells are primarily used to prevent or fight infection. The platelet is an important component of the blood clotting mechanism. The diagnosis of anemia often is helped by study of all three blood elements, as is made clear in subsequent chapters.

Bone Marrow Examination

A specimen of marrow can be obtained by *aspiration* of spicules through a hollow needle placed in the intramedullary cavity of the anterior or posterior iliac crest or the sternum (see p. 17). If aspiration fails (a so-called *dry tap*); if the marrow is thought to be infiltrated or replaced by granuloma, fibrosis, or tumor; or if hypoplasia of the marrow is suspected, then a bone marrow *biopsy* should be performed. A large bore needle is inserted into the

Table 1-2 : Peripheral Blood (Red Cell) Abnormalities

Abnormality	Description	Associated Diseases
Anisocytosis diameter	Abnormal variation in size (normal diameter = 6–8 μm)	Any severe anemia, e.g., iron deficiency, megaloblastic
Microcytosis (Plate 9)	Small cells, less than 6 μm (MCV < 80 fl)	Iron deficiency and iron-loading (sideroblastic) anemia, thalassemia, lead poisoning
Macrocytosis	Large cells, greater than 8 μm (MCV > 100 fl)	Megaloblastic anemia, liver disease, hypothyroidism, hemolytic anemia (reticulocytes), multiple myeloma, physiologic macrocytosis of newborn, myelophthisis
Macroovalocytosis (Plate 17)	Large (> 8 μm) oval cells	Megaloblastic anemia
Hypochromia (Plate 10)	Pale cells with decreased concentration of hemoglobin (MCHC < 30gm/dl)	Iron deficiency and iron-loading (sideroblastic) anemia, thalassemia, lead poisoning, transferrin deficiency, anemia of chronic disease (inflammatory diseases, e.g., rheumatoid arthritis, collagen diseases, malignancies)
Poikilocytosis (Plate 13)	Abnormal variation in shape	Any severe anemia — e.g., megaloblastic, iron deficiency, myeloproliferative syndrome, hemolytic; certain shapes are diagnostically helpful (see following, Spherocytosis through Teardrop cells)
Spherocytosis (Plate 24)	Spherical cells without pale centers; often small, i.e., microspherocytosis	Hereditary spherocytosis, Coombs'-positive hemolytic anemia; small numbers are seen in any hemolytic anemia and after transfusion of stored blood
Ovalocytosis (Plate 25)	Oval cells	Hereditary eliptocytosis, iron deficiency
Stomatocytosis	Red cells with slit-like, instead of circular, areas of central pallor	Congenital hemolytic anemia, thalassemia, burns, lupus erythematosus, lead poisoning, liver disease, artefact
Sickle cells (Plate 27)	Crescent-shaped cells	Sickle cell hemoglobinopathies
Target cells (Plate 11)	Cells with a dark center and periphery and a clear ring in between	Liver disease, thalassemia, hemoglobinopathies (S, C, SC, S-thalassemia)
Schistocytes (Plate 13)	Irregularly contracted cells (severe poikilocytosis)	Uremia, carcinoma, hemolytic-uremic syndrome, disseminated intravascular coagulation, microangiopathic hemolytic anemia, toxins (lead, phenylhydrazine), burns, thrombotic thrombocytopenic purpura
Helmet cells (Plate 31)	A type of schistocyte shaped like military helmet	Uremia, hemolytic-uremic syndrome, disseminated intravascular coagulation, microangiopathic hemolytic anemia, burns, thrombotic thrombocytopenic purpura

Table 1–2 (Continued)

Abnormality	Description	Associated Diseases
"Spur" cells ("burr" cells) (Plate 26)	Cells with long, sharp, irregularly spaced, spinous processes	Hemolytic anemias, liver disease ("spur cell" anemia), normal infants, uremia, microangiopathic hemolytic anemia, disseminated intravascular coagulation, thrombotic thrombocytopenic purpura, pyruvate kinase deficiency, carcinoma
Acanthocytosis	Small cells with thorny projections; similar to burr cells	Abetalipoproteinemia (hereditary acanthocytosis or Bassen-Kornzweig disease)
Teardrop cells (Plate 12)	Cells shaped like teardrops	Myeloproliferative syndrome, myelophthisic anemia (neoplastic, granulomatous, or fibrotic marrow infiltration), anemia with extramedullary hematopoiesis or ineffective erythropoiesis
Nucleated red cells (Plate 4)	Erythrocytes with nuclei still present; may be normoblastic or megaloblastic	Hemolytic anemias, leukemias, myeloproliferative syndrome, polycythemia vera, myelophthisic anemia (neoplastic, granulomatous, or fibrotic marrow infiltration), multiple myeloma, extramedullary hematopoiesis, megaloblastic anemias, any severe anemia
Howell-Jolly bodies (Plate 30)	Spherical blue bodies (Wright stain) within or on erythrocytes; nuclear debris	Hyposplenism, pernicious anemia
Heinz inclusion bodies	Small round inclusions seen under phase microscopy or with supravital staining	Congenital hemolytic anemias (e.g., glucose-6-phosphate dehydrogenase deficiency), hemolytic anemia secondary to drugs (dapsone, phenacetin), thalassemia (Hb H), hemoglobinopathies (Hb Zurich, Köln, Ube, I, etc.)
Pappenheimer bodies (siderocytes) (Plates 15 and 16)	Siderotic granules, staining blue with Wright or Prussian blue stains	Iron-loading anemias, hyposplenism, hemolytic anemias
Cabot rings	Purple, fine, ring-like, intraerythrocytic structures	Pernicious anemia, lead poisoning
Reticulocytosis (basophilia, polychromatophilia, basophilic stippling) (Plates 5 and 23)	Blue, reticular (RNA) network in erythrocytes stains supravitally with new methylene blue; appear as macrocytes with diffuse basophilia (polychromasia), polychromatophilia, or punctate stippling when Wright-stained	Hemolytic anemia, blood loss, uremia, following treatment of iron deficiency or megaloblastic anemias; punctate stippling seen in lead poisoning (mitochondrial RNA and iron)
Rouleaux (Plate 66)	Aggregated erythrocytes regularly stacked on one another	Multiple myeloma, Waldenström's macroglobulinemia, cord blood, pregnancy, hypergammaglobulinemia, hyperfibrinogenemia, cold agglutinin disease, viral infections, malignancies

Suspected hematologic diagnoses for which bone marrow aspiration should be performed

Acute leukemia
Agranulocytosis
Aplastic anemia
Hypersplenism
Idiopathic thrombocytopenic purpura
Iron deficiency (estimation of iron stores)
Lipid storage disease
Lymphoma
Megaloblastic anemia
Metastatic tumor
Multiple myeloma
Waldenström's macroglobulinemia

marrow and a core of intramedullary bone is cut and removed. The specimen (Plate 69) is decalcified, sectioned, and stained with hematoxylin and eosin (H&E), and if indicated, with special stains for fibrosis, amyloid, or tuberculosis. The suspected diagnoses for which bone marrow biopsy is often performed are listed on page 19.

A bone marrow *examination* should include at least the procedures listed under Aspirate in the outline, page 20. The marrow spicules obtained by aspiration are smeared on either cover slips or glass slides. These preparations are then stained with either Wright or Giemsa stain and with Prussian blue for iron. The clot that remains after preparation of the smears is fixed in Zenker's or formalin solution, and then paraffin sections are made. These are stained with H&E and with Prussian blue for iron (Plate 70). Iron stains are done on both the aspirated specimen and the sectioned clot, because the former is particularly helpful for quantitating intracellular iron and detecting ringed sideroblasts (sideroblastic anemias), and the clot section readily demonstrates extracellular iron stores. If a bone biopsy specimen is obtained, touch preparations should be made on glass slides at the time of the biopsy and stained with Wright or Giemsa stain. The marrow biopsy core is then submitted for sectioning and staining with H&E and Prussian blue for iron. The clot section and bone marrow biopsy sections are particularly useful for determining cellularity of the bone marrow. Other special studies may be required as part of the bone marrow examination (see II–V of the outline). Table 1-3 lists common morphologic abnormalities found in bone marrow specimens.

After all the relevant data are available, an attempt should be made to classify the anemia. Most often this is possible at the time of initial workup, but establishment of a definite and specific etiology may require special studies. In the next section a clinically useful classification scheme is described.

Classification of
Anemias

Many different classifications of anemia have been proposed. In Table 1-4 two widely used classifications, morphologic and physiologic, are outlined, along with a third classification scheme that emphasizes the size of red cells and their degree of hemoglobinization.

According to the morphologic classification (I), anemic patients with normal-sized cells and normal hemoglobinization have *normocytic, normochromic anemia* and usually are found to be suffering from blood loss, hemolytic, aplastic, or myelophthisic anemias. *Hemolytic anemias* are those due to increased red cell destruction and *aplastic anemias* are those due to bone marrow

Suspected hematologic diagnoses for which bone marrow biopsy should be performed

Amyloidosis
Aplastic anemia
Granulomatous diseases (tuberculosis)
Lymphoma
Metastatic tumor
Myeloproliferative syndrome (myelofibrosis)
Thrombotic thrombocytopenic purpura

Bone marrow examination

I.   Aspirate
    A. Glass slide or cover slip smears of marrow particles
       1. Wright or Giemsa stain
       2. Iron (Prussian blue) stain
       3. Special cytochemical stains, if indicated, for tuberculosis, fungi, fibrosis, amyloid, etc.
    B. Paraffin section of clot after fixation in Zenker's solution
       1. H & E stain
       2. Iron stain
II. Biopsy obtained with Westerman-Jensen or Jamshidi needle
    A. Touch prep or imprint stained with Wright or Giemsa stain
    B. H & E stain of paraffin section
    C. Iron stain
    D. Special stains, if indicated, for tuberculosis, fungi, fibrosis, amyloid, etc.
III. Bacteriologic studies
IV. Cytogenetic studies (e.g., Philadelphia chromosome)
V.   Phase microscopy (e.g., wet prep for thalassemic inclusion bodies)

Table 1-3 : Bone Marrow Morphologic Abnormalities

Abnormality	Description	Associated Diseases
Cellularity Hypercellularity	Increased number of cellular elements as determined by paraffin section	Myelophthisic anemia (infiltration by neoplastic, Gaucher, or Niemann-Pick cells), leukemia, tuberculosis, aplastic anemia with ineffective erythropoiesis (see also myeloid, erythroid, and megakaryocytic hyperplasia)
Hypocellularity (aplastic)	Decreased number of cellular elements, except fibroblasts, as determined by paraffin section	Aplastic anemia, paroxysmal nocturnal hemoglobinuria, myeloproliferative syndrome, irradiation, tuberculosis (see also myeloid, erythroid, and megakaryocytic hypoplasia)
Erythroid hyperplasia	Increased number of erythroid precursors; M:E ratio decreased ($<$ 2:1)	Blood loss, iron deficiency, hemolytic anemias, thalassemia, polycythemia vera, megaloblastic anemia, hypersplenism
Erythroid hypoplasia	Decreased number of erythroid precursors; M:E ratio increased ($>$ 4:1)	Red cell aplasia associated with thymoma, myasthenia gravis, leukemia. Dilution with peripheral blood will give appearance of erythroid hypoplasia
Myeloid hyperplasia	Increased number of myeloid cells; M:E ratio increased ($>$ 4:1)	Leukemia, infection, leukemoid reaction, infectious mononucleosis, hypersplenism, destruction of leukocytes in peripheral blood
Myeloid hypoplasia	Decreased number of myeloid cells; M:E ratio decreased ($<$ 2:1)	Agranulocytosis, irradiation, preleukemia; increase in erythroid precursors may give appearance of myeloid hypoplasia
Megakaryocytic hyperplasia	Increased number of megakaryocytes, particularly young forms with few nuclear lobes	Blood loss, idiopathic thrombocytopenic purpura, hypersplenism, granulocytic leukemia, megakaryocytic leukemia, destruction of platelets in peripheral blood
Megakaryocytic hypoplasia	Decreased number of megakaryocytes as determined by paraffin section	Irradiation, infection, drugs or toxins, leukemia, myelophthisic anemia (infiltration with neoplastic cells, granuloma, or fibrosis)
Red cell Vacuolated erythroid precursors	Erythroblasts and normoblasts with clear vacuoles in cytoplasm or nucleus	Chloramphenicol toxicity, phenylalanine deficiency, sideroblastic anemias, alcoholism
Delayed hemoglobinization	Presence of late normoblasts with pyknotic nuclei but blue or gray, not pink, cytoplasm	Iron deficiency anemia
"Tissue paper" normoblasts	Late normoblasts with ragged, vacuolated cytoplasm	Iron deficiency anemia
Megaloblastosis (Plates 19, 20)	Presence of large erythroid precursors with mature pink cytoplasm and an immature nuclear chromatin pattern (stippled appearance to nucleus); nuclear-cytoplasmic dissociation	Megaloblastic anemia, leukemia, drugs

Table 1–3 (Continued)

Abnormality	Description	Associated Diseases
Dyserythropoiesis	Changes in erythroid cell nuclear chromatin pattern similar to those seen in megaloblastosis; multinuclearity, intranuclear bridges, "gigantoblasts," and other bizarre nuclear abnormalities of erythroid precursors	Hemolytic anemia, erythroleukemia, drugs, sideroblastic anemias, alcoholism, liver disease, myelophthisic anemia (infiltration with neoplastic cells), congenital dyserythropoietic anemias

White cell (and other nonerythroid cells)

Abnormality	Description	Associated Diseases
Giant myeloid cells (Plate 21)	Large bands, myelocytes, metamyelocytes	Megaloblastic anemia
Myeloid maturation arrest ("Shift to left")	Myeloid hypoplasia, hyperplasia, or normoplasia, but without polys, metamyelocytes, and myelocytes. Myeloblasts and promyelocytes normal or increased.	Agranulocytosis, destruction of leukocytes in peripheral blood (e.g., hypersplenism)
Lymphocytosis or monocytosis	> 20% lymphocytes or 5% monocytes	Aplastic anemias, leukemia, (e.g., chronic lymphatic leukemia), lymphoma, infectious mononucleosis, viral infections, lymphocytic leukemoid reaction, lymphoid follicle
Mast cell hyperplasia (mastocytosis)	> 5% tissue basophils (leukocytes with large, coarse, purple or black granules)	Osteoporosis, mast cell leukemia, systemic mastocytosis
Leukemic cells (Plate 52)	Increased number of primitive white cells or "blasts" (1% or less is normal)	Leukemias (undifferentiated, acute lymphocytic, chronic lymphosarcoma cell, acute or chronic myelocytic, acute or chronic monocytic, myelomonocytic, promyelocytic), erythroleukemia, myeloproliferative syndrome, leukemoid reaction
Reticulum cell hyperplasia	Increased number of reticulum cells (> 5%)	Infections, tuberculosis, malignant histiocytosis, lymphoma, multiple myeloma, inflammatory or collagen disease
Erythrophagocytosis	Phagocytosis of erythrocytes by reticulum cells	Hemolytic anemia, chronic infectious or inflammatory diseases (e.g., tuberculosis, leukemia), histiocytic medullary reticulosis
Lipid-laden macrophages (Gaucher, Plate 61; Niemann-Pick)	Reticuloendothelial cells distended with vacuoles containing lipids. Gaucher cells have pale, foamy or fibrillar, cytoplasm; Niemann-Picks have honeycombed, vacuolated cytoplasm	Lipid storage diseases, multiple myeloma (Gaucher cells), chronic myelocytic leukemia (Gaucher cells), diseases associated with premature destruction of erythrocytes e.g., thalassemia (Gaucher cells)
Lymphoplasmacytoid cells ("plymphocytes") (Plate 67)	Cells with characteristics of both plasma cells and lymphocytes	Waldenström's macroglobulinemia, lymphoma
Plasmacytosis/plasmablastosis (Plate 65)	> 2% plasma cells; must be distinguished from osteoblasts, whose clear zone is distal to the nucleus	Multiple myeloma; lymphoma; Waldenström's macroglobulinemia; liver disease; carcinomatosis; infectious, allergic, or inflammatory

Table 1-3 (Continued)

Abnormality	Description	Associated Diseases
		diseases; amyloidosis; plasma cell leukemia; hypergammaglobulinemia; tuberculosis; Weber-Christian disease
Irritative bone marrow syndrome	Increased plasma cells, eosinophils, monocytes, and reticulum cells	Any infectious, inflammatory, or malignant disease
Lymphosarcoma cells (Plate 63)	Lymphocytes with clefted or nucleolated nuclei	Lymphoma, chronic lymphosarcoma cell leukemia, viral or chronic inflammatory diseases, infectious mononucleosis
Reed-Sternberg cells (Hodgkin's disease, Plate 64)	Multilobed or multinucleolated reticulum cells that give an "owl's eye" appearance in paraffin sections.	Hodgkin's disease, rarely in other malignancies (e.g., melanoma, sarcoma, thymoma, carcinoma, infectious mononucleosis, rubeola)
Lymphomatous infiltration	Collection of lymphocytes, lymphoblasts, and reticulum cells	Malignant lymphoma
Granulomatous infiltration	Granulomata seen in paraffin sections	Tuberculosis, brucellosis, sarcoid, histoplasmosis, infectious mononucleosis, herpes zoster, lymphoma (Hodgkin's) granulomatous hepatitis, berylliosis, collagen diseases (e.g., rheumatoid arthritis)
Tumor cells (Plate 72)	Clumps of cells, each with a multinucleolated nucleus and pale scant cytoplasm; may have intracytoplasmic mucus containing clear areas (adenocarcinoma), or black pigment granules (melanoma)	Carcinoma, sarcoma, melanoma
Marrow fibrosis (Plates 59, 60)	Fibroblasts infiltrate marrow—seen only on paraffin sections; osteosclerosis may occur	Myeloproliferative syndrome, Hodgkin's disease, irradiation, drugs and toxins, carcinoma
Iron Absent iron stores	No iron particles seen intra- or extracellularly	Iron deficiency anemia
Ringed sideroblasts (Plate 8)	Normoblasts with ring of Prussian blue staining mitochondrial iron arranged around the nucleus	Sideroachrestic anemias, lead poisoning, thalassemia, megaloblastic anemia, leukemia, alcoholism, pyridoxine deficiency, drugs (isoniazid, cycloserine, pyrazinamide, azathioprine, chloramphenicol)

Table 1-4 : Classification of Anemias

I. Morphologic

Normocytic, Normochromic (MCV and MCHC normal)	Microcytic, Hypochromic (MCV low, MCHC low)	Macrocytic, Normochromic (MCV high, MCHC normal)
Blood loss	Iron deficiency	Megaloblastic anemia
Hemolytic anemia	Sideroblastic anemia	Liver disease
Aplastic anemia	Thalassemia	Preleukemia
Myelophthisic anemia	Lead poisoning	

II. Physiologic

Hypoproliferation	Maturation Abnormality	Excessive Destruction or Loss of Red Cells
Aplastic anemia	Megaloblastic anemia	Hemolytic anemia
Myelophthisic anemia	Preleukemia	Blood loss
Toxins	Sideroblastic anemia	
Chronic disease	Thalassemia	
Iron deficiency	Iron deficiency	

III. Proposed Clinical

Hypochromic	Megaloblastic	Hemolytic	Aplastic	Myelophthisic	Normochromic, Normocytic
Iron deficiency	B_{12} deficiency	Coombs'-positive anemia	Drug-induced anemia	Leukemia	Blood loss
Sideroblastic anemia	Folate deficiency	Coombs'-negative anemia	Idiopathic anemia	Lymphoma	Chronic disease
Lead poisoning	Preleukemia			Carcinoma	Secondary diseases
Thalassemia				Fibrosis	
Chronic disease				Granulomatous diseases	
Blood counts					
MCHC low	MCV high	MCHC high	Multiple cytopenias	Variable	MCV, MCHC normal
MCV low					

	Blood smears	Reticulocyte Production Index	Marrow
	Hypochromic Microcytic Dimorphic	Low	Absent iron stores Ringed sideroblasts
	Macroovalocytes Hypersegmented polys	Low	Megaloblastic changes Giant myeloid forms
	Spherocytes Polychromatophilia	High	Erythroid hyperplasia
	Normocytic Macrocytic	Low	Aplasia Hypoplasia
	Teardrop forms Nucleated red cells Immature white cells	Low or normal	Infiltration Replacement
	Normocytic Normochromic	Low, normal, or high (blood loss)	Erythroid hyperplasia (blood loss)

failure. *Myelophthisic anemias* are caused by replacement of the bone marrow by malignant cells, granulomas, or fibrosis. The *microcytic, hypochromic anemias* are characterized by small, incompletely hemoglobinized red cells. These anemias have in common a defective production of hemoglobin. An absence of iron stores or a defect in heme synthesis, such as seen in the sideroblastic anemias or lead poisoning, or defective globin synthesis as seen in the thalassemia syndromes, account for most of the microcytic, hypochromic anemias. *Macrocytic anemias* with large erythrocytes are almost always due to deficiencies in vitamin B_{12} or folic acid, although a few are caused by liver disease or poorly characterized anemias that may be related to leukemia.

The physiologic classification of anemia (II) stresses three pathophysiologic mechanisms. The first, failure of normal proliferation of bone marrow elements, may be due to toxins, replacement of the bone marrow by abnormal cells, iron deficiency, or aplasia (hypocellularity). Some patients with aplastic anemia have normal-appearing or actually hypercellular marrow but suffer from anemia secondary to ineffective erythropoiesis. The second major category, excessive loss or destruction of red cells, covers hemolytic anemias characterized by increased hemolysis or breakdown of red cells. With blood loss anemia, the red cell is lost externally or to an internal extravascular site. The third category, maturation abnormalities, includes the megaloblastic and sideroblastic anemias along with some of the hypoproliferative anemias. Normally maturation of the erythrocyte proceeds in both the nucleus and the cytoplasm. In the nucleus the chromatin becomes more clumped and finally pyknotic, while cell size diminishes. In the cytoplasm the initial basophilia is replaced by pink-staining hemoglobin and finally, with maturity, the red cell cytoplasm becomes completely pink-staining. In the megaloblastic anemias nuclear maturation defects are prominent. The cell cytoplasm becomes normally hemoglobinized, but the nucleus remains large and reticulated rather than clumped and pyknotic. This nuclear-cytoplasmic dissociation is sometimes referred to as *dyspoiesis.* Defects in cytoplasmic maturation are characteristic of iron deficiency, thalassemia, and the sideroblastic anemias. Nuclear maturation proceeds normally, but cytoplasmic hemoglobinization is delayed and often incomplete.

The third classification scheme (III) is used in this text and stresses the morphologic abnormalities found in the peripheral blood and bone marrow. For each of six types of anemia it specifies characteristic blood counts, Wintrobe indices, red cell morphology, and bone marrow abnormalities. This allows for quick and relatively inexpensive initial classification of a patient's anemia. Also the hematologic diseases in each category share common pathophysiologic mechanisms. Succeeding chapters describe these mechanisms in detail and also discuss confirmatory findings and tests for each category of anemia.

Treatment of Blood Loss and Anemia

The effects of blood loss are twofold. First, there is a reduction in hemoglobin and therefore in oxygen-carrying capacity. Second, there is concomitant loss of plasma, decrease in blood volume, and inability to maintain normal blood pressure. In the past, whole blood was used to treat anemia without regard to whether the patient was suffering from decreased oxygen-carrying capacity or from decreased blood volume. Due to the scarcity of blood, component transfusion has now become accepted and is a vital means of meeting the need for blood transfusion. If it can be determined that the patient's major problem is inability to supply oxygen to tissues, and not danger from decreased blood volume, then the appropriate component for therapy is packed red cells. These are prepared by centrifugation or sedimentation of whole blood and removal of plasma components. Packed red cells prepared in this manner contain decreased amounts of free hemoglobin, potassium, and other toxins. They may also have a lower incidence of blood-borne viral hepatitis than whole blood. Furthermore, the plasma removed from the whole blood can be fractionated and used in several patients for treatment of bleeding abnormalities or for blood volume expansion. If the patient's major problem is loss of blood volume, then plasma or albumin prepared from plasma should be used. Albumin prepared from plasma is hepatitis virus-free. With few exceptions, it is only for the acutely bleeding patient that whole blood is needed, to supply both plasma and red cells.

Transfusion of blood as the sole means of treating anemia should be limited to patients who have hematologic diseases that are not presently amenable to treatment. In every case great effort should be expended to define and treat the cause of the anemia. Transfusion may be used to tide the patient over while treatment is being undertaken. In no case should blood transfusion be used in place of an adequate diagnostic workup. In many patients, once the cause of the anemia has been defined, it may be possible to avoid transfusion and its attendant dangers. Technical considerations in typing and crossmatching blood are considered in Chapter 7.

CASE DEVELOPMENT PROBLEM: ANEMIA

A 24-year-old Nigerian foreign exchange student comes to the emergency ward after having passed out twice on the street. He reports having had diarrheal stools which were black and possibly bloody. A nurse orders an emergency hematocrit and it is reported as 0.30 (30%). A peripheral blood smear is ready.

1. How would you proceed with this patient?

The history, physical examination, blood counts, and peripheral blood smear form the basis for the initial workup of any patient with a suspected hematologic abnormality. In this case, however, the order in which these examinations are carried out is most important. Since the history suggests that the syncope is secondary to gastrointestinal bleeding and decreased blood volume, the first step is to obtain his vital signs, particularly blood pressure and pulse. Once these have been established as satisfactory, a brief history and a test for blood in stomach and rectum should follow. In this urgent situation the examination of the blood smear comes last. The nurse reports that she has obtained a blood pressure of 120/80 mm Hg with the patient in a lying position and 90/60 with him in the sitting position.

2. How do you account for this discrepancy?

These findings indicate that the patient has *orthostatic hypotension*. This means that his blood volume has been reduced to the point that his vascular tree is unable to compensate by vasoconstriction for the decreased blood volume. This leads to a marked drop in both systolic and diastolic blood pressures when he assumes the sitting or standing position. It is an important clinical sign of decreased blood volume and usually indicates significant loss of blood volume.

3. What other physical findings are most likely present?

This patient very likely has a rapid pulse; pallor of the skin, mucus membranes, conjunctivae, and nail beds; and a cardiac hemic murmur.

4. The laboratory reports his hemoglobin as 10 gm per deciliter and his red cell count as 3.0×10^{12} per liter. Calculate and interpret his Wintrobe indices.

Mean corpuscular volume is 100 femtoliters, mean corpuscular hemoglobin is 33 picograms, and mean corpuscular hemoglobin concentration is 33 gm per deciliter. This indicates that he has a normocytic, normochromic anemia.

He gives a further history of having had a duodenal ulcer; his gastric aspirate and stool when tested for occult blood are both strongly positive. A repeat hematocrit is 0.29 (29%).

5. Does this stabilization of his hematocrit indicate that he has stopped bleeding?

No, because it may take upwards of 1 to 2 days for extravascular fluid to enter the *intra*vascular space and dilute the remaining red cells. This dilution will ultimately lead to further decrease in his hematocrit. The important point to remember is that the hematocrit may not indicate the degree of blood loss until many hours or days have passed. Signs of orthostatic hypotension are therefore very important in assessing the magnitude of acute blood loss.

6. What blood products would you advise for transfusion? Why?

This patient obviously has two deficits. First, he has lost red cells that are necessary for carrying oxygen to tissues. He has also lost plasma proteins that are necessary to maintain intravascular volume. The components that he needs — namely, red cells and plasma — should therefore be replaced. They can be given as whole blood or as packed red cells and either albumin or single donor units of plasma.

He continues to bleed and requires 15 units of whole blood over a period of only 4 hours. He develops "air hunger," which indicates that tissue oxygenation is unsatisfactory. The blood with which he has been transfused is 3 weeks old.

7. Can you account for the tissue hypoxia despite transfusion?

Blood stored for more than a few days in ACD (acid-citrate-dextrose) anticoagulant loses its 2,3-DPG content rapidly. This patient may be unable to unload oxygen from hemoglobin because his 2,3-DPG level is low. Patients who have been given transfusions of smaller amounts of blood can easily replenish their 2,3-DPG levels.
Blood collected in CPD (citrate-phosphate-dextrose) anticoagulant and red cells stored by freezing have high levels of 2,3-DPG. These products should be used in patients who are having rapid, multiple blood transfusions.

Frozen and fresh red cells are obtained for this patient, and his "air hunger" subsides. His bleeding also suddenly stops before surgical measures can be undertaken. Eight hours after admission to the hospital, his hematocrit is stable at 0.30 (30%) and his reticulocyte count has risen to 9 percent. Macrocytes with bluish or polychromatophilic cytoplasm are present in great numbers in his peripheral blood smear.

8. Calculate and interpret his reticulocyte production index.

$$RPI = \frac{\frac{9 \times 30}{45}}{2} = 3$$

His reticulocyte production index is calculated to be 3. This means that his bone marrow production is approximately three times normal. This has come about in response to his anemia and inadequate tissue oxygenation. Since there are large numbers of polychromatophils, a correction factor of 2 is used. These macrocytes account for the high normal mean corpuscular volume.

9. If you assume a normal red cell mass of 2,000 ml for this patient, how many milliliters of red cells will he produce per day with a reticulocyte production index of 3?

Normal individuals with a reticulocyte count of 1 percent replace about 1 percent of their red cells each day. In his case this would be 20 ml. Since his reticulocyte index is 3, he is able to produce 3 X 20, or 60, ml per day.

TOPICS FOR DISCUSSION: ANEMIA

Topics suitable for term papers or seminars in hematology are listed in each chapter. They concern aspects of hematology that are undergoing change and development at the present time and that are not possible to summarize in a textbook. Students are expected to search primary resources, journal articles, and reviews in order to bring themselves and their classmates up to date in these important areas of hematologic investigation. The bibliographies for each chapter include review articles that should aid in researching these topics.

Morphologic and biochemical development of red blood cells

Microstructure and microenvironment of the bone marrow

Red cell deformability and release of red cells

Stem cells, pluripotential and committed

Ineffective erythropoiesis

Structure and function of erythropoietin

Oxygenation and deoxygenation of hemoglobin

Intracellular phosphate compounds and regulation of hemoglobin oxygen affinity

Particle counters

SELECTED REFERENCES

Bellingham, A. J., and Grimes, A. J. Red cell 2,3-diphosphoglycerate. *Br. J. Haematol.* 25:555, 1973.

Beutler, E., and Srivastava, K. Composition of the Erythrocyte. In W. J. Williams, E. Beutler, A. J. Erslev, and R. W. Rundles (eds.), *Hematology* (2nd ed.). New York: McGraw-Hill, 1977.

Erslev, A. J. Classification of Erythrocyte Disorders. In W. J. Williams, E. Beutler, A. J. Erslev, and R. W. Rundles (eds.), *Hematology* (2nd ed.). New York: McGraw-Hill, 1977.

Erslev, A. J. Renal biogenesis of erythropoietin. *Am. J. Med.* 58:25, 1975.

Finch, C. A., and Hillman, R. S. A Clinical Approach to Anemia. In R. I. Weed (ed.), *Hematology for Internists*. Boston: Little, Brown, 1971.

Gordon, A. S. The current status of erythropoietin. *Br. J. Haematol.* 21:611, 1971.

Gurney, C. Erythropoiesis, Red Cell Maturation, and Stem Cell Kinetics. In C. E. Mengel, et al (eds.), *Hematology: Principles and Practice.* Chicago: Year Book, 1972.

Harris, J. W., and Kellermeyer, R. W. Effects of Anemia; Classification of the Anemias; Normal Red Cell Production. In J. W. Harris (ed.), *The Red Cell-Production, Metabolism, Destruction.* Boston: Harvard University Press, 1970.

Hillman, R. S., and Finch, C. A. *Red Cell Manual* (4th ed.). Philadelphia: F. A. Davis, 1974.

Lajtha, L. G. Haemopoietic stem cells. *Br. J. Haematol.* 29:529, 1975.

Lessin, L. S., and Bessis, M. Morphology of the Erythron. In W. J. Williams, E. Beutler, A. J. Erslev, and R. W. Rundles (eds.), *Hematology* (2nd ed.). New York: McGraw-Hill, 1977.

McDonald, G. A., Dodds, T. C., and Cruickshank, B. *Atlas of Hematology* (3rd ed.). Baltimore: Williams & Wilkins, 1970.

Reich, P. R. *Scope Manual of Hematology.* Kalamazoo, Mich.: Upjohn Company, 1972.

Surgenor, D. M. (ed.) *The Red Cell.* New York: Academic, 1975. Vols. I, II.

Thomas, H. M., Lefrak, S. S., Irwin, R. S., Fritts, H. W., and Caldwell, P. B. The oxyhemoglobin dissociation curve in health and disease. Role of 2,3-diphosphoglycerate. *Am. J. Med.* 57:331, 1974.

Weatherall, D. J. (ed.) Haemoglobin: Structure, function and synthesis. *Br. Med. Bull.* 32:193, 1976.

Williams, W. J. Approach to the Patient; Examination of the Peripheral Blood; Examination of the Bone Marrow. In W. J. Williams, E. Beutler, A. J. Erslev, and R. W. Rundles (eds.), *Hematology* (2nd ed.). New York: McGraw-Hill, 1977.

Wintrobe, M. M., et al The Approach to the Patient with Anemia. In M. M. Wintrobe et al (eds.), *Clinical Hematology* (7th ed.). Philadelphia: Lea & Febiger, 1974.

Wintrobe, M. M., et al The Erythrocyte; Section 2; Morphology, Intrinsic Metabolism, Function, Laboratory Evaluation; Production of Erythrocytes. In M. M. Wintrobe et al (eds.), *Clinical Hematology* (7th ed.). Philadelphia: Lea & Febiger, 1974.

Wintrobe, M. M., et al The Approach to Hematologic Problems; Origin and Development of the Blood and Blood-Forming Tissues. In M. M. Wintrobe et al (eds.), *Clinical Hematology* (7th ed.). Philadelphia: Lea & Febiger, 1974.

2 : Hypochromic Anemias

An important mechanism of anemia is defective hemoglobin synthesis, which results in poorly hemoglobinized peripheral blood erythrocytes. After Wright staining, instead of red cells with pink hemoglobin filling the cytoplasm, the cells are pale with only a rim of hemoglobin. Since hemoglobin is made up of two components, either of two pathophysiologic mechanisms can lead to decreased hemoglobin synthesis — defective heme or decreased globin production. *Heme* is made up of iron and porphyrins; deficiencies in either affect heme production. Deficiency of iron stores, failure to utilize iron properly, and defective heme or porphyrin synthesis are characteristic of iron deficiency anemia, anemia of chronic disease, and porphyrias, respectively. In the thalassemia syndromes, *globin* production is decreased, thereby hindering hemoglobin synthesis and producing a hypochromic anemia. In this chapter the anemias related to iron and porphyrin metabolism are discussed; thalassemias are considered in Chapter 6.

Iron Deficiency Anemia

Iron deficiency anemia secondary to blood loss is the commonest cause of anemia in the world. In order to understand the symptoms, etiology, and treatment of this anemia, it is necessary to review normal iron and heme metabolism.

Iron Storage

Hemoglobin. Iron exists in several compartments within the body (Table 2-1). The largest compartment is hemoglobin iron. Hemoglobin contains 0.34 percent elemental iron by weight. Therefore 500 ml of whole blood contains about 250 mg (15 gm/dl $\times$ 5 dl $\times$ 0.0034) of elemental iron. The iron is complexed to an organic compound, heme, a tetrapyrrole, which is discussed later. Iron in this compartment is preferentially used over and over again in the erythropoietic cycle. Iron released at the time of red cell destruction in reticuloendothelial cells is bound to transferrin and delivered to erythroid precursors in the marrow. There it is incorporated into new cells, thus completing the cycle.

Storage Iron. Storage iron exists in two forms: hemosiderin and ferritin. Hemosiderin is usually assayed by its reaction with Prussian blue stain, with which it produces blue particles (Plate 7). In unstained marrow smears it appears as clumps of golden refractile pigment. The amount of hemosiderin in marrow storage

Table 2–1 : Important Iron Compartments in Normal 70-kg Man

Compartment	Iron Content (mg)
Hemoglobin	2,300
Storage (ferritin, hemosiderin)	1,000
Myoglobin	130
Tissue	8
Transport	4

Adapted from Fairbanks, V. F., and Beutler, E., Iron Metabolism, in Williams, W. J. et al (Eds.) *Hematology,* Chap. 11, p. 125. New York: McGraw-Hill, 1972.

sites reflects the state of iron balance; e.g., in patients with iron deficiency anemia, hemosiderin is absent from the bone marrow.

Ferritin, the other storage form of iron, is a water-soluble complex of ferric hydroxide-phosphate and a protein, *apoferritin.* The ferric hydroxide-phosphate core and apoferritin shell form a semicrystalline structure visible with special stains or through the electron microscope. Ferritin is thought to be a more readily usable storage form of iron than hemosiderin. Ferritin is also found in the intestinal mucosa, where it may help regulate iron absorption and excretion. Both forms of iron are stored primarily in the reticuloendothelial system (bone marrow and Kupffer cells of liver and spleen). Ferritin granules have been found by electron microscopy in hemosiderin, and it is thought that hemosiderin may represent partially denatured, partially deproteinized ferritin.

Ferritin-containing iron is detected and quantitated in the serum by a radioimmunoassay procedure. Serum ferritin iron comes from the reticuloendothelial system, where it derives partly from senescent erythrocytes. It is transported to the hepatocyte, where iron is stored and where the ferritin may regulate transferrin synthesis. The latter possibility has not been verified experimentally. Neither has a role for serum ferritin in signaling intestinal cells to absorb iron been demonstrated in humans. Serum ferritin levels do have a direct correlation with tissue, that is, bone marrow iron stores.

Myoglobin. This heme-containing protein is found in muscle. Following severe muscle injury it may be detectable in serum and urine. Iron loss due to myoglobinuria is not a cause of iron deficiency.

Tissue Iron. This compartment is small, but very important, and consists of heme and iron-containing proteins such as cytochromes, catalase, peroxidases, and flavoproteins. Defective synthesis of some of these proteins may be responsible for the skin, mucus membrane, and nail changes found in patients with iron deficiency anemia.

Transport Iron. The iron-binding protein in serum, *transferrin,* migrates in the β-globulin region when serum is electrophoresed on cellulose acetate. Normally in serum there is 120 to 200 mg per deciliter of transferrin protein, or 250 to 400 μg per deciliter of iron-binding capacity. One-third of transferrin contains bound iron, which is carried from the hepatocyte and intestinal mucosal cells to the hematopoietic cells of the bone marrow.

Iron Absorption

The average daily American diet contains 10 to 15 mg of elemental iron, and a normal individual absorbs 5 to 10 percent of ingested iron, or 0.5 to 1.5 mg per day. The absorption of iron depends on many factors. Food and heme iron may be better absorbed than inorganic iron salts. Foods vary in the availability of iron for absorption, meat protein being a particularly good source. Low iron stores and increased iron requirements often increase the percentage of iron absorbed to 20 percent or more. It may be absorbed from almost any level of the small intestine, but the upper levels, particularly the duodenum, are the most efficient sites. In iron-deficient individuals absorption may occur at lower levels.

Iron complexed in organic compounds, such as the heme in hemoglobin or myoglobin from animal meat, is absorbed by a mechanism different from absorption of inorganic iron salts. Iron salts are absorbed in the mucosal cell in the ferrous or divalent state and then converted to the trivalent ferric form. Absorption is decreased by chelating agents such as *desferriox-amine* and by complexing agents such as phytates and is increased by vitamin C and by hydrochloric acid in achlorhydric subjects. Heme split from hemoglobin or myoglobin is absorbed intact into the mucosal cell as hemin, the ferric form of heme. The iron moiety from hemin is split off within the cell. Intraluminal factors such as chelators of iron salts, ascorbic acid, and hydrochloric acid do not appear to inhibit or facilitate this process.

Iron absorption is primarily regulated by the amount of storage iron and the red cell production rate. Increased production and decreased stores lead to greater absorption, and decreased production and normal or increased stores lower absorption. How production rate and storage iron influence mucosal cell absorption is controversial. It is clear that iron in the mucosal cell is carried across the cell by an active transport mechanism. Regulation of iron transport across the cell is linked to the iron content of the mucosal cell. When body iron stores are high, iron is diverted into ferritin and stored in the intestine, and if stores are low or red cell production high, iron passes directly through the mucosal cell into the plasma. Iron stored as ferritin in the mucosal cell may ultimately be deposited into the intestinal lumen when the epithelial cell is sloughed. This serves as a mechanism for iron excretion. However, only small quantities of iron, about one milligram per day, can be excreted in this manner.

These physiological control mechanisms can be overcome by large doses of therapeutic iron or by ingestion of toxic quantities of iron tablets — e.g., taken accidentally by a child. Some types of clay and the antibiotic tetracycline depress iron absorption. Various factors that influence iron absorption are shown (p. 37).

Iron Transport

Ferrous iron must be oxidized before binding to transferrin. The plasma copper protein, ceruloplasm, catalyzes this reaction. Transferrin moves ferric iron from wherever it enters the plasma (intestinal mucosal or reticuloendothelial cells) to the membranes of normoblasts in the bone marrow. From there iron enters the cytoplasm of the normoblast. It is not known whether transferrin enters the cell before releasing its iron load. In any case the transferrin returns to the plasma and is reutilized. Since iron is complexed into heme in the mitochondria, it is no surprise that siderotic or iron-containing granules are present in the mitochondria of normoblasts. The process, from initial binding to the normoblast to incorporation into hemoglobin, takes 6 to 8 minutes. It appears that intracellular free heme level regulates the normoblast's uptake of iron. If heme synthesis is impaired, as may occur in sideroblastic anemias, iron uptake is enhanced and mitochondria become large and filled with iron. These structures surround the normoblast's nucleus, forming a *ringed sideroblast* (Plate 8).

A second, probably less important, mechanism of transportation of iron into the red cell is called *rhopheocytosis.* A *nurse cell,* or reticuloendothelial cell containing ferritin (or hemosiderin), transfers ferritin into normoblasts by *micropinocytosis,* a process consisting of normoblast membrane invagination of ferritin and then cytoplasmic vacuole formation. Nurse cells surrounded by normoblasts can be identified in Wright-stained bone marrow smears. It is also possible that excess iron is removed from normoblasts by these nurse cells.

Reticuloendothelial cell regulation of iron metabolism is important to the pathogenesis of the anemia of chronic disease. In iron deficiency, iron derived from hemoglobin in damaged red cells is promptly released by reticuloendothelial cells and reutilized. In chronic diseases, infections, and malignancies, the

Factors influencing iron absorption

Causing increased absorption
Alcohol
Anemia
Ascorbic acid
Depletion of iron stores
Hydrochloric acid
Hypoxia
Increased erythropoiesis
Liver disease

Causing decreased absorption
Certain clays
Magnesium trisilicate
Malabsorption syndromes
Phytates
Tetracycline

Table 2-2 : Normal Human Iron Requirements

Individual	Iron Requirement (mg/day)
Normal adult male	0.5–1.0
Normal menstruating female	1.2–2.0
Pregnant female	2.4–4.0
Lactating female (with amenorrhea)	0.5–1.0
Postmenopausal female	0.5–1.0
Infant	1.0

reticuloendothelial cells fail to release iron to transferrin, and this leads to iron deficiency within the primitive normoblasts and often a hypochromic anemia.

Congenital Atransferrinemia. Rare individuals congenitally lack transferrin and suffer from a severe, refractory, hypochromic anemia despite excess iron stores. Studies indicate that their iron is not delivered selectively to early normoblasts and cannot be efficiently utilized for hemoglobin production.

Iron Requirement

Table 2-2 shows the iron requirements for different types of individuals. Iron is lost in the feces as blood, bile, and exfoliated mucosal cells. Small amounts are also eliminated in the urine and in sweat. Humans have a very limited ability to increase excretion of iron, and regulation of iron balance is achieved by changing gut absorption depending on the body's requirement for iron. Patients with excessive iron stores usually cannot correct their imbalance without the help of therapeutic blood removal by phlebotomy.

Iron Kinetics

A dynamic picture of iron metabolism can be obtained by use of trace amounts of radioactive iron. Analysis is best performed by experts, but we will describe certain measurements that are of clinical importance.

Radiolabeled iron bound to transferrin is injected into a patient. Curves based on hourly sampling of the peripheral blood and counts of the radioactivity in the plasma are shown in Figure 4. In the normal person 50% of the injected radioactivity disappears from the circulation in approximately 90 minutes. This iron is taken up by the bone marrow and in 7 to 10 days is found in circulating erythrocytes. Usually the clearance of iron from the plasma is expressed as *plasma iron turnover* (PIT).

$$PIT = \frac{plasma\ iron \times plasmacrit}{T\ 1/2 \times 100}$$

Fig. 4 : Radioiron
clearance from plas-
ma. (Adapted from
Bothwell, T. H., et
al, The study of
erythropoietin using
tracer quantities of
radioactive iron. Br.
J. Haematol. 2:1,
1956.)

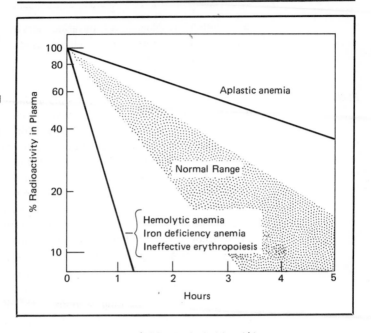

where PIT = mg iron/100 ml whole blood/day
plasma iron is in μg/dl plasma
plasmacrit = 100 − hematocrit (%)
T 1/2 = time (min) to clear 50% of injected radioiron

Normal people clear 0.65 mg of iron from every 100 ml of whole
blood each day, or about 30 to 40 mg of iron leave the plasma
daily. Increased turnover has a correlation with increased effective erythropoiesis (as in hemolytic anemia) or ineffective
erythropoiesis (intra-marrow red cell destruction) and with
deficient iron stores. Decreased turnover is seen with anemias
due to reduced erythropoiesis (as in aplastic anemia).

Another measurement of clinical importance is the percentage
of injected labeled iron that appears in circulating red cells
in 7 to 10 days. In normal people and iron-deficient patients
at least 80 percent of injected radioiron may be counted in
circulating red cells. In patients with marrow aplasia or ineffective erythropoiesis considerably less radioiron is incorporated
into circulating erythrocytes.

Finally, red cell life span can be determined by following red
cell radioactivity over a period of weeks or months. In normal
individuals radioactivity declines rapidly at about 120 days, the
usual life span of red cells. In patients with hemolytic anemia,
erythrocyte life span is foreshortened, and the sharp decline in
radioactivity occurs considerably sooner. As we will see in Chapter 4, determination of red cell life span by labeling hemoglobin
iron in a cohort of erythroid precursors requires more time than

by "random" labeling of cells of various ages with radiochromium. For this reason radioiron is seldom used clinically to assess erythrocyte life span.

Etiology

From a knowledge of normal iron metabolism (outlined p. 41), it is easy to predict the derangements likely to produce a deficiency of normoblast iron. Excessive iron loss, greater than absorption, is the most common cause of iron deficiency anemia. Chronic intestinal or uterine bleeding accounts for most adult cases. Excessive losses occur rarely from microhemorrhages into lung tissue or from hemoglobin released into the bloodstream and excreted through the kidneys. Gastric or duodenal ulcers, esophageal varices, hiatal hernia, colonic diverticula, and tumors often account for bleeding in men and women. Menstrual losses and losses related to pregnancy and delivery are common in young adult women. Bleeding from otherwise silent colon cancers must be considered in all cases of iron deficiency in adults. In warm climates bleeding secondary to intestinal parasites, particularly hookworms, is a common cause of iron loss.

Hereditary hemorrhagic telangiectasia is a rare autosomal dominant disorder that manifests itself, usually in later life, as red or purple nodular, vascular lesions of the skin and mucus membranes. The mucosal lesions in the nose and gastrointestinal tract may chronically rupture and bleed, resulting in blood loss and iron deficiency anemias. This disease is rarely suspected unless the characteristic lesions are seen on the face, lips, tongue, palms, or soles. They blanch when pressure is applied with a glass slide. No effective treatment, except possibly estrogens, is available.

Excessive demand, exceeding iron absorption, is a problem for the 1- to 2-year-old infant, young adolescent, and pregnant woman. In the infant, inadequate iron in the predominantly cow-milk diet accounts for lowered iron stores. This, coupled with an increased demand for iron for erythropoiesis (the full-term infant requires 160 mg, and the premature, 240 mg of iron during the first year of life) often leads to iron deficiency anemia at about age 1 or 2. Although 50 mg of iron is supplied by physiologic destruction of fetal red cells, more is required from the diet. For this reason iron supplementation is recommended for infants, especially premature ones.

The young adolescent is faced with increased demands for iron because of rapid growth and need for increased erythropoiesis. On top of that requirement, the female adolescent begins to menstruate, losing approximately 45 ml of blood per menstrual period. Since 100 ml of blood contains 50 mg of elemental iron, there is an increased requirement of about 25 mg of iron per

Important normal values relevant to iron metabolism

I. Iron balance
   Iron requirement: 1–1.5 mg/day
   Absorption of elemental iron: 10% (can increase to 20% or more)
   Dietary iron content: 15 mg
   Ferrous sulfate tablets (300 mg): 60 mg elemental iron
   Total storage iron: 1000 mg in males; 400 mg in females
   Whole blood elemental iron content: 50 mg/dl

II. Serum levels
   Iron: 80–160 μg/dl (new SI units: 14–29 μmol/L = μg/100 ml ×
   0.179)
   Total iron-binding capacity (TIBC): 250–400 μg/dl (SI units:
   45–72 μmol/L)
   Percent saturation of TIBC: 15–45
   Ferritin: 12–250 μg/L

III. Ferrokinetic values (radioiron)
   Plasma iron turnover: 0.65 mg/dl whole blood/day
   Percent of injected radioiron in circulating erythrocytes: ⩾80%
   (8–10 days after injection)
   Red cell life span: 120 days

IV. Marrow
   Sideroblasts: ⩾30% of normoblasts
   Ringed sideroblasts: none

month or 1 mg per day in menstruating females. For this reason, unless iron is present in sufficient quantities in the diet or iron supplements are taken, iron deficiency anemia occurs in young females.

Pregnancy also increases demand for iron. There is a saving of about 200 mg of iron due to cessation of menses. However, expansion of the mother's red cell mass requires 400 mg of iron, and the fetus and placenta require another 400 mg. Blood loss at delivery, including blood in the placenta, accounts for another 300 mg. The total requirement for a single pregnancy, therefore, is about 1,100 mg. This is more than the average mother's total iron storage compartment. If iron supplementation is not provided, decreased maternal or fetal iron stores result, thereby increasing the chances of iron deficiency in mother or infant.

Malabsorption of iron is an uncommon cause of iron lack. Diseases of the intestinal mucosa, such as celiac disease in children and tropical and nontropical sprue, are associated with an inability to absorb normal quantities of iron from the diet. It is often possible to increase iron stores in such patients by giving large amounts of iron orally or parenterally, if oral administration is not feasible.

Subtotal gastrectomy often leads to iron deficiency many years after the operation. Multiple mechanisms probably account for the patient's decreased iron stores. Rapid transit through the duodenum, achlorhydria, perioperative blood loss, occult bleeding secondary to recurrent ulceration, and decreased iron in postgastrectomy diets have all been suggested as contributing to this iron lack.

Deficiency secondary to poor dietary intake of iron must be very rare in adults. Given normal or even reduced iron stores, it would take years to develop anemia as long as excretion of iron remains normal at 1 mg or less per day. The investigation of an adult case of iron deficiency should never be delayed or abandoned on the excuse that the patient's anemia is due to a poor diet.

Clinical Manifestations

The symptoms of iron deficiency anemias are the same as for any anemia (see p. 2). Prominent are fatigue, weakness, shortness of breath, and symptoms of heart failure. Some gastrointestinal symptoms are peculiar to iron deficiency: intermittent glossitis manifested by inflammation and soreness of the tongue; in children, *pica,* or craving and ingestion of strange substances such as dirt or paint (often containing lead); and in adults, desire to eat ice (*pagophagia*) or clays or starches.

The physical findings include those associated with any anemia, e.g., pallor and tachycardia. There is atrophy of the tongue papillae, usually associated with intermittent glossitis. Fingernails are often fragile and may assume the shape of the head of a spoon, with central depression and raised borders (*koilonychia*). Mucus membranes are often inflamed, with cracking of the lips, *cheilosis,* and inflammation of the corners of the mouth, or *angular stomatitis.* In chronic, severe cases glossitis is accompanied by sore mouth and dysphagia. This *Plummer-Vinson syndrome* is also rarely associated with a web of mucosa at the junction of the hypopharynx and esophagus. Another rare, unexplained finding in iron deficiency is splenomegaly.

Associations between iron deficiency, atrophic gastritis, and histamine-fast achlorhydria are well known, but the reasons for these associations are not. After stimulation of an iron-deficient patient's stomach parietal cells with intramuscular histamine, little or no hydrochloric acid is detected. Younger patients may have a return of HCl secretion after treatment of their iron deficiency. It is not known whether the atrophy and gastritis are secondary to or a result of iron deficiency.

Two tests for achlorhydria are available; both are preceded by a parenteral histamine injection. In one method a soft rubber tube is passed through the patient's nose and into his stomach. A sample of gastric juice is aspirated and then tested for pH and titratable acid. The second method, tubeless gastric analysis or Diagnex blue test, depends on the characteristics of an ingested dye, which on contact with hydrochloric acid turns blue and is ultimately absorbed and excreted in the urine where it is easily measured. Unfortunately a negative result cannot be accepted as definitive evidence for achlorhydria, and the tube method must be employed for confirmation in Diagnex blue test–negative patients. A positive result, with blue urine excretion, is acceptable evidence that gastric acid is present.

The peripheral blood findings are most helpful. The Wintrobe indices reveal a low MCV (55-74 fl) and MCHC (25-30 gm per deciliter). Red cell morphology is characterized by microcytosis (Plate 9), smaller than normal cells, hypochromia (Plate 10), cells with central pallor, and in some cases, cells with only a rim of hemoglobin near the cell wall. Target cells (Plate 11), characterized by pink centers and periphery with a clear ring in between, are often found along with elliptical and teardrop-shaped erythrocytes (Plate 12) and other abnormal erythroid shapes referred to as *poikilocytes* (Plate 13). Generally, the more severe the anemia, the greater the abnormalities of shape.

The reticulocyte count is variable, sometimes less than 1 percent, in other cases 2 to 3 percent. The reticulocyte production index is low. Platelets may be normal, decreased, or even increased. Some hematologists believe any increase in platelets is secondary to bleeding, but others attribute it to iron deficiency itself.

The bone marrow examination is helpful in making a diagnosis, since Prussian blue staining of marrow aspirates or clot sections will show an absence or near absence of both normoblast and reticuloendothelial (extracellular) iron. Less than 10 percent of normoblasts will have Prussian blue staining particles in their cytoplasm.

With Wright staining poorly hemoglobinized normoblasts with scant cytoplasm are seen; these are sometimes called *tissue paper normoblasts.* Mild erythroid hyperplasia with a decreased myeloid-to-erythroid cell (M:E) ratio is common. Abnormalities similar to those seen in megaloblastic anemia have been described in severe cases and the suggestion made that such patients have a defect in folic acid metabolism secondary to iron lack.

As expected, serum iron levels are low ($<$ 50 μg/dl). These are assayed by a chemical reaction between ferrous iron and a chelating agent that turns pink when complexed with iron. Total iron-binding capacity is elevated ($>$ 400 μg per deciliter), and saturation of this protein is less than 15 percent and in many cases less than 10 percent. Total iron-binding capacity is determined by incubating serum with excess iron, separating unbound iron, and then determining by the previously described chemical method the amount of iron bound to protein.

Serum protoporphyrin levels are high, and serum ferritin levels are low ($<$ 10 μg/L) in iron-deficient patients. Because hemoglobin catabolism is less, serum bilirubin is often low, and the serum appears abnormally clear (low icterus index).

One of the best and least expensive tests for iron deficiency is a trial performed with therapeutic amounts of oral iron. In 5 to 10 days after starting therapy, the reticulocyte count rises to 7 to 10 percent or more, directly proportional to the severity of the anemia. The hematocrit should rise 0.05 (5%) to 0.15 (15%) in three weeks and the hemoglobin 2 to 5 gm per deciliter.

Sequence of Development of Iron Deficiency Anemia

The first response to negative iron balance is the utilization and diminution of iron stores. Tissue iron stores, including bone marrow, are reduced, and serum ferritin levels fall ($<$ 10 μg per liter). With exhaustion of iron stores and reduction of marrow sideroblasts to less than 10 percent, serum iron falls, and total iron binding capacity begins to rise. For the first time there is impairment of hemoglobin synthesis, with a resultant normochromic, normocytic anemia. With continued reduction in hemoglobin synthesis, hypochromic and microcytic erythrocytes are produced. Finally, the tissue changes seen in iron deficiency anemia appear in mucus membranes and nail beds.

As an explanation for the microcytic and hypochromic character of this anemia, it has been suggested that when the serum iron falls below 70 μg per deciliter, or transferrin saturation falls below 15 percent, hemoglobin production is reduced and poorly hemoglobinized cells result. An extra normoblastic mitotic division with production of microcytes occurs in response to the low MCHC. It is not clear how the bone marrow is able to detect intracellular hemoglobin concentration. However, it is common to find erythroid hyperplasia in the marrow of patients with iron deficiency.

Therapy. Therapy for iron deficiency anemia is almost always the administration of iron salts such as ferrous sulfate. Three hundred milligrams of the hydrated salt of ferrous sulfate contains approximately 60 mg of elemental iron. In an iron-deficient subject, approximately 100 mg of iron can be incorporated into hemoglobin per day. Assuming 25 percent absorption of iron given as ferrous sulfate to an iron-deficient patient, a 2-gm dose of dehydrated salt (400 mg elemental iron) should provide 100 mg of absorbed iron. Because many patients have gastrointestinal intolerance to iron, it is often best to start off with 300 mg of ferrous sulfate per day and slowly increase the dose to the point where the patient is taking two tablets three times a day for a total of 1.8 gm of ferrous sulfate. If the patient cannot tolerate this large dose, 300 mg of iron sulfate three times daily is usually sufficient.

Allowing for the fact that iron absorption will decrease as the iron deficiency anemia is corrected, six months of therapy is usually required to correct the anemia and replenish iron stores. Common side effects of iron therapy include heartburn, nausea, abdominal cramps, constipation, and diarrhea. These side effects can be counteracted by decreasing the dose of iron salt, by having the patient ingest the tablets immediately after or with meals, or by switching to a different iron preparation such as ferrous gluconate, ferrous fumarate, or ferrous succinate. Patients should be warned that their stools will turn black while they are taking iron salts. Since iron is severely toxic to children, tablets must be stored in "childproof" bottles out of reach.

Failure to respond to replacement therapy may be due to one of the following:

1. Incorrect diagnosis
2. Continued loss of iron, usually secondary to continuing blood loss

3. Chronic infection or inflammatory conditions suppressing marrow productivity
4. Failure to take iron-containing medication
5. Use of sustained release preparation that fails to release iron into duodenum
6. Malabsorption of iron (rarely seen)

Parenteral iron therapy with iron–dextran complex (Imferon) and iron sorbitol citrate (Jectofer) should be instituted only for one or more of the following reasons:

1. Inability to tolerate side effects of oral therapy
2. Presence of inflammatory bowel or peptic ulcer disease
3. Failure to take iron tablets
4. Malabsorption of iron
5. Too rapid a loss of iron (e.g., hereditary hemorrhagic telangiectasia) due to bleeding

A formula that allows for both hemoglobin and storage iron replenishment is generally used to calculate the dose of parenteral iron:

$$\text{Iron to be injected (mg)} = (15 - \text{Hgb}) \ (\text{gm/dl})$$
$$\times \text{body weight (kg)} \times 3$$

The available parenteral preparations contain 50 mg of iron per milliliter. A test dose of 0.5 ml should be given to test for sensitivity, since anaphylactic, sometimes fatal, reactions can occur. The solution is given by a special injection technique to prevent leakage of fluid from the buttock into the skin, which can leave a permanent stain. Five ml (2.5 ml in each buttock) may be injected daily. Intravenous administration by infusion of 5 to 10 ml of solution over 5 minutes is approved by the United States Food and Drug Administration. Another method, which does not have FDA approval, involves dilution of the total calculated dose in 100 ml of saline for each 5 ml of iron dextran solution and infusion at an initial rate of 20 drops per minute and at a maintenance rate (if no reaction occurs) of 40 to 60 drops per minute.

The added cost and risks of parenteral injection, and the few indications for its use, make parenteral injection of iron salts a procedure to be avoided. Generally, adequate study of the patient or a change in oral iron salt dose or method of administration will eliminate the need for parenteral therapy. The rapidity of response to therapy is similar with oral and with parenteral treatment.

Porphyrias

Heme Synthesis

The biosynthesis of heme is a complex process. A simplified outline of this process is presented in Figure 5 in order to explain the pathophysiology of the porphyrias and other hematologically important diseases. Succinyl CoA and glycine condense in the presence of pyridoxal phosphate (vitamin B_6) and the inducible, rate-limiting enzyme Δ-aminolevulinic acid (Δ-ALA) synthetase to form Δ-ALA. The activity of Δ-ALA synthetase is controlled in part by its ultimate product, heme. Another enzyme, Δ-ALA dehydrase, helps form porphobilinogen (PBG), a monopyrrole with a heterocyclic structure. Four PBG molecules are assembled into a large ring-shaped molecule, uroporphyrinogen III. Further changes in the side chains of the pyrroles culminate in the formation of protoporphyrin III, which chelates with iron under the influence of heme synthetase, or ferrochelatase, to form heme. The final and initial steps in heme production occur primarily in the mitochondria of erythroid cells; the intermediate steps take place in the cytoplasm.

Pathophysiology

Although the porphyrias are usually not associated with hypochromic anemia, their pathophysiology is related to that of the sideroblastic anemias and lead poisoning. For this reason three porphyrias of concern to hematologists are discussed here.

Acute intermittent porphyria (AIP), an inherited, autosomal dominant disease, is characterized by acute attacks of abdominal pain sometimes accompanied by severe neurological deficits, including motor and respiratory paralysis, or by severe psychiatric disturbances. Acute attacks may be precipitated by barbiturates, sulfa drugs, ergot, estrogens, griseofulvin, alcohol, and many other drugs that induce Δ-ALA synthetase production. Increased quantities of ALA and PBG are found in the urine. Increased urinary excretion of PBG is revealed by the Watson-Schwartz test. Urine, sodium acetate, and Ehrlich's reagent are mixed, and in the presence of PBG a red compound forms. To confirm its identity as PBG, the reaction mixture should be extracted with chloroform. PBG will remain in the upper aqueous layer, while urobilinogen will be extracted into the lower chloroform layer. A further butanol extraction step will remove other Ehrlich-reacting compounds, leaving only PBG in the aqueous layer.

The primary abnormality in AIP is a defect in porphobilinogen deaminase (PD) activity. Presumably this defect would interfere with heme production and lead to a compensatory rise in Δ-ALA synthetase activity. Enough heme would be synthesized to prevent anemia, but Δ-ALA and PBG would be overproduced. There would be no increase in porphyrin excretion, since PD

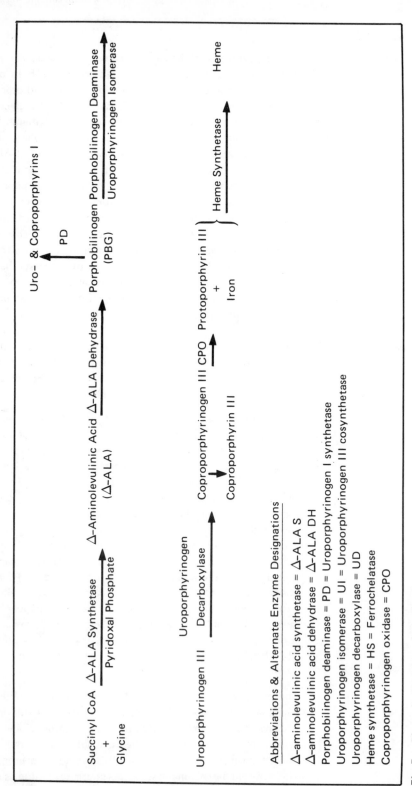

Fig. 5 : Biosynthesis of heme (simplified)

also catalyzes PBG to porphyrins. These proposed pathophysiologic mechanisms do not account for the clinical manifestations of AIP, which remain unexplained. Treatment is symptomatic with avoidance of drugs. In some female sufferers, suppression of ovulation has given relief from attacks. Phenothiazines, codeine, and other narcotics can be used in most patients to treat symptoms. Hematin given intravenously has been successfully used to treat AIP.

The second clinically important type of hepatic porphyria is variegate porphyria. Afflicted patients have skin photosensitivity (due to excessive deposition of light reactive porphyrins) along with episodic abdominal pain and neurologic symptoms sometimes associated with ingestion of barbiturates. ALA and PBG are elevated in the urine, and increased levels of protoporphyrin and coproporphyrin are continually excreted in the feces. The disease runs in families, is found particularly in South Africa, and is inherited as an autosomal dominant. Its etiology is unclear. Treatment is similar to that given for AIP along with protection from sunlight.

Acquired symptomatic porphyria or porphyria cutanea tarda is associated with alcoholic or toxic liver disease and dermal photosensitivity. Increased amounts of porphyrins are excreted in the urine and feces, but there is little or no increased excretion of ALA or PBG. A defect in uroporphyrinogen decarboxylase activity is probably responsible for this disorder. Drugs such as estrogen and alcohol precipitate attacks and should be avoided. Protection from the sun and therapeutic phlebotomies to relieve iron overload may prevent skin manifestations.

Iron-Loading Anemias

The second major type of hypochromic anemia is associated with tissue iron overload. These iron-loading anemias have the following characteristics:

1. Impaired erythropoiesis related to defective heme synthesis and not to iron deficiency
2. Increased plasma iron and saturation of transferrin ($>$ 50 percent)
3. Presence of ringed sideroblasts (Plate 8) in the marrow, usually associated with increased reticuloendothelial as well as normoblast iron
4. Dimorphic peripheral blood picture with normal-sized or small cells seen along with macrocytes (Plate 14) — only some of the cells appear hypochromic

The following classification has been found helpful in differentiating between the various types of iron-loading anemias.

Classification of iron-loading anemias

  I. Congenital or hereditary (sex-linked) sideroblastic anemia
 II. Acquired
    a. Primary
      1. Acquired sideroblastic anemia
      2. Pyridoxine-responsive sideroblastic anemia
    b. Secondary
      1. Alcoholism
      2. Chronic disease and infections
      3. Drugs, including isoniazid and cycloserine (?chloramphenicol)
      4. Hemolytic anemia
      5. Lead poisoning
      6. Leukemia
      7. Megaloblastic anemia
      8. Thalassemia

Noticeably lacking from this list are two diseases, *hemochromatosis* and *transfusion-induced siderosis,* both of which are characterized by tissue iron load. Anemia is rarely associated with these diseases, and when present is not due to defective heme metabolism. Hemachromatosis is a disease characterized by hepatic cirrhosis, large deposits of iron in hepatocytes, diabetes mellitus, and an increased melanin deposition in the skin, giving it a bronze hue. Transfusion-induced siderosis is found in patients who have received multiple blood transfusions and whose organs have iron-overloaded reticuloendothelial cells.

Hereditary (Sex-linked) Sideroblastic Anemia

Hereditary sideroblastic anemia is inherited as a sex-linked recessive disease and therefore clinically affects males. The diagnosis is usually made in adolescence and is characterized by a mild-to-moderate anemia with all the features of an iron-loading anemia. Partial improvement of the anemia results from treatment with vitamin B$_6$ or pyridoxine. Liver and spleen enlargement and a clinical picture resembling hemochromatosis have also been described.

The iron loading seen in these patients has been attributed to two factors: decreased utilization of iron for heme synthesis and, secondarily, increased gastrointestinal absorption of iron. Although heme synthesis is impaired, gut mucosal cell iron is depleted (iron continues to move from the mucosal cell to the marrow), and this leads by an unknown mechanism to increased iron absorption. If normoblast heme concentration regulates iron absorption, impaired heme production would explain why iron continues to enter the normoblast despite the cellular iron overload. The excess iron is deposited in mitochondria, thereby rendering them relatively immobile and fixing them in the perinuclear position that they assume during mitosis. These normoblasts are called *ringed sideroblasts* (Plate 8).

Decreased activity of key enzymes in heme synthesis, most commonly Δ-aminolevulinic acid synthetase (Δ-ALA-S) and rarely heme synthetase (ferrochetolase), has been implicated as the primary defect in hereditary sideroblastic anemia. Pyridoxal phosphate, formed from pyridoxine, is the active coenzyme for Δ-ALA-S and stimulates Δ-ALA-S activity, measured in vitro, in some patients with hereditary sideroblastic anemia. This observation may explain the responsiveness of this disease to high doses (100 mg three times a day) of pyridoxine. However, true vitamin B$_6$ deficiency has never been documented in conjunction with this disease.

Besides treatment with pyridoxine, therapeutic phlebotomies to remove excessive tissue iron stores have been tried as treatment for inherited sideroblastic anemia. Rises in red cell mass followed the removal of 10 gm or more of iron. This observation suggested that relieving mitochondrial iron load improves heme synthesis (perhaps by an effect on heme synthetase activity). However, the defect in heme synthesis remained despite phlebotomy, and iron removal did not affect pyridoxine dependency. In adults, iron removal with chelators such as desferrioxamine has not been successful, since the amount of iron mobilized was relatively small and tolerance to the drug's effect developed with chronic use.

Primary Acquired Sideroblastic Anemia (Sidero-achrestic Anemia)

Primary acquired sideroblastic anemia is a disease of the elderly. It presents with the usual symptoms of anemia but tends to be mild and chronic. It should be suspected when an elderly patient has a hypochromic anemia but is not iron deficient and does not have evidence of chronic disease. Except for pallor and occasionally splenomegaly the physical findings are unremarkable.

The laboratory features of this disease lead to its diagnosis. The peripheral blood smear reveals a population of hypochromic cells, (Plate 14) many normal or small and others that are macrocytic. Staining peripheral blood cells for iron may reveal Pappenheimer bodies (Plate 15) or iron-containing inclusions in mature red cells or *siderocytes.* These siderocytes can also be seen after Wright staining (Plate 16), when they appear as clusters of small, irregular inclusions. Pappenheimer bodies are seen in a number of disorders besides iron-loading anemias, including hyposplenism and some hemolytic anemias. Other blood abnormalities include neutropenia, immature red and white cells, and mild thrombocytopenia or thrombocytosis.

The bone marrow is characterized by erythroid hyperplasia and abnormalities in the normoblasts. There may be nuclear abnormalities, including binucleated cells and cell nuclei reminiscent of those seen in the megaloblastic anemias. The cytoplasm of these cells is often vacuolated or poorly hemoglobinized. Most important, the iron stain shows increased amounts of reticuloendothelial iron and ringed sideroblasts. A "shift to the left" of the myeloid series may be seen, and it is sometimes difficult to distinguish this anemia from the early stages of acute leukemia.

The saturation of the total iron-binding capacity is usually 50 percent or more and is often 100 percent. Besides the iron-loading anemias discussed in this chapter, severe hemolysis, extensive blood transfusions, hepatic necrosis, recent oral ingestion of iron tablets, and marrow hypoplasia may cause saturation of the total iron-binding capacity.

This anemia is usually resistant to all forms of therapy. In most cases folic acid (1 mg per day) is tried, since in a number of patients the serum folic acid level is low and there may be megaloblastic changes in the bone marrow. In some the bone marrow reverts toward normal and the reticulocyte count rises. Anemia is ameliorated in a few cases, but in most, folic acid has little effect. Patients are treated with blood transfusions as needed, and often live for many years without a significant change in transfusion requirements. Pyridoxine, in a dose of 100 mg three times a day, and an androgen such as oxymethalone (50 to 100 mg per day) are often prescribed but unsuccessful. Treatment with adrenocorticosteroids or splenectomy is not advised. Despite treatment, most of these patients die, often from diseases unrelated to their anemia. A few develop severe tissue iron overload secondary to multiple transfusions, and others go on to develop acute myelocytic leukemia, which is often rapidly fatal. In the latter case it is not clear whether the iron loading anemia is the first manifestation of leukemia or whether this type of anemia is associated with a leukemic predisposition.

Pyridoxine-Responsive Sideroblastic Anemia

The clinical findings of pyridoxine-responsive sideroblastic anemia are identical to those of primary acquired sideroblastic anemia. Because of this, the only way to make the diagnosis is to treat all patients suffering from unexplained sideroblastic anemias with large doses of pyridoxine. Those that respond are labeled *pyridoxine-responsive sideroblastic anemia*. A rare patient will respond to pyridoxal phosphate, but not pyridoxine, suggesting that a defect in the conversion of pyridoxine to its active coenzyme form, pyridoxal, may be the cause of this anemia.

Secondary Sideroblastic Anemia

The association of ringed sideroblasts with chronic diseases, infections, leukemia, and hemolytic or megaloblastic anemia is unusual and unexplained. In megaloblastic anemia, if the vitamin B_{12} or folic acid deficiency is successfully treated, the sideroblastic changes will disappear. Similarly, the successful treatment of any other primary underlying disease usually results in disappearance of ringed sideroblasts and other evidence of iron overload.

Drugs such as cycloserine or isoniazid have been associated with iron loading anemia. The mechanism by which they produce ringed sideroblasts is unknown. There have also been reports implicating azathioprine and chloramphenicol (an inhibitor of heme synthetase) as causes of sideroblastic anemia.

The anemia associated with the inherited disease thalassemia is primarily due to a defect in globin rather than heme synthesis. A metabolic abnormality of heme synthesis has been poorly characterized in some thalassemic patients. Iron loading, manifested by saturation of transferrin, hypochromia, and microcytosis, is a prominent finding in thalassemics, but ringed sideroblasts are found infrequently. The presence of iron in the bone marrow, family history, and the presence of increased quantities of hemoglobins such as A_2 and F distinguish thalassemias from both iron deficiency and iron-loading anemias.

Lead Poisoning

Anemia secondary to lead intoxication is characterized by hypochromic red cells, hyperferremia, ringed sideroblasts, ineffective erythropoiesis, and mild hemolysis. The last may be a result of inhibition of membrane cationic pumps. Additionally, in the peripheral blood there is an increased number of coarsely stippled red cells (Plate 68). The stippling is produced by aggregations of altered ribosomes. As a result of the inhibition by lead of sulfhydryl-containing enzymes Δ-ALA DH, coproporphyrinogen oxidase, and heme synthetase in the heme synthetic pathway, there is impaired conversion of Δ-ALA to PBG, coproporphyrinogen to protoporphyrin, and protoporphyrin to heme. As a result, patients with lead intoxication excrete in the urine large amounts of Δ-ALA and coproporphyrins, and free erythrocyte protoporphyrin is increased. In contrast to acute intermittent porphyria, PBG excretion is not greatly increased. Other effects of lead on cellular metabolism probably occur, including damage to mitochondria and impaired globin synthesis.

The diagnosis of lead intoxication is suspected when coarse stippling along with evidence of iron loading is found. Symptoms of lead poisoning include abdominal colic, peripheral neuropathy, and neuropsychiatric disorders. Poisoning is confirmed by lead levels of 70 μg per deciliter or greater in the blood, or greater than 50 μg per day in the urine. Mass screening programs detect either elevations in the red cell protoporphyrin levels or increased serum or urine lead levels. It should be recalled that free red cell protoporphyrin levels will be elevated not only in lead intoxication and iron-loading anemias but also in iron deficiency anemia.

Chelating agents, such as calcium or sodium ethylenediaminetetraacetate (EDTA) and removal of the patient from exposure to lead are the only available treatment. Ghetto children are particularly affected by this disease, since lead-containing paint chips are freely available in their environment and they are especially likely to have an iron-deficient diet that will lead them to eat these.

Alcoholism

Abnormal heme metabolism contributes to the anemia found in alcoholics. Disordered heme synthesis is manifested, particularly after "binge" drinking, by vacuolization of erythroid precursors, ringed sideroblasts, and increased reticuloendothelial iron stores.

These disappear after withdrawal of alcohol and within ten days reticulocytosis and a return of hematocrit to normal are seen. Parenteral administration of pyridoxal phosphate will also correct the disordered iron metabolism, even if alcohol intake continues. Pyridoxine is not effective, which suggests that in alcoholics defective conversion of pyridoxine to its active coenzyme form leads to impaired heme synthesis.

Anemia of Chronic Disease

A moderately severe anemia often accompanies infection, inflammatory disease, disseminated cancer, or tissue necrosis. This third major type of hypochromic anemia also complicates the response of bone marrow to replacement therapy in the presence of iron, folic acid, or vitamin B_{12} deficiency. The hematocrit usually ranges between 0.20 and 0.30. This anemia is often normochromic and normocytic; but because it may be hypochromic and occasionally microcytic, and because it involves a disordered iron metabolism, it must be considered in the differential diagnosis of hypochromic anemias. The anemia of chronic disease is extremely common and is characterized not always by hypochromia but by low serum iron, low total iron-binding capacity, normal or low transferrin saturation, and normal or elevated serum ferritin levels. Although the bone marrow is morphologically normal and is filled with reticulo-endothelial iron, the red cell production index is either decreased or not increased enough considering the severity of the anemia.

The pathogenesis of the anemia of chronic disease is unclear. The factors responsible for the decreased bone marrow function are almost totally unknown. Reticulum cell hyperplasia may contribute to a reduction in red cell life span. There appears to be a basic, unexplained disturbance in the mobilization of iron from marrow reticuloendothelial cells. These cells are filled with Prussian blue-staining iron (hemosiderin), but normoblast iron is reduced. Recent studies suggest that, in chronic diseases, both iron and transferrin are taken up by reticuloendothelial cells, which would account for their decreased levels in the plasma. Decreased transferrin levels seen in acute infections may be related to the observation that removal of iron from the environment of certain bacterial species can be fatal. This implies that transferrin may have a protective role in acute bacterial infections. More evidence is required before this theory can be accepted. Other studies in patients with rheumatoid arthritis, chronic infections, and malignancies have suggested that insufficient amounts of erythropoietin are produced in patients with the anemia secondary to these chronic diseases.

Serum iron levels and total iron-binding capacities are not very helpful in distinguishing the anemia of chronic disease from iron deficiency anemia. In both cases, serum iron is quite low, even less than 20 μg per deciliter, and transferrin saturation may be less than 15 percent. The total iron-binding capacity is usually elevated in iron deficiency anemia and decreased in anemia of chronic disease, however. Bone marrow examination can easily distinguish between the two entities. In iron deficiency, reticulo-endothelial iron is absent, and less than 10 percent of the normo-blasts contain Prussian blue–staining inclusions. In anemia of chronic disease, reticuloendothelial iron is plentiful, even though there is a reduction in normoblast iron. Serum ferritin levels assayed by a radioimmune assay are low in iron deficiency but normal or elevated in patients with anemia and normal or in-creased tissue iron stores. In practice there is another way of distinguishing these diseases — by a trial of iron therapy. Patients with the anemia of chronic disease respond little, if at all, to therapeutic amounts of iron. Iron-deficient patients show a rise in peripheral blood reticulocyte count and hematocrit.

Anemia associated with chronic disease rarely demands therapy, since the hematocrit is usually 0.25 to 0.30. Even if therapy is required, there is none available except supportive treatment with transfusions. These patients require only red cells, not plasma volume; therefore, packed red cells, and not whole blood, should be used for transfusion therapy. Treatment with iron is obviously not indicated.

Cobaltous chloride increases red cell counts in patients with the anemia of chronic disorders. However, it interferes with cell respiration, thereby producing tissue hypoxia, and for this reason cobalt therapy has been abandoned. It does stimulate erythropoietin production, either because of renal tissue hypoxia or perhaps due to the respiratory alkalosis produced by the cen-tral nervous system effects of this compound with a resultant increase in hemoglobin oxygen affinity.

Desferrioxamine

The drug *desferrioxamine* has been found to chelate iron, leading to its excretion in the urine. It has proved partially successful in treating acute iron toxicity in children and has also been sug-gested as a test for iron deficiency and iron-loading anemia. Patients with iron deficiency anemia excrete little iron in the urine after administration of this drug, but patients with iron-loading anemia initially excrete large amounts. Since a great deal of overlap exists between iron-deficient patients and normals, the test is not clinically useful. When a patient is suspected of suffering from iron-loading anemias, this test may provide sup-portive evidence. Desferrioxamine has no therapeutic value in adult forms of sideroblastic anemia, because tolerance develops to its iron-excreting effect.

Approach to patient with hypochromic anemia

I. History
   A. Adults
      1. Menstrual: menorrhagia, metrorrhagia
      2. Pregnancy: deliveries, miscarriages
      3. Blood loss
         a. Gastrointestinal: peptic ulcer symptoms, change in bowel habits, hemorrhoids, hematemesis, melena, hematochezia
         b. Drug-induced: aspirin, Indocin, phenylbutazolidin
         c. Urinary: hematuria
         d. Respiratory: hemoptysis
      4. Chronic disease
         a. Infections
         b. Inflammatory diseases
         c. Malignancy
         d. Fever, weight loss
      5. Diet
      6. Family history: thalassemia, hereditary hemorrhagic telangiectasia, sideroblastic anemia
   B. Infants and children
      1. Diet
      2. Perinatal: prematurity, multiple births, maternal iron lack
      3. Blood loss: gastrointestinal
      4. Chronic disease
      5. Family history
II. Physical examination
   A. Mucus membranes: cheilosis, angular stomatitis
   B. Tongue: glossitis, atrophy
   C. Skin: telangiectasia, evidence of chronic liver disease, koilonychia
   D. Breasts, abdomen, pelvic, rectal, etc.: evidence of infections, inflammatory or malignant disease
III. Laboratory tests
   A. Blood counts and smear (Wright stain)
   B. Reticulocyte count and production index
   C. Stool examination for occult blood
   D. Serum iron and total iron-binding capacity
   E. Bone marrow examination for iron stores
   F. Serum ferritin
   G. Erythrocyte sedimentation rate
IV. Special tests
   A. Gastrointestinal x-rays or endoscopies
   B. Stool examination for parasites
   C. Urine or sputum stained for hemosiderin
   D. Small intestinal biopsy, chemical tests for malabsorption syndromes
   E. Hemoglobins A_2 and F for thalassemia
   F. Therapeutic trial with oral iron supplementation
   G. Therapeutic trial with pyridoxine

APPROACH TO PATIENT WITH HYPOCHROMIC ANEMIA

On the basis of the historical and physical findings, serum iron, total iron-binding capacity (TIBC), and bone marrow examination, it is usually possible to distinguish anemias due to iron lack, iron overload, or chronic disease. Unusual causes of hypochromic anemia, such as thalassemia with poikilocytosis or lead poisoning with coarsely stippled red cells, are suspected on examination of the blood smear.

The characteristic low serum iron and high TIBC distinguish iron deficiency anemia from iron-loading anemia with saturation of iron-binding capacity. Anemia of chronic disease may be confused with iron deficiency, since serum iron levels may be quite low in both; however, usually the TIBC is low or normal and there is evidence for chronic disease and adequate marrow iron stores. Serum ferritin determinations, performed by radioimmunoassay, when available, clearly separate iron deficiency from anemia of chronic disease. Ferritin levels are normal in the face of chronic disease but low in iron-deficient patients. Ferritin levels are usually elevated in iron-loaded patients.

In some cases bone marrow examination of hemosiderin stores is required for differential diagnosis. Adequate iron stores rule out iron deficiency anemia, and ringed sideroblasts are characteristic of sideroblastic anemias. Often blood loss anemia, chronic disease, and iron deficiency are all suspected in one patient. In such a case bone marrow examination or therapeutic trial of oral iron supplementation is required for diagnosis.

Once the diagnosis of iron deficiency anemia is established, the possibility of blood loss from the intestine or uterus must be investigated. Only after blood loss has been ruled out should such rare causes of iron lack be considered as malabsorption syndrome, hemoglobinuria secondary to defective or prosthetic cardiac valves or immunohemolytic anemias, and pulmonary hemosiderosis (an "autoimmune" disease associated with microhemorrhages and hemosiderin-laden macrophages).

Iron-loading anemias are subclassified on the basis of family history, response to pyridoxine, and the presence of primary diseases known to cause transferrin saturation and ringed sideroblast formation.

Usually when anemia of chronic disease is suspected, malignant, inflammatory, or infectious diseases are apparent. Occasionally none of these can be demonstrated, but the *erythrocyte sedimentation rate (ESR)* is elevated. Using the Westergren method, a blood sample is anticoagulated with sodium citrate and drawn up into vertical sedimentation tubes 150 mm or longer. After an hour the length of the plasma column above the sedimented red cells is measured. The rate at which the erythrocytes sediment (millimeters per hour) depends on the serum fibrinogen concentration and to a lesser extent on the concentration of certain globulins. Male patients with ESRs greater than 15 and females with greater than 20 often have occult chronic diseases. The list of chronic diseases that cause hypoferremia and low TIBC is large, but infections, arthritis, and malignant tumors are the most common. Such diseases may cause anemia or prevent a normal response to iron in a patient with both iron deficiency anemia and chronic disease.

CASE DEVEL- OPMENT PROBLEM: HYPOCHROMIC ANEMIA

A 60-year-old man who underwent removal of the lower half of his stomach for ulcers 10 years ago was seen and treated yesterday at his neighborhood health center for acute kidney infection and has been referred to you for further examination. His hematocrit was 0.21 (21%); hemoglobin, 5.0 gm/dl; red blood cell count, $3.2 \times 10^{12}/L$; and reticulocyte count, 3 percent.

1. Calculate and interpret his Wintrobe indices. What would you find on his peripheral blood smear?

   Mean corpuscular volume; 70 fl
   Mean corpuscular hemoglobin; 16 pg
   Mean corpuscular hemoglobin concentration; 24 gm/dl
   You would expect to find microcytosis, smaller than normal cells, and hypochromic, pale-staining cells whose ring of hemoglobin would extend less than two-thirds of the distance between the cell's membrane and center.

2. His peripheral blood smear shows no polychromatophilia. Calculate his reticulocyte production index and interpret the value obtained.

   Reticulocyte production index = $(3 \times 21/45)/1$ = approximately 1.5.
   The production index indicates his bone marrow is 1½ times more active than normal. Considering his very low hematocrit, this response is inadequate. What appears to be an elevated reticulocyte count really represents an inadequate response to his anemia.

After an appropriate history and physical examination are obtained, you order determinations of serum iron and total iron-binding capacity and a stool examination. Three different sets of laboratory values are listed below. For each, describe what you would most likely find in the patient's bone marrow.

a. Serum iron: 20 μg/dl
  Total iron-binding capacity: 450 μg/dl
  Stool for occult blood: positive

Bone marrow examination would reveal erythroid hyperplasia with many poorly hemoglobinized erythroid precursors. The stain for iron would show no reticuloendothelial (extracellular) iron or normoblast (sideroblast) iron.

b. Serum iron: 190 μg/dl
  Total iron-binding capacity: 200 μg/dl
  Stool for occult blood: negative
  Serum ferritin: 500 ng/ml

Bone marrow would show mild erythroid hyperplasia and vacuolization of erythroid precursors. Sideroblastic and extracellular iron would both be increased, and there might be ringed sideroblasts.

c. Serum iron: 20 μg/dl
  Total iron-binding capacity: 180 μg/dl
  Stool for occult blood: negative
  Serum ferritin: 300 ng/ml

Bone marrow examination would be unremarkable, except that intracellular normoblastic iron might be low relative to the normal or increased stores of extracellular iron (anemia of chronic disease).

The serum iron and ferritin of the patient referred to you was low, and his total iron-binding capacity very high. His bone marrow revealed mild erythroid hyperplasia and absent stainable iron.

3. What findings are likely on physical examination?

This patient has iron deficiency anemia, so signs of anemia including pallor of skin, nails, and mucus membranes are present. Angular stomatitis, cheilosis, glossitis, tongue atrophy and koilonychia may be present if the iron deficiency is long-standing. It is also important in such a case to look for a source of blood loss. It is common in this age group for a colonic or stomach neoplasm to present with bleeding or an abdominal mass.

Gastrointestinal x-rays done on your patient revealed a recurrent ulcer at the site where his duodenum had been reattached to the remnants of his stomach. It is believed that he has had intermittent bleeding from this site. No neoplasm or other lesion is demonstrated. Ferrous sulfate, 300 mg orally three times a day, is begun.

4. What response would you expect to these therapeutic doses of iron?

In most cases an elevation in the reticulocyte count begins 3 to 5 days after oral iron therapy is started and reaches a peak in 5 to 10 days. The reticulocytosis depends on the severity of the anemia. Severely anemic patients often have reticulocyte counts above 10 percent. Within 2 to 3 weeks his hematocrit should rise.

5. Assuming he has exhausted his tissue iron stores (1,000 μg) and requires replacement of one-half his red cell mass (2,000/2 = 1,000 ml of red cells), assuming iron absorption averages approximately 10 percent, and knowing that 300 mg ferrous sulfate contains 60 mg elemental iron, calculate how long it would take to replace his red cell mass and depleted tissue iron stores.

Each 100 ml of red cells requires 100 mg elemental iron, so he will require 1,000 mg elemental iron to replace his red cell mass. A total of 2,000 mg iron will be needed to replace the red cell mass and tissue stores. Assuming 10 percent absorption of the 180 mg elemental iron in the 900 mg ferrous sulfate, he will take in about 18 mg of elemental iron per day. Therefore it will take him 2,000 divided by 18 or approximately 3½ months to replace his red cell mass and iron stores. Actually it may take longer, since iron absorption will decrease as iron deficiency is corrected.

Your patient has started iron therapy and has an initial reticulocyte response. However, his hematocrit fails to rise.

6. In this patient, what possible explanations exist for failure to respond adequately to therapy?

First, he may not be taking his iron pills. Stools will turn black if adequate amounts of iron have been ingested. Second, he may be bleeding again and therefore losing blood as fast as he is making it. A follow-up examination of his stools, looking for blood, should be done. Third, his urinary tract infection may prevent adequate response of the bone marrow. It is not known why infections adversely affect bone marrow function, but they do. Fourth, rare patients, particularly those who have undergone gastrectomy, inadequately absorb iron. If this is true of this patient, it may be necessary to treat him with intravenous or intramuscular iron.

Your patient makes a complete recovery from his iron deficiency anemia and his ulcer heals. Ten years later he again presents with a hypochromic anemia, but this time his serum iron is 200 μg/dl and his TIBC is 210 µg/dl. A bone marrow specimen, after staining with Prussian blue, reveals small blue cytoplasmic inclusions surrounding the nuclei of pronormoblasts and normoblasts. Serum ferritin is 700 ng per milliliter.

7. What is the most likely diagnosis? How should he be treated?

Most likely this patient has developed an iron-loading or sideroblastic anemia. A close study of his bone marrow for leukemia is necessary. If a complete workup reveals no etiology, then treatment with pyridoxine should be undertaken. Some patients will respond to this with an elevated hematocrit and reduced blood transfusion requirement, but for the great majority the only treatment is blood transfusion.

TOPICS FOR DISCUSSION: HYPOCHROMIC ANEMIAS

Gastrointestinal absorption of iron

Role of hydrochloric acid, phytates, chelating agents, ascorbic acid, and molybdenum in iron absorption

Red cell inclusions (stippling, Pappenheimer bodies, etc.)

Ferrokinetics

Mechanism of action and use of desferrioxamine

Iron storage compounds, ferritin, and hemosiderin

Heme and hemoglobin synthesis

Bilirubin production and excretion

Tissue changes in iron deficiency anemia

Achlorhydria and atropic gastritis in iron deficiency anemia

Subtotal gastrectomy and its effects on iron absorption

Iron fortification of food

Pathophysiology of secondary sideroblastic anemias

Anemia of chronic disease, infections, inflammatory diseases, malignancy

Alcohol and sideroblastic anemia

Hemachromatosis and hemosiderosis

Porphyrin synthesis

Porphyrias

Lead poisoning

SELECTED REFERENCES

General Considerations

Wintrobe, M. M., et al Iron Deficiency and Iron-Deficiency Anemia. In M. M. Wintrobe, et al (eds.), *Clinical Hematology* (7th ed.). Philadelphia: Lea & Febiger, 1974.

Iron Metabolism

Balcerzak, S. P., and Wheby, M. S. Iron Metabolism: Normal and Abnormal. In C. E. Mengel, et al (eds.), *Hematology: Principles and Practice.* Chicago: Year Book, 1972.

Fairbanks, V. F., and Beutler, E. *Iron Metabolism.* In W. J. Williams, E. Beutler, A. J. Erslev, and R. W. Rundles (eds.), *Hematology* (2nd ed.). New York: McGraw-Hill, 1977.

Finch, C. A., Deubelbeiss, K., and Cook, J. D., et al Ferrokinetics in man. *Medicine* (Baltimore) 49:17, 1970.

Harris, J. W., and Kellermeyer, R. W. Iron Metabolism and Iron-Lack Anemia. In J. W. Harris (ed.), *The Red Cell-Production, Metabolism, Destruction.* Boston: Harvard University Press, 1970.

Wintrobe, M. M., et al Production of Erythrocytes. In M. M. Wintrobe, et al (eds.), *Clinical Hematology* (7th ed.). Philadelphia: Lea & Febiger, 1974.

Iron Deficiency Anemia

Dagg, J. H., and Goldberg, A. Detection and treatment of iron deficiency. *Clin. Haematol.* 2:365, 1975.

Fairbanks, V. F., and Beutler, E. Iron Deficiency. In W. J. Williams, E. Beutler, A. J. Erslev, and R. W. Rundles (eds.), *Hematology* (2nd ed.). New York: McGraw-Hill, 1977.

Herbert, V. Drugs Effective in Iron-Deficiency and Other Hypochromic Anemias. In L. S. Goodman and A. Gilman (eds.), *The Pharmacological Basis of Therapeutics* (5th ed.). New York: Macmillan, 1975.

Jacobs, A., and Worwood, M. Ferritin in serum: Clinical and biochemical implications. *N. Engl. J. Med.* 292:951, 1975.

Wintrobe, M. M., et al Anemias Characterized by Deficient Hemoglobin Synthesis and Impaired Iron Metabolism. In M. M. Wintrobe, et al (eds.), *Clinical Hematology* (7th ed.). Philadelphia: Lea & Febiger, 1974.

Porphyria

Harris, J. W., and Kellermeyer, R. W. Heme Biosynthesis, the Porphyrias, and Porphyrinuria. In J. W. Harris (ed.), *The Red Cell-Production, Metabolism, Destruction.* Boston: Harvard University Press, 1970.

Robinson, S. Disorders of Heme Metabolism: Porphyria and Hyperbilirubinemia. In D. G. Nathan and F. A. Oski (eds.), *Hematology of Infancy and Childhood.* Philadelphia: W. B. Saunders, 1974.

Tschudy, D. P. Acute intermittent porphyria: Clinical and selected research aspects. *Ann. Intern. Med.* 83:851, 1975.

Waldenstrom, J. G. The Porphyrias. In W. J. Williams, E. Beutler, A. J. Erslev, and R. W. Rundles (eds.), *Hematology* (2nd ed.). New York: McGraw-Hill, 1977.

Wintrobe, M. M., et al The Porphyrias. In M. M. Wintrobe, et al (eds.), *Clinical Hematology* (7th ed.). Philadelphia: Lea & Febiger, 1974.

Iron Loading Anemia

Bottomley, S. Porphyrin and iron metabolism in sideroblastic anemia. *Semin. Hematol.* 14:169, 1977.

Eichner, E. R. The hematologic disorders of alcoholism. *Am. J. Med.* 54:621, 1973.

Kushner, J., Lee, G., Wintrobe, M., and Cartwright, G. Idiopathic refractory sideroblastic anemia. Clinical and laboratory investigation of 17 patients and review of the literature. *Medicine* (Baltimore) 50:139, 1971.

Miescher, P. A., and Jaffe, E. R. (eds.) Iron excess: Aberrations of iron and porphyrin metabolism. *Semin. Hematol.* 14:1, 1977.

Sears, D. A. Sideroblastic Anemias. In R. I. Weed (ed.), *Hematology for Internists.* Boston: Little, Brown, 1971.

Valentine, W. N. Sideroblastic Anemias. In W. J. Williams, E. Beutler, A. J. Erslev, and R. W. Rundles (eds.), *Hematology* (2nd ed.). New York: McGraw-Hill, 1977.

Weintraub, L., Conrad, M., and Crosby, W. Iron loading anemia. Treatment with repeated phlebotomies and pyridoxine. *N. Engl. J. Med.* 275: 169, 1966.

White, J. M., and Selhi, H. S. Lead and the red cell. *Br. J. Haematol.* 30:133, 1975.

Wintrobe, M. M., et al Sideroblastic Anemias. In M. M. Wintrobe, et al (eds.), *Clinical Hematology* (7th ed.). Philadelphia: Lea & Febiger, 1974.

Anemia of Chronic Disease

Barret-Conner, E. Anemia and infection. *Am. J. Med.* 52:242, 1972.

Cartwright, G. The anemia of chronic disorders. *Semin. Hematol.* 3:351, 1966.

Kremer, W. B., and Laszlo, J. Hematologic Effects of Cancer. In J. F. Holland and E. Frei (eds.), *Cancer Medicine.* Philadelphia: Lea & Febiger, 1973.

Wintrobe, M. M., et al Anemia of Chronic Disorders. In M. M. Wintrobe, et al (eds.), *Clinical Hematology* (7th ed.). Philadelphia: Lea & Febiger, 1974.

3 : Megaloblastic Anemia

Defective deoxyribonucleic acid (DNA) synthesis underlies the megaloblastic anemias. As a result of this defect in DNA synthesis, the bone marrow contains large erythroid precursors with immature nuclei and mature, hemoglobin-containing cytoplasm (megaloblasts). Also present are large white cell precursors with atypical nuclear chromatin structure. Cytopenias, large oval erythrocytes, and neutrophils with six or more lobes are found in the peripheral blood. In all but a few megaloblastic anemias, the defective DNA synthesis is secondary to vitamin B_{12} or folic acid deficiency. In a small minority. of patients the megaloblastic changes are secondary to serious defects in DNA metabolism due to diseases such as leukemia.

Pathophysiology The anemia seen in association with megaloblastosis is due to ineffective erythropoiesis, that is, death of erythroid cells before release from the marrow, and early destruction of circulating erythrocytes. It is not entirely clear, however, how the deficiency in vitamin B_{12} or folic acid leads to defective DNA synthesis or how defective DNA synthesis results in premature cell death. (The biochemical events that result from vitamin B_{12} and folic acid deficiency are discussed under those headings, pp. 68 and 82.) It is known that a state of unbalanced growth exists in the marrow cells of patients with magaloblastic anemia. The megaloblasts contain a substantially increased amount of RNA and a normal or slightly increased amount of DNA. This imbalance comes about because there is a delay in cell division due to impaired synthesis of one or more deoxyribonucleotides, the precursors of DNA, while RNA production proceeds normally. It is possible that premature cell death results from this unbalanced cell maturation — a concept that, although not yet experimentally confirmed, is helpful in understanding the morphologic and clinical manifestations of megaloblastic anemia. Presumably the degree of impairment of DNA synthesis varies from cell to cell and is more prominent among erythroid cells than among granulocytes.

Laboratory Findings As a result of ineffective erythropoiesis, granulopoiesis, and thrombopoiesis, and premature destruction of defective cells in the peripheral blood, it is unusual to find a patient with megaloblastic anemia who does not have depression of all three cell lines in the peripheral blood. Despite this pancytopenia, the bone marrow is morphologically hyperplastic — a finding that lends support to the theory that ineffective production of blood cells with early death in the marrow is an important pathophysiologic mechanism in megaloblastic anemia.

The megaloblastic bone marrow produces macrocytic, oval red cells. Their MCH and MCV are both increased, so that the MCHC is normal and the cells appear normochromic. Macroovalocytosis (Plate 17), as seen in the peripheral blood smear, is a very important hallmark of megaloblastic anemias. Although the reticulocyte count is often 2 to 3 percent, the reticulocyte production index is low, a reflection of a functionally defective marrow.

Marked abnormalities in the shape of red cells also occur in megaloblastic anemias. It has been suggested that these abnormalities result from fragmentation of abnormal red cells as they pass through small arterioles. Although this explanation is not accepted by everyone, it is clear that, as the megaloblastic anemia becomes more severe, bizarre shapes such as triangles, helmets, and teardrops increase proportionately. In severe megaloblastic anemia the poikilocytosis approaches that seen in microangiopathic hemolytic anemias due to mechanical fragmentation of erythrocytes.

The megaloblastic process also leads to abnormalities in white cells. Cell size and average number of lobes in the mature granulocyte (*poly*) are increased. Normally no more than 1 percent of polys have six nuclear lobes, but in megaloblastic anemia many have six or more, even ten, lobes (Plate 18). There is disagreement about how lobes should be counted. Most observers insist that there be a definite constriction between separate lobes, with only a thin chromatin strand separating them. Disagreement also exists as to whether the hyperlobulation is due to hypermaturity of the megaloblastic neutrophil or to abnormal nuclear division.

Elevated levels of serum lactic acid dehydrogenase (LDH), bilirubin, and urinary urobilinogen are believed to be related to ineffective erythropoiesis. The LDH isoenzyme that is elevated in patients with megaloblastic anemia is characteristic of bone marrow erythroid precursors. Serum LDH elevation is believed to be secondary to premature destruction of red cell precursors within the bone marrow. Similarly, the increase in serum bilirubin and urinary urobilinogen is a reflection of an increase in heme degradation products due to marrow destruction of erythrocyte precursors. Radiolabeled heme is produced in bone marrow cells after injection of radioactive glycine. In patients with megaloblastic anemia, an "early peak" of radiolabeled bilirubin appears within a few days, indicating early destruction of hemoglobin-containing erythroid cells. This observation lends further support to the concept of ineffective erythropoiesis in megaloblastic marrows.

Studies of iron kinetics also suggest ineffective erythropoiesis. Plasma iron turnover and marrow iron are both increased despite decreased incorporation of iron into mature red cells. Elevated plasma iron levels, which fall to normal or low after successful treatment with vitamin B_{12} or folic acid, are often found in patients with megaloblastic anemia.

Hemolysis, or premature death of erythrocytes, in the peripheral blood, as measured by radioiron or radiochromium red cell life span assays, is thought to be due to intrinsic erythrocyte defects caused by unbalanced nucleic acid synthesis in the marrow. Enlargement of the patient's spleen with sequestration or destruction of erythrocytes may also contribute to hemolysis. Laboratory indicators of hemolysis, such as decreased plasma haptoglobin and presence of serum methemalbumin, confirm that hemolysis plays an important role in causing megaloblastic anemia. Despite hemolysis the reticulocyte production index is reduced.

Megaloblastic anemia is characterized by macroovalocytosis, hypersegmented polys, megaloblastic erythropoiesis, and giant myeloid forms in the bone marrow, along with evidence of ineffective erythropoiesis and hemolysis. Morphologically the megaloblastic erythropoiesis (Plates 19 and 20) is characterized by the presence of large cells with pink or gray cytoplasm, whose nuclei, however, have a "clock-face" arrangement of the chromatin network. The chromatin of these hemoglobin-containing normoblasts is stippled or lacy in appearance, an exaggeration of the appearance of normal pronormoblast nuclei. Thus the morphologic appearance — an immature nucleus associated with mature cytoplasm — parallels the biochemical abnormality whereby DNA synthesis and maturation of the cell nucleus is impaired while cytoplasmic RNA and hemoglobin synthesis proceed normally. It is important to remember that the nuclear–cytoplasmic dissociation is best recognized in the late, hemoglobinized normoblast, for in the early basophilic normoblast the nucleus is normally immature. Concomitant iron deficiency, resulting in delay of hemoglobinization, may make it difficult to recognize megaloblastic erythropoiesis. Infection, recent transfusions, and inappropriate treatment — for example, the use of folic acid to treat vitamin B_{12} deficiency — may obscure or normalize the nuclear–cytoplasmic dissocation, thereby making the diagnosis of megaloblastic anemia difficult or impossible.

The term *megaloblastoid* should not be used, since its meaning is unclear. Mild megaloblastosis, megaloblastic marrow features not responsive to vitamin B_{12} or folic acid therapy, and equivocal abnormalities suggestive of megaloblastic anemia have all been called megaloblastoid.

Giant white cell precursor forms (Plate 21), abnormal megakarocytes, and hypercellularity of all three cell lines are almost constant features of megaloblastic marrows. The increased size of the granulocytes is most noticeable at the myelocyte, metamyelocyte, and band stages. These granulocytes also have open chromatin patterns and bizarre lobulations or twists to their nuclei. Megakaryocytes may be distinctly abnormal, with many lobes to their nuclei, sometimes without the normal connection between lobes. The platelets produced by these megakaryocytes tend to be large but functionally normal.

Vitamin B_{12} Deficiency

Although the molecular mechanisms are not understood, it is clear that deficiency of vitamin B_{12} leads to megaloblastic erythropoiesis and anemia. The metabolism of vitamin B_{12} and pathways by which its deficiency may interfere with DNA synthesis will be reviewed here. Since vitamin B_{12} is common in human diets, almost all deficiencies of vitamin B_{12} are a result of malabsorption, and for this reason we shall discuss in some detail the normal absorption of vitamin B_{12}. Clinical features of vitamin B_{12} deficiency, its common causes, and an approach to its diagnosis will also be described.

Biochemistry of Vitamin B_{12}

In simplest terms vitamin B_{12} is made up of a porphyrinlike structure attached to a nucleotide. This structure is analogous to the porphyrin structure of heme, with the position of the heme iron being occupied by a cobalt atom. *Cobalamin* refers to a vitamin B_{12} that lacks a ligand covalently bound to the cobalt atom. Cyanide binding yields a compound called *cyanocobalamin,* and if a hydroxyl group is bound to cobalt, it is called *hydroxycobalamin.* Vitamin B_{12} is usually isolated by first stabilizing the molecule with cyanide. Cyano- and hydroxycobalamin are probably inactive and must be converted to active compounds such as $5'$-deoxyadenosylcobalamin or methylcobalamin.

Three reactions dependent upon vitamin B_{12} may be important to human metabolism. In bacteria and mammalian tissues, deoxyadenosylcobalamin (and methylmalonyl CoA mutase) is required for conversion of methylmalonyl CoA to succinyl CoA. The excretion of methylmalonic acid is increased in vitamin B_{12} deficient humans. In certain bacteria the reduction of purines and pyrimidines to deoxypurines and deoxypyrimidines requires vitamin B_{12} as well as ribonucleotide reductase. This requirement for vitamin B_{12} for the synthesis of DNA precursors has not been demonstrated in man but has been found in the organisms used to assay vitamin B_{12}, namely, *Lactobacillus leichmannii.* Vitamin

B_{12}-starved organisms undergo unbalanced growth and acquire forms that are analogous to the megaloblasts of human vitamin B_{12} deficiency. Methylcobalamin is required for the synthesis of methionine in bacteria and probably in man. This synthesis of methionine also leads to the conversion of N^5-methyltetrahydrofolate (N^5-methyl-FH_4) to tetrahydrofolate (FH_4):

$$\text{Homocysteine} + N^5\text{-methyl-}FH_4 \xrightarrow[\text{methylcobalamin}]{\text{methyltransferase}} \text{methionine} + FH_4$$

Unless methylcobalamin is present, N^5-methyltetrahydrofolate will accumulate, leading to a deficiency of tetrahydrofolate, which is required for thymidine synthesis. This would presumably lead to a defect in DNA synthesis. This entrapment of methyltetrahydrofolate in the absence of vitamin B_{12} may account for the defective synthesis of DNA seen in vitamin B_{12} deficiency and for the partial reversal by folic acid of the megaloblastosis associated with vitamin B_{12} deficiency. Again, it should be emphasized that only the methylmalonic CoA–to–succinyl CoA metabolic pathway has been conclusively demonstrated in animal tissues. Thus the role of vitamin B_{12} in the production of megaloblastic erythropoiesis is not fully defined. Furthermore, none of these metabolic pathways adequately accounts for the defective myelin synthesis and neurologic symptoms prominent in severe human vitamin B_{12} deficiency.

An alternative to the "methylfolate-trap" hypothesis has recently been proposed. Folate is present in cells in two forms. One form has a single glutamic acid residue (monoglutamate), and the other has a chain of up to six residues (polyglutamate). The monoglutamate is the transport form in the serum, and cellular polyglutamates are probably the active coenzymes. The levels of folate polyglutamates in vitamin B_{12}-deficient red cells are lower than normal. Possibly vitamin B_{12} deficiency leads to failure of folate polyglutamate synthesis, which in turn slows entry of folate monoglutamate into cells and increases folate levels in serum. The deficient folate polyglutamate synthesis impairs nucleic acid synthesis. This theory has not been experimentally confirmed.

Vitamin B_{12} Requirements and Stores

The ultimate source of vitamin B_{12} in man is from microbial synthesis. The vitamin B_{12} synthesized by microbes is deposited in animal tissues, such as liver, eggs, and milk, and is therefore plentiful in fish and meat products. The average diet contains 5 to 30 μg of vitamin B_{12} daily, 1 to 5 μg of which usually is absorbed. In the adult a storage pool of 3,000 to 5,000 μg is present, of which 1,000–3,000 μg is stored in the liver. There is some disagreement about the human daily requirement for vitamin B_{12}. It once was put at 0.6 to 1.2 μg, but, according to studies of the loss of vitamin B_{12} in feces and urine and of the amount of vitamin B_{12} required to completely correct megaloblastic anemia due to vitamin B_{12} deficiency, a higher value of 2 μg or possibly up to 10 μg may represent the true daily requirement. The amount of vitamin B_{12} lost per day has been reported as 0.1 percent of total body stores. This might account for the variability in the reported amounts of vitamin B_{12} required daily. These numbers are clinically important for two reasons. First, it is clear that the average American diet contains enough vitamin B_{12}, so that deficiency should not result unless there is a defect in absorption of this vitamin. Also, it is clear that should malabsorption of vitamin B_{12} occur, it will take 2 to 5 years before body stores are exhausted and megaloblastic erythropoiesis supervenes.

Vitamin B_{12}
Absorption

Since vitamin B_{12} deficiency is almost always due to malabsorption, it is necessary to understand the normal physiologic mechnisms involved in the intestinal absorption of this vitamin. In brief, vitamin B_{12} binds with a glycoprotein called *intrinsic factor* (IF), which is secreted by the parietal cells located in the body of the stomach. The intrinsic factor–B_{12} complex is absorbed in the ileum, and the IF removed. Vitamin B_{12} without IF is then transferred to a binding protein in the plasma, which transports the vitamin to the liver, where it is stored. The most common disease associated with vitamin B_{12} malabsorption, *pernicious anemia,* is caused by failure to secrete adequate amounts of IF.

Human gastric IF is secreted by the same cell that produces hydrochloric acid. This parietal cell is stimulated into producing acid and IF by histamine and the histamine analogue betazole hydrochloride and by insulin and gastrin. Healthy subjects secrete about 900 to 8,300 units (1 unit binds 1 nanogram of vitamin B_{12}) per hour, with a mean of 3,000 units. With a single 0.5-mg dose of histamine given parenterally, the concentration of IF increases from 36 to 44 units per milliliter and approximately 4,500 units is produced per hour. Intrinsic factor reaches a peak in the first 15 minutes following injection of histamine, while acid and pepsin secretion reach a peak in 30 to 45 minutes after histamine stimulation. In general the output of IF is paralleled by the amount of acid secreted. There are a few patients who secrete very little acid but continue to secrete adequate amounts of IF. Approximately 500 to 1,000 units of IF is required for maximal absorption of 1 μg of vitamin B_{12}.

Some patients with pernicious anemia produce an antibody to IF which will precipitate human IF. This property is used in a radioimmunoassay for IF. As the assay is usually unavailable clinically, it will not be described here.

In man vitamin B_{12} is absorbed only in the lower ileum. Removal of as little as two feet of ileum may impair vitamin B_{12} absorption, and when more than six feet is removed, absorption is invariably abnormal. The uptake in the ileum is 70 percent of dietary vitamin B_{12} to a limit of 10 μg per day. The vitamin IF–B_{12} complex attaches to the microvilli of the brush border of the cells lining the ileum. Calcium ions and neutral pH must be present, but there appears to be no energy requirement. Transport through the mucosal cell is poorly understood but probably involved as an energy-requiring step. Vitamin B_{12} enters the mitochondria of the mucosal cell, remains there for six hours, and then appears in the blood. Vitamin B_{12} in blood is not attached to IF. It is not clear whether IF is cleaved before entry of the complex into the mucosal cell, or whether IF is removed after the complex has entered the cell.

In the absence of IF there is a second mechanism by which vitamin B_{12} can be absorbed through the ileum. Oral doses of 1,000 μg per day completely reverse the hematologic and neurologic abnormalities found in patients with IF deficiency. The mechanism for this nonphysiologic absorption of large doses of vitamin B_{12} is probably simple diffusion from a high concentration in the intestine into the mucosa. It is probably this mechanism that accounts for responses to oral, high dose, liver therapy in patients with pernicious anemia who were treated before vitamin B_{12} was available for therapy.

Transport of Vitamin B_{12} in Plasma

Three to four hours after oral ingestion, vitamin B_{12} is detected in the blood. A peak level is obtained in 8 to 10 hours. The vitamin is attached to three protein binders named transcobalamin (TC) I (an α_1-globulin present in granulocytes), to TC II (a β-globulin), and TC III. Both TC I and TC II have a half-life of 9 to 10 days. Initially it was believed that TC II was cleared within hours from the serum, but this may have been due to partial denaturation during its preparation.* Studies also suggest that transcobalamin III and transcobalamin I are immunologically related. From studies in man it appears that transcobalamin II is most important, since one infant lacking this protein developed severe megaloblastic anemia. It is probably responsible for all vitamin B_{12} transportation in the body. TC I may serve a storage rather than a transport function. It has been suggested that at least some of these vitamin B_{12} protein binders are produced in leukocytes, which explains their elevation in myeloproliferative diseases and in diseases associated with leukocytosis.

*For most recent rebuttal see R. H. Allen, The Plasma Transport of Vitamin B_{12}. *Br. J. Haematol.* 33:161, 1976.

Schilling Test

One of the most useful means of making the diagnosis of vitamin B_{12} deficiency and determining its etiology is the Schilling test, which measures the absorption of orally administered radiolabeled vitamin B_{12}. The simplest and most commonly employed method is to give the patient a 0.5- or 1 μg-dose of radiocobalt-labeled cyanocobalamin and either immediately after or 2 hours later to administer a 1-mg dose of nonradioactive cyanocobalamin intramuscularly. This "flushing" dose is used to saturate vitamin B_{12} binding sites in the plasma and liver. A 24-hour collection of urine is begun after the radioactive B_{12} has been ingested. Normal subjects will excrete in their urine 7 percent or more of the radioactivity taken orally, whereas patients with pernicious anemia or other causes of vitamin B_{12} malabsorption will excrete less than 5 percent.

Certain precautions must be observed. If the patient's renal status is not satisfactory; a 48-hour or 72-hour collection of urine will be required, since the excretion of vitamin B_{12} will be delayed. If the patient uses a bedpan, contamination with fecal material can sometimes give artifactually high recoveries in the urine collection. If, for one reason or another, a urine collection cannot be obtained, then either whole body radioactivity counting is done, or a serum radioactive B_{12} level is obtained approximately eight hours after an oral dose of radiolabeled vitamin. In the latter case the normal values depend upon the dose of vitamin B_{12} given and the time at which blood samples are drawn. These must be standardized, and normal values made available to the clinician. If whole body radioactivity or plasma radioactivity is measured, a flushing dose of vitamin B_{12} is not used. For unexplained reasons some patients with vitamin B_{12} deficiency following a partial gastrectomy give normal or near-normal results to the Schilling test. It should be remembered that this test can be used to measure vitamin B_{12} absorption even after the patient has been treated for B_{12} deficiency and has fully recovered. On the other hand the administration of the 1-mg flushing dose will treat the megaloblastic anemia and make the hematologic findings revert toward normal.

The second part of the Schilling test is performed only if the first part gives abnormal results. In the second part 60 mg of hog IF is given orally along with the radioactive vitamin B_{12}. If there is a defect in the absorption of the vitamin IF-B_{12} complex, then abnormally small amounts of B_{12} will be excreted. However, if the patient's gastric secretions lack IF, the addition of hog IF to the vitamin B_{12} oral dose leads to normal urinary excretion of the vitamin B_{12}. Thus, the part one and part two Schilling tests distinguish IF deficiency from ileal malabsorption of IF-B_{12} complex. A third part of the Schilling test may be performed if the patient suffers from malabsorption of the IF-B_{12} complex secondary to small intestinal bacterial overgrowth. In this part of the Schilling test a two-week course of antibiotic therapy with tetracycline, 250 mg four times a day, is prescribed. If bacterial overgrowth was responsible for the abnormal second part of the Schilling test, then tetracycline treatment should normalize vitamin B_{12} absorption. In practice, the third part of the Schilling test is seldom performed.

Finally, it should be emphasized that the hog IF used in the Schilling test must be tested for activity. This means that each new lot of IF must be tested by giving a sample to a patient with known IF deficiency and finding that it corrects the vitamin B_{12} malabsorption. If this is not done, it is possible for inactive hog IF to cause a falsely abnormal second part Schilling test.

Clinical Findings in Vitamin B_{12} Deficiency

Anemia secondary to vitamin B_{12} deficiency is associated with low serum vitamin B_{12} levels, abnormal Schilling test results, response of the anemia to physiologic doses of vitamin B_{12} but not to folic acid, and, sometimes, neurologic defects. *Subacute combined system disease* is due to degeneration of myelin in the dorsal and lateral columns of the spinal cord in association with vitamin B_{12} deficiency. It is characterized by paresthesias or tingling in the extremities and by decreased vibratory and position sense. An abnormal gait and loss of bladder and rectal control are characteristic of the chronic, severe form of this disease. In modern times it is unusual to encounter more than the paresthesias and loss of position and vibratory senses, probably because most patients with unexplained anemia or neurologic findings are very quickly treated with massive doses of vitamin B_{12}. Occasional patients may have combined systems disease in the absence of noticeable anemia. Other nervous system abnormalities include changes in the patient's personality, giving rise to *megaloblastic "madness"*. The patient may be demented, disoriented, irritable, or depressed or have memory and intellectual impairment.

The ability to assay the concentration of serum vitamin B_{12} has greatly simplified the diagnostic approach to patients with megaloblastic anemia. The first reliable tests utilized organisms such as *Euglena gracilis* or *Lactobacillus leichmannii*, which require vitamin B_{12} for growth. A standard curve was developed by incubating several suspensions of these organisms, each with a different amount of vitamin B_{12}. After allowing sufficient incubation time for growth, the resultant suspensions were assayed by optical density methods for turbidity. If large amounts of vitamin B_{12} were present, the optical density was high. After a standard curve had been developed, then unknown serum samples could be similarly assayed and, by use of the standard curve, a serum B_{12} value determined. These microbiologic assays, however, were difficult to perform. The organisms behaved unpredictably, and contamination with vitamin B_{12} from distilled water or other sources sometimes occurred. More frequently certain antibiotics and drugs inhibited the growth of the organisms, giving falsely low results. Today most vitamin B_{12} assays are done by radioisotope dilution methods. Aliquots of pooled serum containing vitamin B_{12} binders are incubated with radiolabeled vitamin B_{12} and increasing amounts of unlabeled vitamin B_{12}. The more unlabeled B_{12} present, the more radioactive vitamin B_{12} will be released from the B_{12} binders and then absorbed by charcoal or DEAE-cellulose (diethylaminoethyl cellulose). The amount of radioactivity remaining bound to transcobolamins is inversely proportional to the amount of unlabeled radioactive vitamin B_{12} present. By plotting known amounts of vitamin B_{12} added against radioactivity remaining after absorption with charcoal or DEAE-cellulose, a curve is obtained from which the amount of vitamin B_{12} in a serum sample, can be determined. In normal sera, 200 to 1,000 ng per liter is detected. There are technical difficulties with this test, but, when performed properly, it gives quick and reliable results that are not affected by drugs or antibiotics.

A therapeutic trial is sometimes undertaken to determine whether patients with megaloblastic anemia have vitamin B_{12} or folic acid deficiency. Physiologic amounts — 5 μg or less — of vitamin B_{12} are given parenterally. If the patient has vitamin B_{12} deficiency, a reticulocytosis is seen in three or four days and reaches a peak in five to ten days. With a complete response the hematocrit rises to normal, usually within three to four weeks. The amount of time required to perform this trial inclines clinicians to use, instead, the serum B_{12} level assay or Schilling test. It should be emphasized that patients undergoing this therapeutic trial must be on a folic acid–deficient diet. For, if they were to receive large amounts of folic acid in their diet and be folic acid–deficient rather than vitamin B_{12}–deficient, they would have a reticulocyte response that might be attributed to the parenteral vitamin B_{12}. Large doses of folic acid, 5 mg or more, may produce a reticulocyte response in patients with vitamin B_{12} deficiency, but the hematocrit will not return to normal. Administration of large amounts of folate to patients who have neurologic involvement may lead to further impairment.

Conditions Associated with Vitamin B_{12} Deficiency

The causes of vitamin B_{12} deficiency follow (p. 75).

Pernicious Anemia. Pernicious anemia (PA) is the disease most often associated with vitamin B_{12} deficiency. It is defined as anemia resulting from defective secretion of IF by the gastric mucosal cells. Characteristically patients with PA are of Northern European extraction and have fair complexions and blue eyes. Long earlobes, prematurely gray hair, and blood group A are

Causes of vitamin B_{12} deficiency

Common Causes
Partial gastrectomy
Pernicious anemia
Sprue

Uncommon Causes
Blind loop syndromes
Cancer
Deficiency of folate or vitamin B_{12}
Drugs
Fish tapeworm
Poor diet (vegetarianism)
Pregnancy
Regional ileitis, particularly with ileal resection
Selective malabsorption of vitamin B_{12}
Severe chronic pancreatitis
Thyroid disease

other clinical features associated with PA. The patients are usually elderly and are seldom blacks or orientals. Not all patients fit this description, and many patients who have these clinical findings do not suffer from PA. Female and male patients may be infertile secondary to vitamin B_{12} deficiency, and for this reason pernicious anemia is seldom associated with pregnancy.

Patients with PA invariably do not secrete hydrochloric acid, even after parenteral stimulation with histamine or betazole. Their defective IF secretion means they give abnormal results to part one of the Schilling test and normal results to part two. The correction of the Schilling test by oral IF is the most important laboratory confirmation of this diagnosis. Two types of antibodies to IF may be detected in the serum or gastric juice of a large percentage of patients. One type of antibody blocks the binding of vitamin B_{12} to IF and is called *blocking antibody*. The second type, *precipitating antibody,* attaches to and precipitates IF or IF–B_{12} complex, thereby blocking the attachment of the IF–B_{12} complex to the ileal mucosa.

The presence of these antibodies and the ability of corticosteroids to reverse defective parietal cell function early in pernicious anemia (presumably by suppressing antibody production or function) support an autoimmune theory for the etiology of PA. According to this theory, injury to the gastric mucosa, perhaps initiated by a virus, leads to production of antibodies directed against the parietal cell or IF. Parietal cell antibodies are relatively common and are found not only in patients with pernicious anemia but also in those with gastritis and many other diseases. Although not demonstrated experimentally, it has been presumed that these parietal cell antibodies are cytotoxic and able to destroy parietal cell function. The antibodies to IF are effective in neutralizing IF function, but only when they are present in gastric juice. Seventy-five percent of PA patients have detectable IF antibodies in the gastric juice. It cannot be overemphasized that this autoimmune theory has not been proved since the observations on which it is based are few and contradictory.

Pathologic examination of the stomach of PA patients reveals only atrophy of the mucosa with some inflammatory cells. Megaloblastic epithelial cells may be present and occasionally are mistaken for neoplasia. For this reason caution should be exercised in examining exfoliated, epithelial, gastric cells for malignancy before correcting megaloblastic anemia. There does appear to be a small but definite increased incidence of gastric carcinoma in patients with pernicious anemia.

All the features of megaloblastic anemia have been described in association with pernicious anemia, e.g., pancytopenia, glossitis, atrophy of the tongue, and evidence of ineffective erythropoiesis. Abnormalities specific for vitamin B_{12} deficiency are also present. Serum vitamin B_{12} level is low, usually less than 150 ng per liter. Neurologic symptoms, particularly paresthesias and loss of position and vibratory sense, are common. When parenteral vitamin B_{12} therapy is instituted, there is a typical response. It should be emphasized that such a response is not characteristic of PA alone but will occur in patients with vitamin B_{12} deficiency due to any cause.

The diagnosis of PA is confirmed by a low serum B_{12} and typically abnormal results of the Schilling test. With the growth of nuclear medicine the Schilling test can now be performed in most parts of the country. Where it cannot, a therapeutic trial with vitamin B_{12} will suffice. Assays for methylmalonic aciduria and antibodies to IF or parietal cells are in general difficult to obtain, and assays for IF in gastric juice can be obtained only in research centers. The tube test or the Diagnex blue test for achlorhydria are readily available, but most patients with pernicious anemia are in the elderly age group, so a finding of achlorhydria is not unusual. If gastric acid is present, the diagnosis of pernicious anemia is effectively ruled out. Vitamin B_{12} deficiency can exist even in the presence of gastric acidity, but not with a PA etiology.

Incidentally, gastric hydrochloric acid is now measured by determining the pH of gastric juice with a pH meter. Achlorhydria is present if the pH is not less than 3.5 pH units and does not decrease by more than 1 pH unit following maximal stimulation with histamine. When the pH drop after histamine is more than 1 pH unit, even though the initial pH is above 3.5 pH units, the condition is called *hypochlorhydria*.

Congenital IF Deficiency. Congenital IF deficiency is a rare disease of children and is characterized by a selective defect in IF secretion. The resultant vitamin B_{12} malabsorption is correctable with oral IF. Gastric mucosa and gastric acidity are both normal. Autoantibodies to IF and parietal cells are not present. Congenital qualitatively abnormal intrinsic factor production is another very rare cause of vitamin B_{12} deficiency.

Selective Vitamin B_{12} Malabsorption. Selective vitamin B_{12} malabsorption, another rare disorder of children, runs in families and is associated with persistent proteinuria of unknown etiology. IF secretion is normal, and there are no antibodies against IF or against ileal receptors for the IF–B_{12} complex. Recent studies suggest a defect occurring somewhere in the chain of events after IF–B_{12} attaches to the surface of the ileal cell and before the absorbed vitamin binds to transcobalamin II. There appears to be no morphologic lesion, and the absorptive defect does not appear to result from lack of ileal receptors for IF-B$_{12}$. Antibodies to IF are not found in these patients. Congenital transcobalamin II deficiency and vitamin B$_{12}$ deficiency secondary to maternal deficiency, both very rare diseases, can be confused with this disorder.

Partial or Total Gastrectomy. Ultimately, removal of the stomach in toto results in vitamin B$_{12}$ malabsorption due to lack of IF. After body stores of vitamin B$_{12}$ have been exhausted, megaloblastic anemia occurs in five or six years, unless the patient is treated with parenteral vitamin B$_{12}$. Vitamin B$_{12}$ deficiency may also occur in partially gastrectomized patients. Untreated patients can develop frank megaloblastic anemia, but in most cases they have only depressed serum B$_{12}$ levels or abnormal reactions to part one of the Schilling test. As mentioned previously, some patients with partial gastrectomies will have difficulty absorbing vitamin B$_{12}$ bound to food but not the purified vitamin. These patients have a normal Schilling test but have depressed serum levels of vitamin B$_{12}$. The vitamin B$_{12}$ deficiency seen after partial gastrectomy is attributed to surgical loss of IF-producing cells, but probably more important is continued gastritis and loss of parietal cells in the remaining stomach. The gastritis may be related to concomitant iron deficiency. Although only a small percentage of patients with partial gastrectomy develop frank megaloblastic anemia, some surgeons administer vitamin B$_{12}$ prophylactically after gastrectomy. Other surgeons treat postgastrectomy patients only when the vitamin B$_{12}$ level becomes depressed or the Schilling test abnormal. Iron and folic acid deficiency are both also associated with gastrectomy (See Interrelationships between Vitamin B$_{12}$, Folic Acid, and Iron, p. 92.

Malabsorption Syndromes. Various intestinal defects and diseases can lead to vitamin B$_{12}$ deficiency. These diseases are relatively uncommon compared to pernicious anemia. Nontropical sprue (celiac disease) and tropical sprue are diseases characterized by villous atrophy, which causes malabsorption of various substances, including vitamin B$_{12}$. Nontropical sprue is thought to be due to sensitivity to gluten, a substance found in many grains. The etiology of tropical sprue is unknown, but it appears to respond to folic acid or antibiotic therapy. Patients with malabsorption syndromes have abnormal part one and part two Schilling tests. Patients with the form of tropical sprue that responds to antibiotics have a normal part three Schilling test.

The blind loop syndrome occurs in patients who have a portion of the small intestine isolated from the mainstream of the gut. Isolated duodenal and ileal loops result, respectively, from partial gastrectomies and operative procedures for inflammatory bowel diseases. In these blind loops or in intestinal diverticuli, bacterial overgrowth occurs due to failure of drainage and stasis of intestinal contents. Although these bacteria do not require vitamin B_{12} for their growth, binding sites on their cell walls compete with their host's IF for vitamin B_{12}, thereby reducing vitamin B_{12} absorption. The patient's absorption improves after surgical removal of the diverticuli or loop or after the blind pouch is returned to the main gastrointestinal stream.

A rare but interesting cause of vitamin B_{12} deficiency is fish tapeworm infestation with *Diphyllobothrium latum,* an intestinal parasite present in freshwater fish such as pike. When insufficiently cooked fish is ingested, tapeworms ultimately develop in the intestines. Some Finns and makers of gefilte fish in the United States have a habit of tasting raw fish and thereby become infected by this tapeworm. The worm competes in the jejunum with the host for vitamin B_{12}. The diagnosis can be suspected only on the basis of the patient's history. Confirmation depends on demonstration of the tapeworm ova in feces. Once this is demonstrated, appropriate antihelminth therapy will cure the patient.

Other Unusual Causes for Vitamin B_{12} Deficiency. Vitamin B_{12} malabsorption is sometimes associated with regional ileitis, an inflammatory disease of the ileum of unknown etiology. Most often this occurs after the ileum has been resected as part of the therapy for this disease. Since the disease usually does not involve the intestinal mucosa, it is unlikely by itself to cause vitamin B_{12} malabsorption.

Vitamin B_{12} malabsorption has also been associated with thyroid disease, particularly hypothyroidism, and the presence of thyroid autoantibodies. Drugs such as colchicine, para-aminosalicylic acid, alcohol, metformin, phenformin, anticonvulsants, slow release potassium chloride, and neomycin have been shown to interfere with vitamin B_{12} absorption, usually without severe deficiency. In the case of para-aminosalicylic acid, folic acid therapy may reverse the malabsorption.

Patients with severe, chronic pernicious anemia may have a decreased ability to absorb vitamin B_{12} even in the presence of IF. This ileal defect usually disappears after months of parenteral therapy with vitamin B_{12} for the pernicious anemia.

Dietary deficiency of vitamin B_{12} is rare, since there are high concentrations of this vitamin in foods of animal origin. Vegetarians, particularly in India, may have a diet so deficient in vitamin B_{12} that they develop mild megaloblastic anemia.

Severe folic acid deficiency can, in rare cases, interfere with vitamin B_{12} absorption.

Patients with Zollinger-Ellison syndrome, which results in hypersecretion of acid in the stomach and a low intestinal pH, have difficulty in the binding of B_{12}-IF complex to the ileal mucosa. Correction of the hypersecretion of acid has led to improved vitamin B_{12} absorption.

Chronic pancreatic insufficiency has also been associated, in a few patients, with vitamin B_{12} malabsorption. Pancreatic extract reverses this defect, but the precise constituent of the extract that enhances vitamin B_{12} absorption has not been determined.

Finally, vitamin B_{12} deficiency may occur as a result of increased demands of pregnancy, hyperthyroidism, hyperactive erythropoiesis, neoplastic growth including multiple myeloma, and myeloproliferative disorders. A few patients with multiple myeloma also have frank pernicious anemia, but many others have only macrocytosis or unexplained decreased serum vitamin B_{12} levels.

Treatment of Vitamin B_{12} Deficiency

Since most vitamin B_{12} deficiency is due to malabsorption of the vitamin, parenteral injection of vitamin B_{12} is required for therapy. For patients who have reversible diseases such as fish tapeworm, sprue, and blind loops, treatment of the primary disease should be undertaken after initial replacement with parenteral vitamin B_{12}. If treatment is successful, these patients will not require maintenance therapy. However, the vast majority of patients with vitamin B_{12} deficiency have pernicious anemia or other diseases that cannot be cured by drugs or surgical procedures, and these patients will require lifelong injections of vitamin B_{12}.

Initially 100 μg per day of hydroxycobalamin should be injected intramuscularly or subcutaneously for 5 to 7 days. Hydroxycobalamin is preferable to cyanocobalamin, because it binds better to proteins and therefore remains in the body three times longer than cyanocobalamin. Only a small fraction of this material will be retained, but it will begin to replace body stores. Parenteral administration, 100 μg monthly or bimonthly, should then be carried out to maintain the hematocrit and vitamin B_{12} level. It is probably easiest to try bimonthly injection and follow the hematocrit. If a patient's hematocrit falls, and the serum B_{12} level is low, then monthly injections should be administered. It is true that pernicious anemia patients respond to treatment with animal IF; but they rapidly become resistant and will ultimately require parenteral vitamin B_{12}. A massive dose of 1,000 μg per day given orally to PA patients who will not accept parenteral therapy gives an adequate hematologic response and probably repletes body stores. However, this treatment cannot be relied upon to maintain normal erythropoiesis, and for this reason it is not recommended.

Transfusion therapy can be quite dangerous for patients with moderate to severe megaloblastic anemia. These patients have a normal or often increased blood volume and transfusion may cause them to go into severe, irreversible congestive heart failure. Therefore blood should not be given to patients with megaloblastic anemia unless there is evidence of tissue hypoxia manifested by angina or symptoms of the central nervous system. In most cases it is possible to withhold transfusions and to treat with vitamin B_{12} or folic acid. Patients who need transfusions should be given packed red cells along with a diuretic and their fluid balance closely monitored.

Elevated levels of uric acid in serum and urine may occur in response to a physiologic or pharmacologic dose of vitamin B_{12} administered parenterally to deficient patients. In some cases uricosuria is severe enough to precipitate kidney damage. Another very rare complication is sudden, unexplained death that may be due to potassium levels low enough to precipitate cardiac arrythmias. It is presumed that the extracellular (serum) potassium level becomes low because of production of new red cells, which requires intracellular potassium. Patients with severe megaloblastic anemia, therefore, require close observation of serum uric acid and potassium levels during therapeutic trials and therapy.

There is conflicting evidence concerning the association of pernicious anemia with an increased incidence of stomach cancer (reported as high as 10 percent). In many cases of gastric carcinoma, surgical treatment is unsuccessful, perhaps because the carcinoma is detected too late. For this reason gastric cytologic examinations, rather than 6-monthly or yearly gastrointestinal x-rays, have been recommended for patients with pernicious anemia. If cytologic results are positive, gastroscopy and x-ray studies are done, and if indicated, a surgical procedure is performed. If cytologically malignant cells are detected without gastroscopic or x-ray evidence of a tumor, it may be necessary to perform a partial gastrectomy despite inability to demonstrate frank gastric carcinoma. This problem has not yet been resolved. At the very least, PA patients should have x-ray examinations of the upper gastrointestinal tract done at yearly intervals, and it is not unreasonable to perform gastric cytologic examinations at 6-month intervals.

*Biochemistry of
Folic Acid*

The terms *folic acid* and *folate* refer to a large group of compounds consisting of three moieties, pteridine, para-aminobenzoic acid, and a variable number of glutamic acid units. The first two moieties in combination are sometimes called *pteroyls*. The number of glutamic acid moieties attached to the pteroyl determines the name of the compound. There are pteroyl monoglutamates, pteroyl triglutamates, and pteroyl polyglutamates. The addition of four hydrogen groups to the pteroyl results in a compound called tetrahydrofolic acid, which participates in many cellular enzymatic reactions. The reduction of folic acid (pteroyl monoglutamate) to dihydrofolic acid and then to tetrahydrofolic acid is catalyzed by an enzyme, dihydrofolate reductase. Compounds structurally resembling folic acid — for example, aminopterin and amethopterin (methotrexate) — may inhibit this enzyme and are called *antifols*.

One-carbon fragments may be bound to various sites on the pteridine moiety of tetrahydrofolic acid. These one-carbon fragments participate in many reactions, particularly those involving the synthesis of purines, pyrimidines, and DNA. Methylation of deoxyuridylate to form thymidylate is effected, in part, by one-carbon transfer from a tetrahydrofolate compound. Limitation of thymidylate synthesis leads to impairment of DNA synthesis and megaloblastosis.

Folic acid coenzymes are also important in methionine, serine, and histidine metabolism. In regard to the last, an insufficiency in tetrahydrofolic acid leads to the accumulation of formiminoglutamic acid (FIGLU). FIGLU is a product of histidine metabolism and requires tetrahydrofolate for its conversion to glutamic acid. Patients who are folic acid–deficient will excrete elevated amounts of FIGLU, particularly when challenged with large oral doses of histidine. Normal people excrete little or no FIGLU, but no symptoms or abnormalities result from its accumulation in the body. Other enzymatic reactions depend upon folates for their metabolism but are not central to the problem of folic acid deficiency.

*Measurement of
Folic Acid*

Most of the physiologic and clinical investigations of folic acid metabolism have been performed by using microbiologic assays with *Lactobacillus casei,* a folic acid–requiring organism. These assays measure all metabolically important folic acid derivatives. Tubes containing culture medium deficient in folic acid are inoculated with *L. casei.* Known amounts of folic acid are added to some of these tubes, and growth, measured by turbidity, is determined after a specified period of time. With this data a standard curve can be drawn that relates concentration of added folic acid to the turbidity or growth of the organisms. This curve can then be used to determine the amount of folate in a serum or tissue sample added to the remaining tubes. In practice serum and red cell folic acid levels are most often determined. For research purposes levels in tissues such as the liver can also be measured. Antibiotics interfere with this microbiologic assay by causing falsely low values.

Recently a folic acid-binding protein (FBP) has been found in condensed milk. Using this folic acid binder and radiolabeled folic acid it is now possible to perform a radioisotope displacement assay similar to that used for vitamin B_{12} measurements. First a standard curve is determined by adding known amounts of unlabeled folic acid to a mixture of binder and radiolabeled folic acid. The amount of radioactivity on the binder is inversely proportional to the amount of unlabeled folic acid added. Serum or tissue homogenates with unknown amounts of folic acid can then be assayed. This method is not affected by antibiotics or other drugs.

Leukocyte lysates from patients with chronic myelocytic leukemia, serum from pregnant women and women taking oral contraceptive drugs, and human milk all contain FBP. Barely measurable amounts are present in normal serum and larger quantities in sera from folic acid–deficient patients. FBP in serum prevents the cellular uptake of the folate it binds and as such is not a serum folate delivery protein. The site of synthesis and the function of FBP are currently under investigation.

Absorption of Folic Acid

Folates are widely distributed in a variety of foods, including green vegetables, liver, kidney, and dairy products. A daily diet contains fifty to several hundred micrograms (normal Western diet, 600–700 µg) of folates. Cooking, particularly boiling, destroys this thermolabile vitamin. Food folate is presented to the intestine largely conjugated to glutamates. The polyglutamates are broken down in the intestinal lumen by *folate conjugases* that convert polyglutamate to monoglutamate. It is not clear whether this cleavage occurs in the brush border of the intestinal cell or within the cell itself. In any case the monoglutamates appear to be absorbed best in the proximal jejunum. Some duodenal, but no ileal or colonic, absorption occurs. Folic acid (monoglutamate) is detected in the serum minutes after an oral dose of unconjugated folic acid, and peak values are obtained in 1 to 2 hours. The peak of activity after an oral dose of conjugated folates occurs later, at 2 to 3 hours.

The monoglutamate forms of folic acid can be absorbed against a concentration gradient. This suggests the existence of an active transport mechanism. Other data suggest that passive transport occurs as well. There may also be some absorption of folates in the form of diglutamates or triglutamates. During the process of intestinal absorption the folates are converted to 5-methyltetra-hydrofolate, which is the main transport and storage form of folate in man.

Folates are excreted by way of the urine and feces and are also destroyed by catabolism, which involves oxidative splitting of the parent molecules into pteridine and para-aminobenzoyl-glutamic acid. About 50 to 100 μg of folic acid are required daily from food to balance these losses. Normally 5 to 20 μg of folic acid are stored in the liver and other tissues. For this reason it may take 3 to 6 months for tissue stores to be completely exhausted in the absence of folate replacement.

The rapid uptake of folic acid into tissues has made it difficult to devise absorption tests similar to the Schilling tests for vitamin B_{12} absorption. It also appears that the rate of folate absorption is dependent upon the amount of folic acid in tissue stores. Even with the use of tissue-saturating doses of folic acid, the variable influence of folate stores makes it difficult to interpret folic acid absorption experiments that employ oral doses of radioactive folic acid.

Clinical Findings Experimental folic acid deprivation leads initially to reduced serum folate levels. Hypersegmentation of neutrophils, low red cell folate levels, excretion of FIGLU following histidine administration, macroovalocytosis, megaloblastic bone marrow, and finally anemia developed after 4½ months of deprivation.

Clinically patients with folic acid deficiency present with morphologic features of megaloblastic anemia and low serum and red cell folic acid levels. Often they have diseases associated with folic acid deficiency, such as alcoholism or cirrhosis. Neurologic abnormalities are not caused by folate deficiency but may be present due to alcoholism or liver disease.

The diagnosis is usually confirmed by a finding of low concentrations of serum folate — less than 3 μg per liter (normal, 5-20 μg per liter). The serum levels are a more sensitive test for folate deficiency than red cell levels and fall before the red cell folate levels (normal, 160-640 μg per liter) become depressed. Therefore low serum folate levels indicate folate deficiency, while low red cell folate levels confirm folic acid deficiency as the cause of megaloblastic anemia. Subnormal red cell folate levels are also found in vitamin B_{12}-deficient patients (p. 69). FIGLU and radioactive folic acid absorption tests are not usually available to the clinician.

In some diagnostically difficult cases a therapeutic trial with folic acid is performed by first putting the patient on a folic acid-deficient diet, then injecting physiologic doses of folic acid (200 μg per day). A tetrahydrofolic acid compound — folinic acid, or citrovorum factor — is available in a liquid, injectable form that is easily diluted so that 200 μg can be injected each day. In a folic acid-deficient patient the reticulocyte response should occur in 3 to 5 days and reach a peak in 5 to 10 days. A vitamin B_{12}-deficient patient will not respond to this dose of folic acid. Large doses, 1 to 5 mg daily, will cause a patient with vitamin B_{12} deficiency to respond with reticulocytes, but the anemia will be only partially, if at all, corrected. Furthermore there is evidence that large pharmacologic doses of folic acid administered to patients with pernicious anemia and combined system disease will lead to neurologic deterioration (see p. 86).

Dietary Deficiency. Many individuals have an inadequate dietary intake of folic acid: the elderly person who is unable to obtain proper foods, the chronic alcoholic who rarely eats, the poverty-stricken patient whose diet lacks vegetables, eggs, and meat. Premature infants and children on synthetic diets also have a decreased dietary intake of folic acid. Prolonged cooking of vegetables results in destruction of folic acid compounds, and the person who eats vegetables prepared only in this way may have dietary deficiency.

Alcoholism and Liver Cirrhosis. Alcoholics and patients with chronic liver disease suffer from folic acid deficiency, probably because of poor diet and impaired hepatic storage of folates. There is some evidence, furthermore, that alcohol and liver disease interfere with absorption and metabolism of folates. Deficiencies of other B vitamins and vitamin C are commonly associated with folic acid deficiency in these patients.

Malabsorption Syndromes. As in the case of vitamin B_{12} malabsorption, nontropical, gluten-sensitive sprue and tropical sprue may be causes for folate malabsorption and deficiency. Biopsy of the jejunum to look for villous atrophy is indicated if a patient has unexplained folic acid deficiency and symptoms or tests indicative of intestinal malabsorption. The absorption of D-xylose, a nonmetabolizable sugar, by the jejunum has proved to be a valuable screening test for sprue. Fat absorption studies and gastrointestinal x-rays may also establish a diagnosis. Monoglutamic folic acid, in contrast to food folates, is absorbed by patients with malabsorption syndromes. In the case of tropical sprue, folic acid therapy improves intestinal symptoms and villous atrophy as well as correcting the folate deficiency.

Folic acid deficiency thought to be secondary to malabsorption

Causes of folic acid deficiency

Common Causes
Alcoholism
Cancer chemotherapy with folic acid antagonists
Hemolytic anemia
Liver disease
Myeloproliferative diseases
Poor diet or overcooking of folate-containing foods
Pregnancy
Sprue and malabsorption syndromes

Uncommon Causes
Drugs such as anticonvulsants and oral contraceptives
Infiltrative lesions of the small intestine
Renal dialysis
Skin diseases including psoriasis and exfoliative dermatitis
Vitamin C deficiency

has also been found in patients following subtotal gastrectomy, resection of the jejunum, and infiltration of the small intestine by lymphoma, leukemia, amyloid, or Whipple's disease. It has also been described in association with scleroderma and diabetes mellitus. Treatment of folic acid deficiency due to intestinal malabsorption requires only 1 mg of monoglutamic folic acid. Some patients with mild disease will respond to the amount of folate present in a normal American diet.

Drug-Induced Folic Acid Deficiency. Antifols, inhibitors of dihydrofolate reductase, result in deficiency of active folate compounds which, if persistent, leads to megaloblastic anemia. The antifols include aminopterin (methotrexate), used in cancer chemotherapy; antimalarial drugs such as pyrimethamine; a diuretic, triamterene; an antiparasite drug, pentamidine; and a drug used for treating urinary tract infections, trimethoprim.

Certain drugs such as the anticonvulsants diphenylhydantoin, phenobarbitol, and primidone are also associated with folic acid deficiency. It is thought that these drugs, along with glutethemide, isoniazid, cycloserine, and oral contraceptives, interfere with folic acid absorption, possibly by inhibiting intestinal folate conjugases.

In the case of anticonvulsant and oral contraceptive users, increased requirements due to microsomal enzyme induction in the liver, changes in folate-binding protein, and, in the case of oral contraceptives, increased urinary excretion of folic acid have also been proposed as the pathogenesis of folate deficiency. Folic acid therapy given to patients with anticonvulsant-induced deficiency may increase the frequency of seizures, but this phenomenon has not been experimentally confirmed.

Folic Acid Deficiency Secondary to Increased Folate Demand. Low folic acid levels are common in pregnancy but are often overlooked because in many nondeficient patients hemoglobin levels normally fall below 10 gm per deciliter in the third trimester. Lactation, multiple pregnancies, poor diet, and any concurrent conditions that result in abnormal folic acid metabolism may further increase requirements for folic acid during pregnancy. During the latter stages of pregnancy 400 μg per day of folic acid is required — eight times the normal 50 μg per day requirement. Pregnant women should therefore be given 400 μg per day of folic acid. It was formerly said that supplementation at this level might be deleterious to patients with undiagnosed pernicious anemia. It is true that this amount of folic acid would mask pernicious anemia and possibly make any neurologic symptoms worse. Pernicious anemia usually renders the patient sterile, however, and pregnancy associated with vitamin B_{12}

deficiency is very rare. Furthermore if folic acid is not given to pregnant women, there will be an increased incidence of megaloblastic anemias. It has been argued that folic acid deficiency leads to complications such as abruptio placentae, spontaneous abortions, and bleeding; but a causal relationship between these complications and folic acid deficiency has not been demonstrated. Megaloblastic anemia of pregnancy should be avoided, in any case, however, since extreme fatigue, shortness of breath, glossitis, and diarrhea all increase the burden of pregnancy.

Anemia associated with hyperproliferation of marrow erythroid cells, as seen in sickle cell anemia, congenital spherocytosis, immunohemolytic anemia, thalassemia, and other hemolytic anemias, may cause folic acid deficiency. This should be suspected when a patient's reticulocyte count has been high but then falls at the same time that the anemia unexpectedly worsens. If folic acid deficiency is the cause, the patient will respond with an outpouring of reticulocytes following folic acid therapy.

Patients with psoriasis and exfoliative dermatitis may lose 5 to 20 μg of folic acid per day. Folic acid deficiency may develop because of the chronic cell exfoliation.

Occasionally individuals with neoplastic diseases, including carcinoma, leukemia, and lymphoma, will develop reduced levels of serum folate, presumably due to increased demand by tumor tissues. In a very few cases, usually when there are other reasons for the development of folic acid deficiency, a frank megaloblastic anemia responsive to folic acid will arise. Interestingly, folic acid deficiency may accompany various myeloproliferative diseases, including myelocytic leukemias and agnogenic myeloid metaplasia, but is rarely, if ever, seen in polycythemia vera. Chronic diseases such as rheumatoid arthritis and infections are also associated with folic acid deficiency, which may be due to increased folate requirement as well as poor dietary intake.

Removal of folate from plasma during renal dialysis was a frequent cause of folic acid deficiency until this loss was recognized and routine prophylactic administration of folic acid prescribed.

Therapy of Folic Acid Deficiency

Despite the many causes of folic acid deficiency, 1 mg of oral folic acid per day is sufficient in all cases to restore serum levels and reverse megaloblastic anemia, even in malabsorption syndromes. Parenteral folic acid is seldom used except to reverse the effect of antifols during cancer chemotherapy or when microgram quantities of folic acid are required for a therapeutic trial. Folic acid supplementation as prophylaxis against deficiency is indicated for pregnancy, liver disease, hemolytic anemia, alcoholism, skin diseases, and, if the patient is undergoing dialysis, uremia.

APPROACH TO PATIENT WITH MEGALOBLASTIC ANEMIA

In clinical practice megaloblastic anemia is suspected when examination of the peripheral blood smear or Wintrobe indices (MCV > 100 fl), performed as part of an investigation of anemia, suggests that macrocytosis or macroovalocytosis is present. In some cases abnormally low serum folate or vitamin B_{12} levels are the first evidence of deficiency; and sometimes a patient comes to the hematologist because of neurologic signs and symptoms suggestive of vitamin B_{12} deficiency or because of a history of illness often associated with vitamin B_{12} or folic acid deficiency. Historical or physical evidence suggestive of diseases associated with vitamin B_{12} or folic acid deficiency should be obtained. Dietary history, alcohol intake, and confirmation of diarrhea, pregnancy, or drug ingestion are most important. Careful attention must be given to nervous system involvement as manifested by paresthesias, ataxia, difficulty with bladder or bowel, and loss of position or vibratory sense. Peripheral neuropathy with "stocking-glove" sensory loss is not uncommon in association with folic acid deficiency but is due to concurrent alcoholism or liver disease and not to folate lack. Patients with severe folic acid deficiency may have glossitis and diarrhea, in contrast to patients with pernicious anemia, who may have lemon yellow skin, blue eyes, long earlobes, and prematurely gray hair. (See p. 90.)

Careful examination of the peripheral blood usually reveals macroovalocytosis and hypersegmented polys. A bone marrow sample showing megaloblasts and giant myeloid forms confirms the diagnosis of megaloblastic anemia. Laboratory studies, such as measurement of serum B_{12} and folate levels and gastric analysis for acid, should be performed to establish etiology. Conditions other than vitamin B_{12} or folate deficiency can also be associated with macrocytosis, as follows (see p. 91).

If vitamin B_{12} deficiency is suspected as a cause of megaloblastic anemia, then a Schilling test should be performed, even if the patient has received prior treatment with vitamin B_{12}. Finally, in some cases it may be necessary to follow the reticulocyte and hematocrit responses to small doses of vitamin B_{12} or folic acid. With measurement of serum B_{12} and folic acid levels readily available, therapeutic trials are seldom performed.

In a few cases of very severe anemia and tissue hypoxia, particularly if manifested by angina, it may be necessary to treat the patient with both folic acid and vitamin B_{12} before the etiology of the deficiency is discovered. By obtaining serum levels and

Approach to patient with megaloblastic anemia

Historical findings

Abdominal operations, particularly if a surgical bypass or blind loop was created
Alcohol intake
Ataxia (Abnormal gait)
Bladder and bowel dysfunction
Diarrhea or fatty stools
Dietary history
Drug therapy, particularly anticonvulsants, antituberculosis drugs, cancer chemotherapy
Family origins, in particular Northern European background
Glossitis
Loss of position or vibratory sense
Paresthesias
Pregnancy, past and present
"Stocking–glove" distribution of sensory loss

Physical Examination

Evidence of acute or chronic glossitis or atrophy of tongue
Evidence of peripheral neuropathy or combined systems disease
Lemon yellow skin
Scleral icterus

Laboratory Tests

Tests to establish whether or not the anemia is megaloblastic

Bone marrow examination
Examination of the peripheral blood
Serum lactic acid dehydrogenase assay

Investigations to establish etiology

Gastric analysis for acid
Malabsorption tests for example, D-xylose absorption
Red cell folate
Schilling tests
Serum folate
Serum vitamin B_{12}

Investigations to determine complications or prevent them

Serum potassium
Serum uric acid

Therapeutic Trial

Hematocrit and reticulocyte response to physiologic amounts of vitamin B_{12} or folic acid

Causes of macrocytosis other than megaloblastic anemia

Aplastic anemia
Arsenic intoxication
Hypothyroidism and hypopituitarism
Liver disease
  ("thin macrocyte" or "target cell" results from excessive membrane
  lipids)
Marrow infiltration with neoplastic tissue
Neonatal macrocytosis
Preleukemia
Protein malnutrition
Reticulocytosis
  (intense erythropoietin stimulation due to hemolysis or bleeding)
Scurvy
Splenectomy

saving extra aliquots in the freezer in case the originals are lost, it is possible to make a definitive diagnosis in retrospect. Even when this fails, a Schilling test can be used to separate megaloblastic erythropoiesis due to folate deficiency from that due to vitamin B_{12} deficiency.

Response to Vitamin B_{12} or Folate Replacement Therapy

The changes in symptoms, peripheral blood, bone marrow, and neurologic status associated with treatment of folate or vitamin B_{12} deficiency are as follows:

1. Symptoms and mucus membrane abnormalities improve (48 hours).
2. Serum uric acid level rises and serum potassium falls (48 hours).
3. Bone marrow erythroid morphology reverts to normal (24-48 hours).
4. There is reticulocytosis and increased neutrophil and platelet counts (5-10 days).
5. Macroovalocytes and hypersegmented polys disappear (2-3 weeks).
6. Evidence of ineffective erythropoiesis, elevated bilirubin and LDH levels, etc., disappears (1-3 weeks).
7. Neurologic improvement occurs (80-90 percent of patients improve in 6 months to 1 year, but some chronic neurologic manifestations of vitamin B_{12} deficiency may be irreversible).

Gastric atrophy, achlorhydria, and IF secretion usually do not improve unless the vitamin B_{12} deficiency is of short duration.

Interrelationships Between Iron, Folic Acid, and Vitamin B_{12}

Chronic iron deficiency is associated with impairment of parietal cell function. Often achlorhydria and occasionally diminished IF secretion are documented in patients with iron deficiency anemia. Iron absorption may be less efficient, since hydrochloric acid facilitates absorption of iron. Patients with iron deficiency may have hypersegmented polys in their blood and giant myeloid forms in their marrow. These abnormalities are not reversed by iron or vitamin therapy. Only occasionally do patients develop frank vitamin B_{12} deficiency in association with iron deficiency and impaired parietal cell IF secretion.

A few patients have been described who apparently do not have tropical sprue but have severe folate deficiency and abnormal iron, folic acid, and IF-B_{12} complex absorption. These unusual individuals must be distinguished from patients with tropical sprue-induced intestinal malabsorption who respond to folic acid therapy. Most likely tropical sprue is due to microorganisms in the gut and not to primary folic acid deficiency.

Chronic vitamin B_{12} deficiency in some patients with PA leads to difficulty in absorbing the $IF-B_{12}$ complex. This observation explains why some patients with PA have abnormal part two Schilling test reactions that return to normal after several months of parenteral vitamin B_{12} therapy. A few patients with PA have folate malabsorption, which also becomes normal after vitamin B_{12} therapy.

Dyserythropoietic Anemias

Although approximately 95 percent of anemias characterized by megaloblastic erythropoiesis are due to either vitamin B_{12} or folic acid deficiency, in a number of diseases at least some of the abnormalities seen with megaloblastic anemia are present but there is no demonstrated lack of vitamin B_{12} or folic acid. Some of these diseases are inherited, others are iatrogenic, and some have no explanation but may be neoplastic. All fail to respond to replacement therapy with vitamin B_{12} or folic acid.

Hereditary orotic aciduria is a rare congenital disease secondary to reduced activity of the enzymes required to convert orotic acid to uridylic acid. Because of this defect the synthesis of pyrimidine ribonucleotides, precursors of both RNA and DNA, is impaired. For reasons that are not entirely clear this enzyme deficiency is manifested by megaloblastic anemia, growth impairment, and renal excretion of orotic acid in large quantities. Therapy with uridine ameliorates these abnormalities.

Another rare disorder of infancy is due to decreased activity in the liver of formiminotransferase, the enzyme that catalyzes the breakdown of FIGLU. As a result there is excessive urinary excretion of FIGLU, megaloblastic anemia, and extreme elevation of serum folate levels. The very few patients reported appear to respond partially to pyridoxine therapy.

Besides the antifols, which impair DNA synthesis, a number of antimetabolites, used in treating cancer, block the synthesis of nucleic acids and lead to morphologic abnormalities indistinguishable from those of megaloblastic anemia. Unlike the antifols, those drugs produce effects that are not reversed by administration of folinic acid. The drugs include the purine analogues, 6-mercaptopurine, thioguanine, and azathioprine, and they interfere with the metabolism of nucleic acids by their incorporation into purine nucleotides. This interference leads to the development of megaloblastic changes in the bone marrow that are not reversed by vitamin B_{12} or folic acid therapy but are reversed by discontinuation of the antimetabolite. Similarly, drugs such as 5-fluorouracil interfere with pyrimidine and DNA synthesis and can lead to mild megaloblastic anemia. Another inhibitor of pyrimidine synthesis, 6-azauridine, inhibits the enzymatic catabolism of orotic acid and causes a mild megaloblastic anemia. Cytosine arabinoside, hydroxyurea, and possibly daunomycin may also cause megaloblastic changes secondary to interference with DNA synthesis.

Megaloblastic dyserythropoiesis in the bone marrow may be seen in patients suffering from aplastic anemia, myelosclerosis, iron deficiency, sideroblastic anemias, infections, myelocytic leukemias — in particular erythroleukemia — and congenital dyserythropoietic anemias. Dyserythropoiesis is defined by certain morphologic and functional characteristics. A common finding is asynchrony of nuclear-cytoplasmic maturation, along with nuclear lobulation and fragmentation, karyorrhexis, pyknosis, binuclearity, and multinuclearity with budding and internuclear bridging. In some cases there are frank megaloblastic changes, particularly in the leukemias, erythroleukemias (plate 22), and sideroblastic anemias. Again it should be stressed that this megaloblastic dyserythropoietic morphology does not respond to vitamin B_{12} or folic acid administration. There may also be cytoplasmic abnormalities in the erythroid series, including vacuolization, basophilic stippling, and excessive amounts of iron in lysosomes or mitochrondria.

Functionally the dyserythropoietic state is characterized by ineffective erythropoiesis. The marrow appears hypercellular, but the reticulocyte production index is low. Iron kinetic studies reveal rapid plasma clearance of radioiron into the bone marrow but diminished radioiron in circulating erythrocytes. Increased hemoglobin catabolism is indicated by unconjugated bilirubinemia, increased fecal urobilinogen, and high endogenous carbon monoxide production, which cannot be accounted for by peripheral blood hemolysis. It is therefore assumed that hemolysis is occurring within the bone marrow before release of the mature red cells. In many cases the red cells that are produced are defective and have shorter than normal survival time. Lactic dehydrogenase may be released from the bone marrow cells into plasma as a result of intramedullary destruction of erythrocytes. In some cases folic acid deficiency may also result because of the hyperactive erythropoiesis.

It should be stressed that in iron deficiency, thalassemia, aplastic anemia, and myelosclerosis, the dyserythropoietic component may be minimal. On the other hand erythroleukemia, in some cases of acquired sideroblastic anemia, and in many cases of acute myelocytic leukemia, dyserythropoiesis may be quite prominent.

As previously mentioned, folic acid antagonists, antimetabolites, irradiation, and spindle inhibitors such as colchicine or vincristine may, by their effect on DNA or RNA metabolism, cause dyserythropoiesis.

Recently three types of rare, usually familial, dyserythropoietic anemias have been described. They have in common characteristic morphologic alterations of dyserythropoiesis, ineffective erythropoiesis, increased peripheral erythrocyte turnover, disturbances of iron metabolism usually leading to iron loading, and nonresponsiveness to the usual hematinics. Although these anemias are often inherited, they may go undetected until adulthood. *Type I* congenital dyserythropoietic anemia (CDA) is characterized by megaloblastoid erythroblasts and erythroblasts with internuclear chromatin bridges — that is, strands of chromatin connecting the nuclei of two adjacent erythroblasts. The anemia is macrocytic in type, chronic, and unresponsive to any known therapy. In some patients it is inherited as an autosomal recessive.

Congenital dyserythropoietic anemia *type II,* sometimes called HEMPAS (*h*ereditary *e*rythroblastic *m*ultinuclearity with a *p*ositive *a*cidified *s*erum test), is characterized by a normoblastic, refractory anemia with multinucleated erythroblasts. Anisocytosis and poikilocytosis are found in the peripheral blood, along with inappropriately low reticulocyte counts. In the bone marrow erythropoiesis is essentially normoblastic, but many of the mature normoblasts have two or more nuclei or multilobulated nuclei. There are increased iron stores, but ringed sideroblasts are unusual. Most importantly, in almost all cases the patient's erythrocytes can be hemolysed by certain sera from normal individuals after acidification of the sera to pH 6.8. This "normal" sera contains a naturally occurring, IgM, complement-binding, cold isoantibody. HEMPAS erythrocytes are strongly agglutinated by antibodies to I and i blood group antigens and have an increased sensitivity to complement. Large numbers of Gaucher-like (Plate 61) cells are found in the marrow of some HEMPAS patients. This type of CDA may be inherited as an autosomal recessive. Although it is the most common type of CDA, it is extremely rare.

Type III CDA is characterized by erythroblastic multinuclearity and the presence of *gigantoblasts* (Plate 22). These are large, erythroid-appearing cells with multiple or lobulated nuclei and have nuclear–cytoplasmic asynchrony. Macrocytosis in the peripheral blood is not prominent, nor is internuclear bridging. There is increased agglutination of the patient's red cells by anti-i and anti-I sera but no lysis by acidified serum. This CDA may be inherited as an autosomal dominant.

There have been a few reports of apparently acquired dyserythropoietic anemia. These patients appear to have an increased susceptibility to lysis by anti-i and anti-I antibodies but do not have positive acidified serum lysis tests. In most cases the anemia is not severe enough to require transfusions. White cell and platelet counts are usually normal. Congenital and acquired dyserythropoietic anemia should be considered in the differential diagnosis of refractory, iron-loading, and hemolytic anemias and in patients with thalassemia syndromes.

CASE DEVELOPMENT PROBLEM: MEGALOBLASTIC ANEMIA

A 78-year-old man had a subtotal gastrectomy 6 years ago for benign bleeding gastric ulcers. At that time one-half of his stomach was removed and the remaining upper half was joined to the second part of the small intestine, the jejunum. The end of the small intestine that normally connects to the outlet of the stomach was sewn closed. Since then the only medication he has taken is multivitamins containing 1 μg vitamin B_{12}, 0.1 mg folic acid, and no iron salts. His hematocrit at present is 0.17 (17%); hemoglobin, 4.8 gm per deciliter; mean corpuscular volume, 130 fl; and reticulocyte count, 3 percent.

1. On the basis of the laboratory findings, can you predict the morphologic abnormalities to be found in his peripheral blood smear?

   By dividing his mean corpuscular volume into his hematocrit, the red blood cell count is calculated to be 1.3 million per deciliter. Dividing this result into his hemoglobin yields a mean corpuscular hemoglobin of 37 pg. Finally, by dividing his hemoglobin by his hematocrit, a mean corpuscular hemoglobin concentration of 28 gm per deciliter is obtained. Since the MCV is elevated, and the MCH and MCHC are low, the peripheral blood smear should reveal macrocytosis and hypochromia.

His peripheral blood smear showed macrocytosis and oval-shaped large erythrocytes. There was hypochromia and variation in the size and shape of his cells, along with teardrop forms, target cells, and an abnormally low number of platelets. A white blood cell count was taken and found low.

2. List the possible causes of his anemia on the basis of the history and laboratory findings and suggest physical findings that would confirm one or more of these diagnoses.

   Macroovalocytosis, depression of all three blood counts, and the history of gastrointestinal surgery suggest the diagnosis of megaloblastic anemia. If this is correct, the patient might have lemon yellow skin, which is due to a combination of anemia and hyperbilirubinemia secondary to ineffective erythropoiesis; intermittent bouts of glossitis; atrophy of the tongue; neurologic disturbances, such as paresthesias, ataxia, and loss of position sense; and premature graying of the hair.

The hypochromia seen on the peripheral blood smear and the low MCHC suggest concurrent iron deficiency anemia, which might be manifested by glossitis, cheilosis, angular stomatitis, atrophy of the tongue, or spooning of the fingernails.

Aplastic anemia is a third possibility, since all three blood counts are depressed and macroovalocytosis is sometimes seen in aplastic anemia. Aplastic anemia is often idiopathic or due to drugs or toxins. Usually there are no helpful physical findings.

The high reticulocyte count and anemia suggest the diagnosis of hemolytic anemia. Except for hyperbilirubinemia and jaundice, physical findings do not help confirm this diagnosis. Some cases of hemolytic anemia are due to an enlarged spleen, and it would be well to look for a mass in the left upper quadrant of the abdomen.

Finally, the teardrop forms and severe poikilocytosis suggest replacement of the bone marrow by fibrosis or a malignant infiltration, although in this case these abnormalities are more likely to be due to megaloblastic or iron-deficiency anemia. Except for bone tenderness, there would be little in the way of physical findings.

On physical examination this patient did have lemon yellow skin, atrophy of his tongue papillae, and loss of vibratory sense, but there was no splenomegaly and no neurologic findings. There was no exposure to toxins or drugs other than vitamins and no evidence of malignant disease.

Following is a list of tests available at your hospital and the charge for each (billed to the patient).

Bone marrow examination, $25
Serum folate, $15
Serum vitamin B_{12} level, $15
Gastric aspiration for acid, $50
Intrinsic factor assay on gastric contents, $100
Serum antibodies against intrinsic factor and parietal cells, $100
FIGLU test, $30
Schilling test (each part), $30
Hospitalization for therapeutic trials, $150 per day
Serum iron and total iron binding capacity, $10

3. Leaving therapeutic considerations aside, what is the most cost-effective approach to diagnosing this patient's anemia?

There is more than one correct answer to this question. One possible approach might be to start with a bone marrow examination, which would make the diagnosis of megaloblastic anemia or iron deficiency anemia, provided the bone marrow was stained for hemosiderin. It would also exclude aplastic anemia and anemia secondary to marrow replacement by fibrosis or tumors. If megaloblastic anemia was found, then a Schilling test should be performed. Since vitamin B_{12} deficiency results from malabsorption of the vitamin, either because of lack of IF or ileal malabsorption, vitamin B_{12} deficiency is unlikely if the Schilling test results are normal. The Schilling test would also determine whether vitamin B_{12} deficiency, if present, was due to lack of IF or ileal malabsorption. A serum vitamin B_{12} level would not be more helpful. Assaying the folic acid level is also unnecessary, since the patient is taking 100 μg of folic acid. The relatively low reticulocyte response in the face of a severe anemia suggests that, at most, mild hemolysis is occurring. The total expenditure of funds using this approach would be approximately $85. A therapeutic trial, unless it could be reliably performed at home, would be a very expensive procedure and, unlike the Schilling test, would not determine the mechanisms of any vitamin B_{12} deficiency. Other approaches are certainly possible, and we leave them to the student to consider.

4. This patient's bone marrow revealed changes diagnostic of megaloblastosis. What abnormalities of the red cells, white cells, platelets, and megakaryocytes, other than those previously described, might be found in his bone marrow and peripheral blood?

Often associated with megaloblastosis are pancytopenia and a low reticulocyte production index. The peripheral blood shows hypersegmented polys, and immature red and white cells are sometimes present. Some of the immature red cells are recognizable as products of megaloblastic erythropoiesis. Platelets are decreased and large. Changes in the bone marrow include giant metamyelocytes and myelocytes with characteristic chromatin abnormalities, abnormal megakaryocytes with hyperlobulation of their nuclei, nuclear abnormalities in the normoblasts with small pieces of DNA seen in the cytoplasm (Howell-Jolly bodies), increased mitoses, and bizarre abnormalities of nuclei including fragmentation and binuclearity and multinuclearity.

This patient had a normal serum folic acid level, a low serum vitamin B_{12} level, abnormal part one Schilling test results, and absent marrow iron stores. Results of the part two Schilling test were entirely normal.

5. What is the most likely diagnosis? Are there any other possibilities? How would you treat the most likely diagnosis?

Almost certainly the patient has pernicious anemia with acquired absence of IF secretion. There have been some reports of children who fail to secrete IF but do not show evidence of further parietal cell malfunction, and a few patients have been described who have had abnormal quantitative or qualitative IF secretion. Such cases are extremely rare, however, and since treatment is the same as for pernicious anemia, further workup is not justified.

Loading and then maintenance doses of parenteral vitamin B_{12} will adequately treat pernicious anemia. If angina or other evidence of severe tissue oxygen lack is present, then slow transfusion with packed red cells and concurrent diuretic therapy is indicated. Remember, treatment is actually initiated at the time the Schilling test is done.

Loading doses of vitamin B_{12} were given along with transfusion of two units of packed red cells because the patient developed angina.

6. How would you follow this patient's response to therapy, and what would you consider if he responds only partially?

The reticulocyte count reaches a peak 5 to 10 days following the first injection of vitamin B_{12}. The rise in reticulocyte count might be blunted by the transfusion of 2 units of red cells. Over a period of 3 weeks the hematocrit should rise rapidly toward normal. If the anemia is only partially corrected, then consideration should be given to the following factors: First, there is hypochromia and absent iron stores, so concomitant iron deficiency exists. Patients with pernicious anemia often initially have normal or elevated serum iron levels that fall to subnormal levels with treatment but ultimately become normal. In a few cases the serum iron level remains low and the patient has a partial response to vitamin B_{12} therapy. These patients require investigation and treatment for iron deficiency. Another reason for failure to respond is the presence of an intercurrent infection, particularly of the urinary tract. Correction of infectious or inflammatory diseases is required before the bone marrow is able to respond optimally.

TOPICS FOR DISCUSSION: MEGALOBLASTIC ANEMIA

Biochemistry of vitamin B_{12}

Gastric intrinsic factor

Antibodies to intrinsic factor

Intestinal absorption of vitamin B_{12}

Newer assays of vitamin B_{12}

Schilling test and its variants

Vitamin B_{12} binding proteins

Pathogenesis of pernicious anemia

Treatment of pernicious anemia (complications)

Inherited forms of vitamin B_{12} deficiency

Biochemistry of folic acid

Absorption and malabsorption of folic acid

Folic acid assays

Drug-induced folic acid deficiency

Folic acid-binding proteins

Neurologic disease and vitamin B_{12} and folic acid

Malabsorption, gastrectomy, and megaloblastic anemia

Intestinal bacterial flora and megaloblastic anemia

Pregnancy and megaloblastic anemia

Megaloblastic anemia associated with drugs such as anticonvulsants, birth control pills, and anticancer agents

Dyserythropoietic anemias

Differential diagnosis of vitamin B_{12} and folate deficiency

Culture of megaloblastic marrow — use in diagnosis

Interrelationships between B_{12}, folate and iron

Nutritional requirement for vitamin B_{12} and folate

Hypersegmented poly and its significance

Macrocytosis and its significance

Serum and red cell enzyme changes in megaloblastic anemia

Ferrokinetic studies in megaloblastic erythropoiesis

Ineffective erythropoiesis and decreased red cell life span in megaloblastic anemia

Leukemia, sideroblastic anemia, and megaloblastic anemia

SELECTED REFERENCES

General Considerations

Beck, W. S. Erythrocyte Disorders: Anemias Related to Disturbance of DNA Synthesis (Megaloblastic Anemias). In W. J. Williams, E. Beutler, A. J. Erslev, and R. W. Rundles (eds.), *Hematology* (2nd ed.). New York: McGraw-Hill, 1977.

Chanarin, I. *The Megaloblastic Anaemias*. Philadelphia: F. A. Davis, 1969.

Harris, J. W., and Kellermeyer, R. W. Pernicious Anemia and the Non-Addisonian Megaloblastic Anemias. In J. W. Harris (ed.), *The Red Cell-Production, Metabolism, Destruction: Normal and Abnormal*. Boston: Harvard University Press, 1970.

Herbert, V. Drugs Effective in Megaloblastic Anemias. In L. S. Goodman and A. Gilman (eds.), *The Pharmacological Basis of Therapeutics* (5th ed.). New York: Macmillan, 1975.

Hoffbrand, A. V. (ed.) Megaloblastic anemia. *Clin. Haematol.* 5:1, 1976.

Klipstein, F. A. The Megaloblastic Anemias. In R. I. Weed (ed.), *Hematology for Internists*. Boston: Little, Brown, 1971.

Stebbins, R., Scott, J., and Herbert, V. Drug-induced megaloblastic anemias. *Semin. Hematol.* 10:235, 1973.

Sullivan, L. W. The Megaloblastic Anemias. In C. E. Mengel, et al (eds.), *Hematology: Principles and Practice*. Chicago: Year Book, 1972.

Wintrobe, M. M., et al Macrocytic Anemias. In M. M. Wintrobe, et al (eds.), *Clinical Hematology* (7th ed.). Philadelphia: Lea & Febiger, 1974.

Wintrobe, M. M., et al Production of Erythrocytes-Nutritional Requirements for Red Cell Production. In M. M. Wintrobe, et al (eds.), *Clinical Hematology* (7th ed.). Philadelphia: Lea & Febiger, 1974.

Vitamin B_{12}

Allen, R. H. The plasma transport of vitamin B_{12}. *Br. J. Haematol.* 33:161, 1976.

Chanarin, I. New light on pernicious anemia. *Lancet* 2:538, 1973.

Sullivan, L. W. Vitamin B_{12} metabolism and megaloblastic anemia. *Semin. Hematol.* 7:6, 1970.

Folic Acid

Herbert, V. Folate forms, functions, and fate. *N. Engl. J. Med.* 286:214, 1972.

Streiff, R. R. Folic acid deficiency anemia. *Semin. Hematol.* 7:23, 1970.

Waxman, S. Folate binding proteins *Br. J. Haematol.* 29:23, 1975.

Wu, A., Chanarin, I., Slavin, G., and Levi, A. J. Folate deficiency in the alcoholic — its relationship to clinical and haematological abnormalities, liver disease and folate stores. *Br. J. Haematol.* 29:469, 1975.

4 : Hemolytic Anemia

Increased red cell breakdown, *hemolysis,* is a far too common cause of anemia. Some acceleration of erythrocyte destruction occurs in practically every disease state. When erythrocyte survival is shortened to less than 15 to 20 days, *hemolytic anemia* results. In some patients erythrocyte survival may be one-sixth to one-eighth of normal, but there is no decrease in red cell mass and therefore no anemia. This *compensated hemolytic state* occurs because the unsuppressed bone marrow can compensate for hemolysis by increasing its output of red cells six to eight times. Often, however, marrow suppression combines with increased red cell destruction to produce an anemia which is said to have a *hemolytic component.* This chapter will be concerned with the biochemical changes that result from increased erythrocyte destruction and with the approach to the diagnosis of hemolytic anemia.

Physiologic and Biochemical Abnormalities Associated with Hemolysis

This section discusses the sequence of events that occurs when red cells rupture and release hemoglobin. Normally, senescent erythrocytes are destroyed in the reticuloendothelial system (RES), particularly in the spleen, without release of hemoglobin (see pathway (1) in Figure 6). However, if hemolysis is severe, no matter whether it occurs in the circulation (intravascular breakdown) or in the RES (extravascular breakdown), hemoglobin will appear in the plasma and urine. The severity, chronicity, and site of hemolysis determine which hemoglobin breakdown products are detectable.

Haptoglobins

Figure 6 shows the pathway for the disposal of hemoglobin once released from the red cell. Hemoglobin in plasma is normally bound to an α_2-glycoprotein called *haptoglobin.* Haptoglobin is produced in the liver, and its structure is genetically determined, having three principle phenotypes with varying ability to bind hemoglobin. Once the haptoglobin–hemoglobin complex is formed, it is too big to be excreted by the kidney and is taken up by hepatic parenchymal cells, where the hemoglobin is converted to bilirubin. Up to 1.5 gm per liter of hemoglobin may be present in the plasma without free hemoglobinemia or hemoglobinuria. If hemolysis is severe, however, the ability to synthesize and release haptoglobin from the liver cannot keep up with its clearance. In

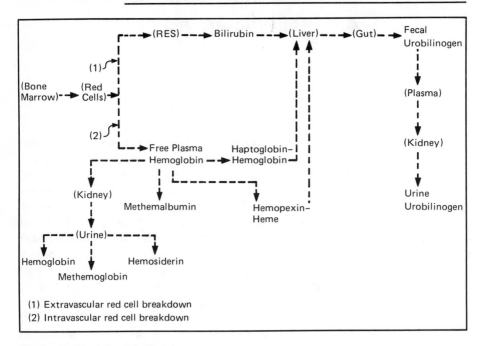

Fig. 6 : Pathways for red cell and
hemoglobin breakdown

this case the haptoglobin level falls, and its disappearance serves as evidence for the presence of abnormally rapid red cell destruction.

Two factors make haptoglobin less than optimal as a test for hemolysis, however. First, certain phenotypes bind hemoglobin poorly and since haptoglobin levels are often determined by their ability to bind hemoglobin, levels as low as .025 gm per liter may be reported in normal individuals. Second, in the presence of inflammation, infection, or malignancy the haptoglobin behaves as an acute phase reactant, and its production is increased to the point where its level may be normal or even high in the presence of mild-to-moderate hemolysis. Low haptoglobin levels seen in association with liver disease are probably a result of chronic hemolysis secondary to hepatic dysfunction rather than decreased hepatic synthesis of haptoglobin.

Plasma haptoglobins may be measured by methods based on their hemoglobin-binding capacity, their peroxidase activity when complexed with hemoglobin, or their immunologic specificity. Haptoglobins are able to bind oxyhemoglobin, and methemoglobin, but not myoglobin, deoxyhemoglobin, nor hemoglobin H nor Barts.

The haptoglobin level is diagnostically valuable only if it is very low or absent, in which case it serves as evidence of accelerated red cell destruction. Low haptoglobin levels normally occur when red cell destruction exceeds twice the normal rate. Following cessation of acute hemolysis, plasma haptoglobins return to normal within 3 to 6 days or sooner. Continuous hemolysis results in chronically depressed haptoglobin levels. It should be remembered that haptoglobin binds hemoglobin but not heme nor myoglobin. This means that patients who have myoglobinuria do not have a depressed serum haptoglobin level, although their urine appears red. The serum in patients with myoglobinemia is not colored, since myoglobin is a relatively small molecule that is rapidly excreted by the kidneys. In contrast, hemoglobinuria is associated with pink plasma, because hemoglobin is relatively slowly excreted or degraded. Patients with red urine who have clear serum and normal haptoglobins probably have myoglobinemia, while patients with red urine, pink serum, and depressed haptoglobin levels have hemoglobinemia.

Hemopexin

Hemopexin is a β-glycoprotein that specifically binds heme when haptoglobin has been depleted. The normal concentration is 50 to 100 mg per deciliter. During hemolysis hemopexin levels will fall but never completely disappear. Once heme is bound to hemopexin, it is probably taken up by hepatocytes. Normally very little hemopexin is found in the urine, but in the presence of renal disease hemopexin may be excreted with albumin. Its level is best determined by radioimmunodiffusion. Although mildly elevated levels occur in diabetes mellitus and infections, hemopexin is not an acute phase reactant as is haptoglobin.

Methemalbumin

Albumin is another protein that will bind heme. Free hemoglobin in the plasma is oxidized to *methemoglobin* (trivalent or ferric state of heme iron). Methemoglobin nonenzymatically dissociates into heme and globin. The oxidized heme complexes with albumin to form methemalbumin, which can be measured spectrophotometrically or can be detected on serum electrophoretic patterns after staining for heme-containing compounds. It has about the same electrophoretic mobility as albumin. Because methemalbumin circulates in the plasma for a relatively long period of time, it is useful in diagnosing moderate to severe hemolysis many hours or even days following the acute hemolytic episode. The heme in methemalbumin is probably transferred to hemopexin, which is cleared by the liver.

Free Plasma Hemoglobin

Free, unbound hemoglobin in the plasma can be detected by its pink coloration. In cases of severe hemolysis this may be obscured by the presence of the brown-appearing methalbumin or the dark pigment methemoglobin. Hemoglobin in plasma can be measured by its peroxidase activity. In clinical practice a hematocrit capillary tube filled with blood is rapidly centrifuged and the supernatant plasma dropped onto a tablet containing benzidine. A blue color indicates the presence of free hemoglobin in the plasma. Hemoglobinemia usually occurs only in severe intravascular hemolysis.

Hemoglobinuria and Hemosidinuria

Unbound hemoglobin (molecular weight, 66,000) appears in the urine as a red pigment after saturation of hemoglobin-binding proteins in plasma. Methemoglobin may be present with it and give a brown color to the urine. Methemalbumin does not usually appear in the urine during hemoglobinuria.

Besides excreting free hemoglobin and methemoglobin, the kidney may also excrete hemosiderin. Hemoglobin iron is extracted and stored in renal tubular cells as ferritin and hemosiderin. These epithelial cells are sloughed into the urine. Hemosiderin is detected by concentrating the urine sediment, making a smear, and staining with Prussian blue in the same manner that bone marrow is stained for iron. Large, hard-to-overlook, blue granules of hemosiderin are seen under high power magnification. In normal individuals no hemosiderin is detected. Usually hemosidinuria is present in patients undergoing chronic intravascular hemolysis, particularly if secondary to mechanical lysis of erythrocytes by defective prosthetic or diseased cardiac valves.

Bilirubin

Within the reticuloendothelial system, hemoglobin is degraded to dipyroles and ultimately to bilirubin. During this degradation carbon monoxide is formed. The measurement of this carbon monoxide production can be used to assay the rate of red cell destruction. Bilirubin is transported via the plasma to the liver. There it is conjugated with glucuronide and excreted as a constituent of bile into the small intestine. The bilirubin glucuronides are water-soluble and react with Ehrlich's diazo reagent in the van den Bergh test. The amount of color that develops after addition of Ehrlich's reagent is called *direct bilirubin* and represents the conjugated bilirubin glucuronide. The free, unconjugated, water-insoluble bilirubin does not participate in the color reaction until methanol is added. The portion of color that develops after the addition of alcohol is called unconjugated bilirubin or *indirect bilirubin.* In patients with hemolysis and increased production of bilirubin it may not be possible for the liver to conjugate all the bilirubin produced. Because unconjugated bilirubin is poorly excreted by the kidneys, the level of indirect serum bilirubin can be elevated in patients with moderate to severe hemolysis. On the other hand a normally functioning liver can conjugate large amounts of bilirubin, so that even in the face of moderate hemolysis, serum bilirubin may be within the normal range or only slightly elevated.

Urobilinogen

Bilirubin is further degraded to *fecal urobilinogen* after excretion with bile into the gastrointestinal tract. Fecal urobilinogen measured with Ehrlich's aldehyde reagent is increased in the face of hemolysis. Unfortunately measurement of fecal urobilinogen levels requires a 3-day collection of stool followed by homogenation of the feces and determination of the urobilinogen content. Increased fecal urobilinogen (normal, 190–230 mg per day) is good evidence for hemolytic anemia. However, few laboratories are willing to process the fecal material in order to perform this assay.

Urobilinogen in the intestinal tract is absorbed and excreted into the urine, where it can be measured with Ehrlich's aldehyde reagent. Patients with moderate or severe hemolysis often excrete increased amounts of urine urobilinogen. Of course normal levels do not exclude hemolysis (see summary, p. 108).

Red Cell Survival Time

Up to this point the discussion has concerned tests for hemolysis that depend on detection of hemoglobin breakdown products. Increased erythrocyte destruction can be measured more directly by labeling red cells with radioisotopes and assaying their survival.

Two methods of labeling red cells in order to determine their survival time have been discussed in Chapter 1: radiochromium label-

**Pigmented hemoglobin breakdown productions
found after severe (intravascular) hemolysis**

I. In Plasma
    A. Hemoglobin
    B. Methemoglobin
    C. Bilirubin
    D. Methemalbumin
    E. Haptoglobin–hemoglobin complexes (rapidly removed from
        plasma)

II. In Urine
    A. Hemoglobin
    B. Methemoglobin
    C. Bilirubin

Fig. 7 : Red cell life span as determined with radiochromium-labeled erythrocytes

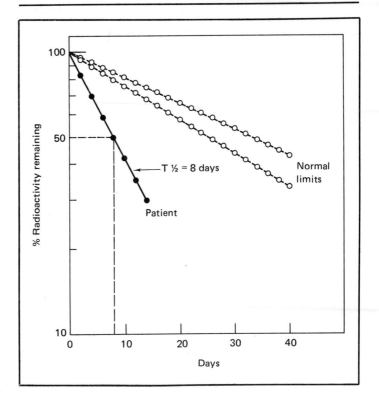

ing of β-chains within the red cell and radioiron labeling of the heme iron in hemoglobin. In the former method a sample of blood is incubated at 37°C with radiochromium and, after washing, is reinjected. This method labels both young and old cells in the blood sample and provides an average red cell survival time. Injection of radioiron, on the other hand, labels a cohort of young marrow red cells. These red cells are released into peripheral blood, their radioactivity measured, and their life span calculated. Thus the survival time of a cohort of red cells all having a similar, young, age is determined.

The radioiron method takes more time because only newly formed cells are labeled, but it provides data on actual red cell life span. Although red cell life span can be derived from radiochromium labeling, assumptions must be made concerning the rate of radiochromium elution from the β-chains of hemoglobin. In practice the radiochromium method is the most frequently used and the time at which one-half the originally administered radioactivity is left is called the T½ (Fig. 7). Normally it is in the range of 25 to 32 days. Patients who have values of less than 25 days are considered to have increased red cell destruction. Both this radiochromium method and the radioiron cohort labeling depend upon certain assumptions. First, the red cells must not be damaged during the period of labeling, either by anticoagulants or by incubation. Second, the patient must be hematologically stable; that is, he cannot be losing blood through hemorrhage or have a predominance of young cells because of recent, acute hemolysis of old erythrocytes.

Techniques such as transfusion with compatible but serologically distinguishable red cells, and labeling with difluorophosphate 32, technetium 99m, glycine ^{14}C, and other substances, have also been used to measure red cell life span. Although seldom done, it is possible to use these radioisotopic techniques to determine whether the hemolysis is due to an intrinsic cellular defect or to the environment surrounding the cell. For example, if a patient's cells after labeling are rapidly hemolyzed when injected back into the patient but have a normal life span when injected into a compatible, normal volunteer, then *extracorpuscular* factors are suspected as the cause for premature destruction. However, if red cell survival is abnormal, both in the patient and in a normal recipient, then an *intracorpuscular* rather than an extracorpuscular defect exists — in other words, the defect causing the hemolysis resides in the red cell.

Using radiochromium methods it is possible to measure red cell mass as well as life span. Furthermore, comparing radioactivity in liver, spleen, and bone marrow by external counting probes can yield information concerning the site of erythrocyte destruction or sequestration.

Classification of Hemolytic Anemia

There is no general agreement on a classification of hemolytic disorders. Classification schemes can be based on whether hemolytic anemia is due to intracorpuscular or extracorpuscular causes as indicated by cross transfusion procedures and the determination of erythrocyte life span (see classification I of outline, p. 112). A valid classification can be based on such causes; however, the means necessary for the procedures are often unavailable to the clinician. Furthermore, some diseases are associated with both intracorpuscular and extracorpuscular causes of red cell destruction.

Other classifications divide the hemolytic anemias according to whether they are inherited or acquired. Interestingly, most inherited disorders lead to intracorpuscular hemolytic anemias, whereas acquired disorders are due mainly to extracorpuscular factors. Therefore an inherited/acquired classification resembles the intracorpuscular/extracorpuscular one. Such a classification can be used, but it is sometimes difficult in clinical practice to decide whether the patient's hemolytic anemia is acquired or inherited. The family and personal history are often insufficient to make a decision.

Another classification (II of outline) depends on whether the hemolytic disease is due to intravascular or extravascular (RES or reticuloendothelial system) hemolysis or to fragmentation of the red cell. It is often difficult to decide whether intravascular or reticuloendothelial hemolysis is occurring, however, and it is difficult to recall which diseases fall within each category.

Experience has led us to use the Coombs' test (see Chapter 5), which determines whether there is antibody-mediated hemolysis or not. A clinically useful classification (III), which is followed in this text, results from separating hemolytic anemias into those that are mediated by antibodies and those that are not.

No matter which classification is used, it should be realized that the number of known mechanisms of hemolysis is limited. Inherited enzyme deficiencies can result in the death of red cells in two ways: through the effects of these deficiencies on cell membranes and metabolism or through producing inclusion bodies made up of precipitated hemoglobin. The production of inclusion bodies results in removal of erythrocytes by the reticuloendothelial system. These inclusions may also be "pitted" from red cells by the spleen, leaving the cell intact but with a loss of membrane that makes the erythrocyte acquire a more spheroidal shape. If this process continues, the cell ultimately undergoes lysis.

Membrane abnormalities may result in loss of red cell deformability, inability to maintain normal permeability to sodium and potassium, or attachment of complement to the membrane, causing premature erythrocyte lysis. Abnormalities associated with the hemoglobin within the red cell may also lead to hemolytic anemia. The best example is sickle cell anemia, in which the abnormal hemoglobin may cause permanent membrane distortion. Such deformations of the red cell membranes lead to premature lysis of the red cell.

Some mechanical factors cause hemolysis, for example, red cell fragmentation due to jet streams within abnormal cardiac valves or fragmentation due to deposition of fibrin within small blood vessels. Infiltration of the RES organs and reticuloendothelial hyperplasia secondary to inflammatory or infectious diseases also lead to premature red cell death. Thermal injury and chemical toxins are less common causes of hemolytic anemia.

The hemolytic anemias covered in later chapters were chosen for

Classification of hemolytic anemias

I. On the Basis of Intracorpuscular (Inherited) Versus Extracorpuscular (Acquired) Factors*
  A. Intracorpuscular abnormalities
    1. Hereditary defects of red blood cells
      a. Hereditary spherocytosis
      b. Hereditary ovalocytosis
      c. Thalassemia
      d. Enzyme deficiencies
      e. Hemoglobinopathies
    2. Acquired defects
      a. Paroxysmal nocturnal hemoglobinuria
      b. Nutritional deficiencies
  B. Extracorpuscular abnormalities
    1. Acquired defects with antibodies
      a. Erythroblastosis fetalis
      b. Transfusion reactions
      c. Acquired hemolytic disease (autoimmune and drug-induced)
    2. Acquired defects not associated with antibodies
      a. Chemical toxins
      b. Physical agents
      c. Infectious agents
      d. Microangiopathic hemolytic anemias
      e. Hypersplenism
  C. Interaction of intracorpuscular and extracorpuscular abnormalities
    1. Favism
    2. Unstable hemoglobins
    3. Lead poisoning
    4. Pernicious anemia
II. On the Basis of Intravascular Versus Extravascular Site of Destruction[†]
  A. Intravascular hemolysis
    1. Mechanical
    2. Osmotic
    3. Chemical
    4. Complement damage
  B. Fragmentation hemolysis
    1. Sickle cell anemia
    2. Arteriolar damage
    3. Consumption coagulopathy
    4. Heart valve prosthesis
  C. Reticuloendothelial or extravascular destruction
    1. Immune hemolysis
    2. Heinz body anemia and hemoglobinopathies
    3. Red cell membrane abnormalities — hereditary spherocytosis
    4. Erythrocyte enzyme deficiencies
    5. Hypersplenism
III. On the Basis of Presence or Absence of Antibody Mediation
  A. Antibody-mediated (Coombs' test–positive)
    1. Autoimmune anemia
    2. Drug-induced autoimmune anemia

*Adapted from Harris, J. and Kellermeyer, R., *The Red Cell Production, Metabolism, Destruction: Normal and Abnormal,* rev. ed. Cambridge, Mass.: Harvard University Press, 1970.
[†]Adapted from Hillman, R. and Finch, C., *Red Cell Manual,* 4th ed., p. 41. Philadelphia, Pa.: F. A. Davis, 1974.

    3. Transfusion reaction anemia
    4. Hemoglobinurias (except PNH)
    5. Erythroblastosis fetalis
B. Not antibody-mediated (Coombs' test–negative)
    1. Hereditary spherocytosis
    2. Congenital nonspherocytic hemolytic anemias (membrane and enzyme abnormalities)
    3. Hemoglobinopathy
    4. Thalassemia
    5. Microangiopathic hemolytic anemia
    6. Hypersplenism
    7. Diseases with an inflammatory component (reticuloendothelial hyperplasia)

discussion on the basis of their frequency in the United States population and the extent of our knowledge of their pathophysiology. In a few cases specific anemias are discussed that are rarely seen but about which we have a good deal of knowledge concerning the mechanism of hemolysis. An understanding of these anemias, despite their rarity, is important as a basis for devising approaches to the mechanisms of hemolysis in more common, but less well understood, hemolytic anemias.

Clinical Findings in Hemolytic Anemia

Unlike the case of iron deficiency and megaloblastic anemia, only limited information can be gained from the history and physical examination of a patient with a hemolytic anemia. A family history of jaundice, anemia, or splenomegaly, when elicited, is helpful, since many hemolytic anemias are inherited. Jaundice, when found, is often intermittent and usually seen in patients suffering from hemolytic anemia due to inherited erythrocyte defects, transfusion reactions, or autoimmune hemolysis. Splenomegaly is a cause of hemolytic anemia and also may result from excessive red cell breakdown. Obviously the appearance of hemoglobin breakdown products in the blood or urine suggests severe hemolysis.

Peripheral Blood

Almost all patients with hemolytic anemia manifest a bone marrow response to increased red cell destruction. In some cases this response is mediated by increased erythropoietin production secondary to anemia and tissue hypoxia. In cases of mild anemia there is no tissue hypoxia, but reticulocyte counts are high. It may be that red cell stroma or membranes stimulate the bone marrow to produce or release reticulocytes; in any case, as a result of marrow stimulation, an increased number of reticulocytes are present. In fact sustained reticulocytosis and an elevated reticulocyte production index are probably the best evidence that hemolysis is occurring. The reticulocytes appear as round macrocytes with pale blue cytoplasm or, in some cases, with very fine blue cytoplasmic stippling, sometimes referred to as *polychromasia*. These *polychromatophils* (Plate 23) will stain supravitally as reticulocytes (Plate 5). In moderate to severe hemolytic anemia there may be enough macrocytosis so that mean corpuscular volume is increased into the range normally found in patients with megaloblastic anemia.

Another abnormality in the peripheral blood which should suggest the diagnosis of hemolytic anemia is *spherocytosis* (Plate 24). In antibody-caused, or immune-mediated, hemolytic anemia, spherocytes are numerous, while in all other types of hemolytic anemias, some are seen, but their number may be small. Spherocytes are usually microcytic and spherical rather than discoidal and biconcave in shape. Although they appear hyperchromic, their mean cell hemoglobin (MCH) is not greater than normal. They are one of the few causes of an elevated mean corpuscular hemoglobin concentration (MCHC), however.

Spherocytes result from damage to cell membranes that causes loss of membrane surface area and hence the spheroidal shape. Spherocytes become trapped in splenic sinuses, where they undergo biochemical changes ultimately resulting in lysis. Similar entrapment may occur in other organs of the reticuloendothelial system. Because of their shape, spherocytes are osmotically fragile and will lyse after exposure to slightly hypotonic solutions. The mechanisms of spherocyte production and the reasons for their premature destruction are discussed in Chapter 5.

Bone Marrow

Unless the patient's bone marrow is suppressed by inflammatory diseases or drugs, normoblastic hyperplasia occurs in response to hemolysis. The M:E ratio is reduced, and the number of fat cells is remarkably less. Many immature, nucleated erythroid forms are often present, with a small increase in the size of the normoblasts. If stores of folic acid have been exhausted due to chronic hemolysis, megaloblastic changes may be seen. Dyserythropoiesis, abnormalities in the erythroid nuclei that resemble changes in megaloblastic anemia, are not uncommon in hyperplastic marrows secondary to moderate-to-severe hemolysis. In some cases nucleated red cells may escape into the peripheral blood.

Abnormalities in erythrocyte shape (for example, fragmented, targeted, or sickled cells) are seen in certain hemolytic anemias. These will be described and discussed later in chapters dealing with specific causes of hemolytic anemia. It should be emphasized, however, that spherocytes, reticulocytosis, and normoblastic hyperplasia of the bone marrow are found in hemolytic anemias due to any cause.

Skeleton

Changes in bone x-rays due to marrow hyperplasia in the medullary cavity of bones are common in congenital hemolytic anemias and rare in acquired disorders. These changes are most marked in thalassemia major and sickle cell anemia. In the skull the space between the bone tables is broadened, the intramedullary cavity is less dense, and the tables, especially the outer, are thinned. Bony trabeculae may develop at right angles to the tables, giving rise to a *hair-on-end* appearance common in thalassemics. In long bones, ribs, vertebrae, and metacarpals, widening of the medullary cavity and thinning of the cortex secondary to marrow hyperplasia may be seen on x-ray examinations. Bony sclerosis as a result of bone infarction may be found in bone x-rays of patients with sickle cell anemia.

In children severely affected with congenital hemolytic anemias some of the skeletal changes are found on physical examination. These patients have "rodent-like" faces secondary to marrow hyperplasia in the facial bones, and skull changes result in elongation or *tower skull.*

APPROACH TO PATIENT WITH HEMOLYTIC ANEMIA

Most patients with hemolytic anemia present with jaundice due to elevated indirect bilirubin levels, anemia with high reticulocyte count, rapidly developing anemia in the absence of blood loss, or abnormal red cell morphology associated with hemolysis. During the initial investigation of an anemic patient, the blood counts, particularly the reticulocyte count, and the examination of the blood smear are by far the most helpful in arriving at a diagnosis of hemolytic anemia. Patients with anemia and a persistently elevated reticulocyte count, not due to treatment of iron, folate, or B_{12} deficiency, who have spherocytosis and polychromatophilia are prime candidates for this diagnosis. Once hemolytic anemia is suspected, many tests are available to confirm the diagnosis (see Table 4-1). Of course the best test is a radioisotopic red cell survival study but this procedure is expensive, time-consuming, and often unavailable. Furthermore patients who are not in a steady state, that is, who are bleeding or have recent hemolysis, are not candidates for this test. For these reasons confirmation of the diagnosis of hemolysis is obtained from tests such as measurements of serum haptoglobin, methemalbumin, or fecal or urine urobilinogen, and bone marrow examination for erythroid hyperplasia. The Coombs' test for antibody-mediated hemolytic anemia

Table 4-1 : Biochemical Abnormalities Associated with Hemolysis*

Test	Mild-to-Moderate Hemolysis (extravascular)	Severe (Intravascular)
Hemopexin	Decreased	Decreased
Haptoglobin	Decreased	Decreased
Plasma hemoglobin	Normal	Increased
Urine hemoglobin	Normal	Increased
Methemalbumin	Normal	Increased
Serum bilirubin	Normal	Increased
Urine bilirubin	Normal	Increased
Fecal Urobilinogen	Increased	Increased
Urine Urobilinogen	Increased (normal)	Increased
Urine Hemosiderin	Normal	Present

*There will almost always be reticulocytosis, spherocytosis, marrow erythroid hyperplasia, and shortened red cell life span.

Approach to patient with hemolytic anemia

I. History
  A. Color of urine and feces
  B. Drugs, toxins, and traumatic exposures
  C. Familial history of jaundice, anemia, or enlarged spleen
  D. History of disease associated with hemolysis
  E. History of intermittent jaundice, anemia, or enlargement of the spleen
  F. Presence of dark urine and its relation to sleep, cold, exercise, or drugs

II. Physical Examination
  A. Enlarged liver
  B. Enlarged spleen
  C. Face and skull abnormalities
  D. Jaundice
  E. Leg ulcerations
  F. Signs of diseases associated with hemolytic anemias, for example, lymph node enlargement or purpura

III. Laboratory Data
  A. Bilirubin, direct and indirect
  B. Bone marrow examination (erythroid hyperplasia)
  C. Coombs' test
  D. Fecal urobilinogen
  E. Laboratory tests on parent's, sibling's, or children's blood
  F. Peripheral blood morphology (spherocytosis, polychromatophilia, nucleated reds, stippling, fragmentation, sickle cells, target cells, etc.)
  G. Red cell life span by radiochromium method
  H. Reticulocyte count (reticulocyte production index)
  I. Serum haptoglobin
  J. Serum hemopexin
  K. Serum methemalbumin
  L. Urine urobilinogen
  M. X-ray of skull, hands, and long bones

is most valuable when it is positive. A description of this test and its interpretation is given in the following chapter.

Once the diagnosis of hemolytic anemia has been confirmed, it is necessary to consider the various types of hemolytic anemia (see Classification, p. 112). In order to do this it is necessary to know the diagnostically helpful characteristics of each clinically important hemolytic anemia, and these are discussed in the succeeding two chapters.

CASE DEVELOPMENT PROBLEMS: HEMOLYTIC ANEMIA

A 70-year-old housewife is admitted to the hospital with severe anemia. A diagnosis of pernicious anemia was confirmed by parts one and two of the Schilling test performed 5 days prior to admission. Her hematocrit on admission was 0.15 (15%). Because of this she was given a transfusion of 2 units of packed red blood cells. Prior to the transfusion the blood bank had reported difficulties in obtaining compatible blood. On the day following admission, after she had received transfusions, the laboratory reported a reticulocyte count of 18 percent.

1. Describe at least two possibilities to account for the reticulocytosis.

   The high reticulocyte count could be a response to treatment of pernicious anemia. She received parenteral vitamin B_{12} as part of the Schilling test. The other possibility is hemolysis, concurrent with pernicious anemia, due to incompatible blood transfusions.

2. What findings on the peripheral blood smear would distinguish between these two possibilities? What findings on the peripheral blood smear might be present but would not distinguish between these possibilities?

   Patients with pernicious anemia often have oval macrocytes (macroovalocytosis), while hemolytic anemia is associated with spherocytosis. The presence of macrocytosis and polychromatophilia would not be helpful. The same large polychromatophilic cells would be seen in patients with pernicious anemia who are responding to vitamin B_{12} injections and in patients with a hemolytic anemia.

3. This patient had quite severe polychromatophilia and both macroovalocytes and macrocytes. On the basis of this information calculate and interpret the reticulocyte production index.

   The reticulocyte count (18 percent), multiplied by the hematocrit (0.15), divided by a normal hematocrit (0.45), and finally divided by 2 (correction factor for severe polychromatophilia) yields a reticulocyte production index of 3. Therefore this patient's bone marrow is three times more active than normal. The reticulocyte production index does not help decide between treated pernicious anemia and hemolytic anemia. In both cases bone marrow is expected to be hyperactive.

4. The serum haptoglobin level is .025 gm per liter. Give several interpretations of this laboratory result.

The first and most obvious interpretation is that the patient is hemolyzing and has saturated the serum haptoglobins to the point where synthesis can no longer keep up with clearance of the haptoglobin–hemoglobin complexes. It is conceivable that the decreased haptoglobin is due to the ineffective erythropoiesis and decreased life span found in pernicious anemia. However, it is rare to find decreased haptoglobins in pernicious anemia patients. Finally, it is possible that the patient has genetically deficient haptoglobins.

5. Assuming she suffered acute hemolysis following incompatible blood transfusions, list the tests that you would order and the results to be expected.

Test	Results
Serum hemopexin	Decreased
Methemalbumin	Present
Plasma hemoglobin	Present
Urine hemoglobin	Present
Fecal urobilinogen	Increased
Urine urobilinogen	Increased
Bilirubin	Increased (particularly indirect fraction)
Coombs' test	Positive
Urine hemosiderin	Present
Bone marrow examination	Erythroid hyperplasia

6. You decide not to perform a radiochromium 51 red cell survival assay. Why would it have been difficult to interpret?

The patient is not in a steady state. She has received a transfusion, and it is possible that she has recently had an acute hemolytic episode due to incompatible blood. In this case the transfused cells would be lysed and cleared quickly, so that the patient's cells of normal life span, and not the incompatible, short-lived donor erythrocytes, would be labeled, and a falsely normal red cell survival would be obtained.

Over a period of 3 weeks her hematocrit returns to normal. Laboratory testing confirms the diagnosis of a severe hemolytic transfusion reaction.

Two years later, she is in an automobile accident and has muscle injuries. A hematoma (collection of blood) develops in the retro-peritoneal space, and she immediately receives multiple blood transfusions. Her plasma and urine are now colored pink. Hapto-globins are absent.

7. How would you distinguish myoglobinuria from hemoglobin-uria in this case?

Both myoglobin and hemoglobin react with benzidine and color urine red, but only hemoglobinemia results in pink plas-ma and binds with haptoglobin. Myoglobin is cleared so rapidly by the kidneys from plasma that it usually does not occur in sufficient concentration to color plasma. Of course myoglobin may be present, along with hemoglobin, in the urine. Immuno-logic tests that can detect the presence of myoglobin are avail-able.

8. How would you distinguish between a hemolytic transfusion reaction and a hematoma that is releasing hemoglobin into the patient's plasma?

This is a very difficult distinction, since in either case hemo-globin and hemoglobin breakdown products will be present in serum and urine for a period of hours or days. The patient might have an antibody in her plasma as a result of the transfu-sion reaction 2 years previously. Recrossmatching the red cells in the transfused blood and the patient's serum should reveal the incompatibility. If there is no incompatibility, then the hematoma is the likely cause for the hemoglobinemia and hemoglobin breakdown products.

Luckily she required no further transfusions and made an un-eventful recovery.

TOPICS FOR DISCUSSION: HEMOLYTIC ANEMIA

Red cell life span measurements, including carbon monoxide production

Radioactive tracers in the diagnosis of hemolysis and for the loca-tion of sequestered red cells

Biochemistry and physiology of haptoglobin and hemopexin

Bilirubin and other hemoglobin breakdown products, their meta-bolic pathways, measurement and clinical usefulness

Determination of intravascular versus extravascular hemolysis

Hemoglobin breakdown products and the kidney

Morphology and function of the marrow in hemolytic anemia

Red cell membrane physiology

Mechanisms of hemolysis

    Immunologic mechanisms

    Membrane abnormalities

    Metabolic abnormalities

    Red cell deformability

    Reticuloendothelial system hyperplasia

    Physical factors in red cell destruction (trauma, fragmentation, heat, etc.)

    Erythrophagocytosis

Ineffective erythropoiesis

Red cell senescence

Repair of injured red cells

Mechanisms of spherocyte production

Classifications of hemolytic anemias

Differential diagnosis of reticulocytosis

Myoglobinemia and myoglobinuria

SELECTED REFERENCES

Berlin, N. I. Laboratory Evaluation of Erythrokinetics. In W. J. Williams, E. Beutler, A. J. Erslev, and R. W. Rundles (eds.), *Hematology* (2nd ed.). New York: McGraw-Hill, 1977.

Cooper, R. A. Destruction of Erythrocytes. In W. J. Williams, E. Beutler, A. J. Erslev, and R. W. Rundles (eds.), *Hematology* (2nd ed.). New York: McGraw-Hill, 1977.

Erslev, A. J. Production of Erythrocytes. In W. J. Williams, E. Beutler, A. J. Erslev, and R. W. Rundles (eds.), *Hematology* (2nd ed.). New York: McGraw-Hill, 1977.

Harris, J. W., and Kellermeyer, R. W. Red Cell Destruction and the Hemolytic Disorders. In J. W. Harris (ed.), *The Red Cell-Production, Metabolism, Destruction: Normal and Abnormal.* Boston: Harvard University Press, 1970.

Hershko, C. The fate of circulating hemoglobin. *Br. J. Haematol.* 29:199, 1975.

Lessin, L. S., and Rosse, W. (eds.) Diagnosis, mechanisms and treatment of hemolytic anemias. *Mod. Treat.* 8:321, 1971.

Mengel, C. E., Kann, H. E., and Carolla, R. L. Hemolytic Anemia: I. General Considerations, Enzymatic and Membrane Abnormalities, and Nonimmune Acquired Disorders. In C. E. Mengel, et al (eds.), *Hematology: Principles and Practice.* Chicago: Year Book, 1972.

Miller, D. R. The Laboratory Evaluation of Hemolysis. In R. I. Weed (ed.), *Hematology for Internists.* Boston: Little, Brown, 1971.

Perrotta, A. L., and Finch, C. A. The polychromatophilic erythrocyte. *Am. J. Clin. Pathol.* 57:471, 1972.

122

Prankerd, T. A. J., and Bellingham, A. J. (eds.) Haemolytic anaemias. *Clin. Haematol.* 4:1, 1975.

Schmid, R. (ed.) Physiology and disorders of hemoglobin degradation I. *Semin. Hematol.* 9:1, 1972.

Szur, L. Surface counting in the assessment of sites of red cell destruction. *Br. J. Haematol.* 18:591, 1970.

Weed, R. I. (ed.) The importance of erythrocyte deformability. *Am. J. Med.* 49:147, 1970.

White, P. Degradation of Hemoglobin. In W. J. Williams, E. Beutler, A. J. Erslev, and R. W. Rundles (eds.), *Hematology* (2nd ed.). New York: McGraw-Hill, 1977.

Wintrobe, M. M., et al The Hemolytic Disorders: General Considerations. In M. M. Wintrobe, et al (eds.), *Clinical Hematology* (7th ed.). Philadelphia: Lea & Febiger, 1974.

5 : Coombs' Test-Positive Hemolytic Anemias

This chapter deals with hemolytic anemias associated with the binding of antibody or complement to red cells. Warm antibodies active at 37°C or cold antibodies active at room temperature or below may arise against erythrocyte antigens. In some cases these antibodies activate a series of proteins referred to collectively as complement; in others, the red cells are coated with antibody alone or with both antibody and complement. As a result of activation or *fixation* of complement by hemolytic antibodies (hemolysins) there may be intravascular red cell lysis and release of hemoglobin; but more frequently immune lysis, if it occurs, is delayed and happens slowly in the reticuloendothelial system, particularly the spleen.

Hemolytic Anemia, Antibodies, and Complement

Antibodies and complement play various roles in the pathogenesis of the immunohemolytic anemias. Five categories of hemolytic anemia are described in Table 5-1. In each category different antibodies and a different role for complement are involved. The human complement system consists of many plasma protein components. A subunit of C1, or the first component of complement, contains a combining site for the Fc portion of immunoglobulins and initiates the complement cascade. This C1 subunit reacts with IgG or IgM antibodies that have combined with their corresponding antigen or have been aggregated. In the case of IgG antibodies, at least two molecules of IgG in close proximity to one another must react with antigen. With IgM antibodies, two subunits of the same IgM molecule may serve to activate the first component of complement. IgG1, IgG2, and IgG3 antibody subtypes are capable of activating complement. IgG4 is not.

In the first category of hemolytic anemia, the antibodies are *hemolysins,* which characteristically fix many complement components and thereby cause frank hemolysis. They may be either IgG or IgM immunoglobulins, but not IgA globulins, as IgA cannot fix complement. The hemolysins may be autoantibodies or may have arisen secondary to sensitization. Most are active in the cold. The Donath-Landsteiner antibody (p. 140) and some cold agglutinins found in cold agglutinin hemolytic diseases are examples of hemolysins. As a result of the initial

Table 5-1 : Characteristics of Antibody-Mediated Hemolytic Anemias

Hemolytic Anemia (antibody type)	Antibody Characteristics	Complement	Immunoglobulin Type	Example
Hemolysin	Hemolytic	Fixed	IgG	Donath-Landsteiner
	Cold		IgM	Autoimmune warm hemolysins
	Rarely warm			Transfusion reaction
Hemagglutinin	Agglutinate	May be fixed	IgM	Isohemagglutinins
	Warm or cold			Cold hemagglutinin hemolytic anemia
Warm-reacting	Requires Coombs' test for detection	Usually not fixed	IgG	Autoimmune hemolytic anemia
	Autoimmune			Transfusion reaction
	Sensitized			Hemolytic disease of the newborn (erythroblastosis fetalis)
Complement coating alone	Dissociates from red cell after fixing complement	Fixed	IgG	Autoimmune hemolytic anemia
	Warm or cold		IgM	
"Innocent bystander"	Directed against drug	Fixed	IgM	Drug-induced (quinidine) hemolytic anemia

activation of C1 components, C4, C2, and then C3 are fixed and activated on the red cell. Complement components 5 through 9 then are activated, and lysis of the red cell results. This usually causes intravascular hemolysis with elevation of plasma hemoglobin levels and decreased whole serum complement levels. Warm-acting hemolysins directed against certain blood group antigens are also known to exist.

Hemagglutinins are usually IgM isoantibodies like anti-A or anti-B that are directed against antigens in the ABO blood group system. They cause a second type of hemolytic anemia by their ability to agglutinate red cells rapidly at warm or cold temperatures, which causes erythrocyte sequestration and destruction in the reticuloendothelial system. Complement may play a role by promoting phagocytosis of these red cells in the reticuloendothelial cells.

A third type of hemolytic anemia is caused by warm-reacting, IgG, 7S antibodies, which, due either to sensitization or to autoimmunity, coat red cells and thereby promote the sequestration of those red cells in the reticuloendothelial system, particularly the spleen. Approximately three hundred molecules of this antibody on a red cell are detected by the usual clinical tests (Coombs' test), but only a few molecules are needed to cause hemolysis. Complement activation is not usually involved in this form of hemolytic anemia.

A fourth type of hemolytic anemia is characterized by the presence of complement alone on the red cells. Presumably small amounts of warm- or cold-reacting IgG or IgM immunoglobulins directed against red cell antigens fix complement on the red cells and then dissociate from them. Complement-coated erythrocytes are then destroyed prematurely, particularly in the spleen. More than 100 molecules of C3 per red cell may be detected, and more than 1,100 molecules of C3 per cell is correlated with overt hemolysis.

Complement components may also be present on red cells in a fifth type of hemolytic anemia, in which red cells serve as *innocent bystanders*. An IgM antibody is produced against a drug. As a result of interaction between the drug and the antibody, possibly on or near the surface of a red cell, complement is fixed to the red cell. The cell may then undergo premature sequestration and destruction.

In summary, activation of the whole complement sequence by hemolysins results in rapid lysis of red cells. More commonly, only partial activation of the complement system occurs, and this results in red cells that are covered by activated complement components, particularly C3. As a result of this complement coating, these erythrocytes are prematurely destroyed in the reticuloendothelial system.

Pathogenesis of Immunohemolytic Anemia

The surface of human red blood cells is covered with substances that are capable of provoking an immune reaction and that are called blood group antigens. The most important groups of red cell antigens are the ABO and Rh systems; and besides these there are many other, less important, systems. A red cell membrane antigen stimulates the production of antibodies in individuals who lack that antigen's blood group. Thus, a normal immune system reacts by producing antibodies to foreign substances. Under certain conditions this system may produce antibodies against the body's own red cell antigens. When this happens, red cells become coated with antibody, complement, or both. These substances can most easily be detected with anti-γ-globulin or anticomplement antibodies by using the Coombs' test which will be described shortly.

There is no generally accepted explanation for why patients produce autoantibodies against their own red cells. Some investigators suggest that minor damage to the red cells leads a normal immune system to sense them as being foreign and therefore produce antibodies against them. It has not yet been demonstrated that the red cells of patients suffering from auto-immune hemolytic anemias actually have abnormal antigenic structures. An alternative explanation is that the immune system becomes deranged, falsely senses normal red cell antigens as foreign, and as a result produces autoantibodies.* The cause of derangement may be acquired, perhaps by infection with certain viruses, or inherited. Animal models provide evidence for the ability of viruses to derange the immune systems, and family studies have yielded some evidence for a genetic predisposition to autoimmune phenomena.

No matter which of these explanations is ultimately proved correct, the hallmark of autoimmune diseases is the presence of antibody or complement on red cell surfaces. In some immuno-hemolytic anemias (incompatible transfusion reactions, for example), the antibodies are not directed against the patient's own red cells but are, rather, correctly aimed at destroying foreign red cells. We refer to both types of antibody-mediated hemolytic anemia as *immunohemolytic* or *Coombs' test–positive hemolytic anemia* and reserve the term *autoimmune hemolytic*

*It has been proposed that previously suppressed "clones" of antibody-producing cells emerge that have not acquired, or have lost through mutation, the ability to recognize some antigens or erythrocytes as native, and that these clones elaborate antibodies against the red cells.

anemia (AIHA) for those cases in which antibodies are directed against the patients' own red cell antigens.

Combs' Testing

The modern-day Coombs' test is designed to detect antibody or complement on human red cells or to detect the presence of an antibody in serum. An important part of this test is Coombs' reagent. Coombs' reagent is produced by injecting human γ-globulins, produced by preparative electrophoresis, into animals such as rabbits and thereby raising an antiserum against human γ-globulin. A β-globulin fraction containing components of complement is injected into other rabbits, and an antiserum raised against complement. The antiserums raised against human γ- and β-globulins are absorbed to remove unwanted antibodies. The *gamma Coombs' reagent* or *anti-human γ-globulin serum* and the *non-gamma Coombs' reagent* or *anticomplement serum* are then assayed, diluted, and for most clinical purposes combined into a *broad spectrum Coombs' reagent* or *antiglobulin serum.* This latter reagent can detect either complement or antibody on red cells.

Actually the Coombs' test consists of a series of steps, only the last of which utilizes the Coombs' reagent. In the *direct antiglobulin (Coombs') test (DAT)* the patient's red cells are washed thoroughly with saline to remove any nonspecifically bound immunoglobulins.* The washed red cells are suspended in albumin, incubated at 37°C for 1 hour, and centrifuged to promote agglutination. Agglutination indicates the presence of antibody on the red cells. In most cases of autoimmune hemolytic anemias, antibody on the red cells is detected by the DAT. The antibodies involved are IgG, warm-reacting (37°C), *incomplete antibodies.* They are not large enough to span the distance between red cells, which are normally repelled by their negative surface changes. For this reason the antiglobulin serum is required: it forms interlocking lattices between red cells and thereby causes agglutination. Albumin, which diminishes the negative charge on red cells, is used to promote agglutination. If the red cells are coated with complement and not antibody, the anticomplement antibody contained in the broad spectrum Coombs' reagent will produce red cell agglutination. Autoimmune hemolytic anemia (AIHA), transfusion reaction, certain drugs, and diseases such as

---

*If IgM, macroglobulin, *complete antibodies* are present on the erythrocytes, direct agglutination of the patient's red cells may occur at room temperature or below. These macroglobulins are sometimes called cold antibodies or *cold agglutinins.* If present in extremely high titer, they can cause a hemolytic anemia. In normal individuals, they are commonly found in low titer, not sufficient to cause direct agglutination in this part of the Coombs' test.

lupus erythematosus, lymphoma, and lymphocytic leukemia are associated with a positive DAT.

The *indirect antiglobulin (Coombs') test* requires the use of *test cells* as well as Coombs' reagent. Red cells from two or more individuals are combined to produce a suspension that contains all the common, clinically important, red blood cell antigens. After reaction of these test cells with the patient's serum, the cells are washed thoroughly, and the same steps as those described for the DAT are performed. Agglutination should occur only if the serum contains an antibody that will coat at least some of the test cells or if the serum contains an antibody that will cause complement fixation to the test cells, even though the antibody itself may not remain attached. In regard to the latter possibility, complement-fixing macroglobulins may be eluted from red cells and not be detected by antiglobulin reagents, but their complement "footprint" is detected by the anticomplement Coombs' reagent.

For most clinical purposes it is important to remember only that a positive DAT with broad spectrum Coombs' reagent indicates that antibody or complement is present on the patient's *red cells* and that a positive indirect antiglobulin test, or *antibody screen,* indicates that an antibody is present in the patient's *plasma.*

Certain antibodies are normally present in humans. The macroglobulin antibodies against group A and B antigens are one important example. Since test cells are usually group O and therefore do not have A or B antigens, and since Coombs' reagent is absorbed so that it does not have anti-A or anti-B antibody, these naturally occurring isoantibodies do not interfere with Coombs' testing. Rarely, antibodies may appear naturally without any apparent stimulus; but usually the presence of an antibody in a patient's serum means that stimulation by a foreign blood group antigen, either because of prior blood transfusion or because of pregnancy with transplacental migration of incompatible fetal red cells, has occurred, or that an autoimmune hemolytic anemia is present.

Classification of Coombs'-Positive Hemolytic Anemias

Those hemolytic anemias for which the direct or indirect Coombs' tests are positive may be classified in many ways. Some classifications are based on whether the antibody involved reacts at 37°C or at room temperature or below (20°C to 4°C). Others divide these anemias into those that are idiopathic and those that are associated with neoplastic, autoimmune, or inflammatory diseases. A clinically useful classification of Coombs' test-positive hemolytic anemias combines these two systems.

Classification of Coombs' test–positive hemolytic anemias

I. Idiopathic Autoimmune Hemolytic Anemia
    A. Warm autoantibody type
    B. Cold autoantibody type
II. Autoimmune Hemolytic Anemia associated with Underlying diseases
        (lupus erythematosus, chronic lymphatic leukemia, lymphoma)
    A. Warm autoantibody type
    B. Cold autoantibody type
III. Drug-induced Coombs' Test-positive Hemolytic Anemias
IV. Transfusion Reactions due to Incompatible Red Cells
V. Paroxysmal Cold Hemoglobinuria

Idiopathic Auto-immune Hemolytic Anemia

Patients with autoimmune hemolytic anemia (AIHA) usually come to the attention of physicians because of anemia or signs of hemolysis. Sometimes the disease is first suspected when the patient develops jaundice and yellow sclera or when blood is found in the serum or urine. Usually the initial investigation reveals a high reticulocyte count and reticulocyte production index. Some of the pigmented hemoglobin breakdown products associated with hemolysis are detected in the urine or serum and confirm the diagnosis of hemolysis. Direct and indirect Coombs' testing is then performed and a diagnosis of AIHA made.

The anemia is usually mild or moderate, but some patients may have severe anemia with hematocrits of less than 0.10 (10%). Examination of the blood smear reveals marked spherocytosis (Plate 24) and polychromatophilia (Plate 23). The latter may not be present if the bone marrow is suppressed by a nutritional deficiency or by an underlying bone marrow–suppressive disease. Often white blood cell counts are elevated, and occasionally the patient has thrombocytopenia. The combination of antibody-mediated hemolysis and thrombocytopenia is known as the *Evans-Duane syndrome.* The Evans-Duane syndrome is rarely encountered and is generally treated the same as an autoimmune hemolytic anemia.

Serology of AIHA

The DAT is positive. By using anti-γ-globulin and anticomplement Coombs' reagents rather than the broad spectrum reagent it is possible to determine whether antibody, complement, or both are present on the patient's red cells. These different patterns of reaction with Coombs' reagents are significant in the differential diagnosis of the immunohemolytic anemias. In many cases the patient's serum will contain antibody and give a positive indirect antiglobulin test. In no case should the indirect antiglobulin test be positive and the DAT negative. Some patients give a positive reaction only to the anticomplement Coombs' test, but usually a complement-fixing IgG antibody can be demonstrated on their red cells by more sensitive tests that are available in research laboratories. A few patients with marked spherocytosis, hemolysis, and no cause for a Coombs' test–negative hemolytic anemia give negative results to the direct and indirect broad spectrum Coombs' tests. In some of these cases a positive test can be obtained by using different reagents from other manufacturers and by being very careful to wash the cells thoroughly. If the cells are not thoroughly washed, small amounts of non-specifically bound immunoglobulin will neutralize the anti-globulin antibodies in the Coombs' reagent and give rise to a false negative Coombs' test. Some other patients with clinical findings strongly suggestive of Coombs' test-positive hemolytic anemia but with negative antiglobulin tests can be shown to have Coombs' test positivity when the DAT is performed at room temperature or $4°C$. Apparently at these temperatures changes in antibody configuration occur that allow agglutination with Coombs' reagent. Finally there are very rare cases in which AIHA is suspected but neither antibodies nor complement can be detected on the patients' red cells. Some of these individuals respond to the therapy used for treating AIHA.

False positive DATs may result if the Coombs' reagent contains antibodies against the β-globulin, transferrin. Reticulocytes bind transferrin and, in the presence of moderate reticulocytosis and a Coombs' reagent containing antitransferrin, a false positive DAT may result. This rarely occurs with modern-day reagents, which have been absorbed to remove antitransferrin antibodies.

Warm Auto-antibody-Type Hemolytic Anemias

Two types of antibody may be responsible for autoimmune hemolytic anemias. Most commonly, warm antibodies reactive at $37°C$ and of the IgG type are present, with or without concurrent complement coating of the red cells. In some cases these warm antibodies are directed against specific antigens on the red cells, usually antigens in the Rh system (for example, anti-c or anti-e). Unfortunately in many cases the antibody is directed nonspecifically against many blood group antigens, usually in the Rh group. Sometimes the antibody will react with all red cells except those of the Rh_{null} type. (Rh_{null} lacks all the known antigens associated with the Rh system.) The antibody may be directed against structural components common to all Rh antigens. When there is only complement coating of the red cells and no demonstrable warm or cold antibodies, it is not entirely clear how the complement fixation occurs. It is possible that antibodies, because of their number or physical characteristics, cannot be detected by the methods usually employed in blood banks. In some cases very sensitive methods for detecting antibody will show their presence despite negative antiglobulin tests.

In general the rate of hemolysis is proportional to the concentration of cell-bound antibody. Patients with little in the way of detectable antibody, and patients whose cells are coated with complement alone, generally have mild hemolytic anemia. Some patients with positive DATs do not hemolyze or hemolyze so slowly that their bone marrows can increase erythrocyte production sufficiently to maintain a normal hematocrit, a so-called *compensated autoimmune hemolytic anemia.*

Antibody- and complement-coated red cells are generally sequestered and destroyed in the RES, particularly in the spleen.

If the spleen is removed or the cell is heavily coated with antibody, the liver may play a clinically significant role in clearance of coated erythrocytes. Many factors determine whether complement-coated red cells are destroyed or converted to spherocytes. The amount of complement fixed, the type of antibody involved in activating complement, the rate of complement sensitization, the inactivation of fixed complement, and other factors determine whether complement-coated red cells are rendered spherocytic, destroyed in the RES, or left to circulate normally.

Antibody-coated red cells bind to splenic macrophages through receptor sites specific for the Fc portion of the IgG molecule, and phagocytosis, red cell fragmentation, and spherocytosis result. The structurally rigid spherocytes and red cell fragments are subsequently destroyed in the RES. Red cell agglutination in the splenic sinusoids may also contribute to hemolysis.

In most cases of AIHA red cell hemolysins are not present. Occasionally, severe cases of autoimmune hemolysis are associated with intravascular hemolysis complicated by hemoglobinemia and hemoglobinuria and with actual lysis of cells during antiglobulin testing.

Cold Autoantibody-Type Hemolytic Anemia

The second type of autoimmune hemolytic anemia is mediated by cold-agglutinating autoantibodies. These antibodies arise in association with diseases such as influenza, infectious mononucleosis, and acute mycoplasmal pneumonia. They also occur in chronic *cold hemagglutin disease* (CHAD) without apparent cause and are associated not only with hemolytic anemia but also with symptoms secondary to agglutination of red cells in the patient's circulation after exposure to cold temperatures. Cold-reactive autoantibodies have several interesting characteristics. First, they are macroglobulins with IgM specificity, which means they are large molecules (sedimentation velocity 19S, as opposed to 7S for warm-reacting antibodies). They are *complete antibodies,* which, if mixed with compatible human red cells, will agglutinate them at 4° to 20°C, since their large size enables them to span the distance between negatively charged red cells. Furthermore, these antibodies have specificity against a blood group antigen, I. This blood group antigen is part of the I-i blood group system. Fetal red cells have i on their surface and react only with antiserum directed against i. As the fetus matures and in early infancy a process takes place by which the i antigen is lost and I antigenicity is gained in the red cell. Almost all adult red cells have only the I antigen on their surface. Therefore, serum from patients with cold agglutinins will clump almost all human red cells. If for some reason the titer of cold agglutinins is particularly high and the patient's environment is cold, red cell agglutination will occur in the patient's microcirculation, leading to pain, blanching, and numbness in toes and fingers. This process also causes hemolysis of some of the agglutinated red cells, if they are subjected to mechanical trauma. As a result of the cold antibody reaction with anti-I, complement is fixed to the red cell and may be detected by the DAT. The IgM cold antibody itself is not detected by antiglobulin testing. Sometimes, enough antibody and complement activity is present at body temperature to cause hemolysis, which is often chronic, but not severe.

Not infrequently patients have a positive DAT due to complement coating alone and have only a low titer of cold agglutinins. In some of these cases the low titer cold agglutinins are enough to cause complement fixation and ultimate splenic destruction of red cells. In other cases, it is possible that an undetected warm-reacting antibody is also present and capable of fixing complement, so that the cold agglutinins are actually insignificant and not etiologically related to the hemolytic anemia.

The clinical findings in patients with chronic cold hemagglutinin disease include acrocyanosis (Raynaud's phenomenon) with cyanosis of skin surfaces exposed to cold, minimal splenomegaly, chronic mild-to-moderate hemolytic anemia, and sometimes mild jaundice. Examination of the blood smear shows spherocytosis and polychromasia. If the blood is cooled to $40°C$, intense autoagglutination occurs but disappears if the blood is then warmed to $37°C$. Cold agglutinin titers are very high, usually greater than 1:10,000. It should be emphasized that, unless the anticomplement Coombs' test is positive and a high titer of cold agglutinins demonstrated, the presence of chronic cold hemagglutinin disease is unlikely.

Therapy of Auto-
immune Hemolytic
Anemia

At least four therapeutic modalities must be considered for the treatment of autoimmune hemolytic anemia. The first, for patients with moderate or severe hemolysis, is transfusion therapy. Transfusion should be avoided if the patient is not symptomatic from his anemia, since patients with hemolysis tend to become sensitized to foreign red cell antigens and develop hemolytic transfusion reactions. Patients with angina, postural hypotension, or other symptoms of severe anemia must be transfused. It is best to used packed red cells rather than whole blood to avoid fever due to antibodies against leukocytes or other plasma components. A fever might be confused with a hemolytic transfusion reaction. An attempt should be made to discover the specificity, if any, of the autoantibody. If the antibodies are directed against only a few kinds of red cell antigens, then compatible blood can often be obtained from a rare donor file. In most cases the antibody is nonspecific and it is not possible to obtain a completely compatible crossmatch. It is then necessary to find red cells that react weakly with the patient's antibody and to infuse these cells slowly while watching carefully for signs of an acute hemolytic transfusion reaction. Usually the cells can be transfused safely, but their life span will be no longer than the patient's own erythrocytes. For this reason, transfusion therapy is a stopgap measure and is used only to tide the patient over until his disease remits spontaneously or responds to therapy.

A more difficult problem is transfusion of patients with cold hemagglutinin hemolytic anemia. Because the cells agglutinate at room temperature, it is difficult to carry out accurate ABO typing of them. Multiple washings of the cells with warm saline will remove enough of the cold agglutinins to permit accurate ABO typing. Crossmatching can be performed at 37°C, although perfectly compatible donor cells may not be found.

High doses of adrenal corticosteroids (prednisone, 100 mg per day) are usually instituted immediately in moderate or severe autoimmune hemolytic anemia. These appear to be more effective in patients with warm- than with cold antibody–mediated hemolysis. Some patients respond within a few days, but often treatment must be continued for weeks before a fall in the reticulocyte count and a slow rise in the hematocrit is seen. When the hematocrit reaches 0.30 (30%), very slow tapering of the steroid dose may be attempted. Generally therapy must be maintained for months, during which time a spontaneous remission may occur.

Approximately 50 percent of patients will respond to corticosteroids. Their hematocrit during steroid therapy will be high enough so that they are not symptomatic, and the dose of steroids is low enough so they will not develop severe side effects such as gastrointestinal bleeding, hypertension, diabetes mellitus, sepsis, edema, severe Cushing's syndrome, and osteoporosis. Anemic patients who do not respond to this therapy or who must be maintained on high doses of corticosteroids should be considered for splenectomy.

About 50 percent of patients undergoing splenectomy for autoimmune hemolytic anemia initially go into complete remission without any further requirement for steroid therapy. Those patients who do not remit or who subsequently relapse can often be kept asymptomatic on prednisone in lower doses than prior to surgery. Patients with small amounts of warm antibodies, those with splenomegaly, and those who show an initial response to prednisone are the most likely to respond to splenectomy. Splenic sequestration studies using radiochromium-labeled red cells have been used to predict response to splenectomy. A high ratio of spleen to liver erythrocyte uptake is associated with a good response. Complications of splenectomy include perioperative infections, postsplenectomy thrombocytosis, thromboembolism, and death from overwhelming sepsis, particularly in children months or even years following the operation.

Splenectomy, as well as corticosteroids, may exert its initial effect by decreasing the number of reticuloendothelial cells that phagocytize antibody-coated or complement-coated red cells. Corticosteroids, and perhaps even splenectomy, decrease the production of red cell antibody. Steroids may also decrease the affinity of the autoantibody for red cell antigens.

A certain number of patients do not respond to splenectomy, corticosteroids, or both together. Some of these patients may die as a result of unremitting hemolysis or complications of steroid therapy or splenectomy. Recently such unresponsive patients have been treated with immunosuppressive drugs like azathioprine (Imuran), cyclophosphamide (Cytoxan), and other alkylating agents known to be immunosuppressive. This therapy is investigational and cannot be recommended unless the patient's prognosis is poor. There is always the danger that these drugs will suppress the bone marrow, make the anemia significantly worse, or cause leukopenia, infections, and thrombocytopenia.

Patients with cold antibody–mediated hemolytic anemia should be given transfusions of only warmed blood devoid of plasma (complement); otherwise the transfused cells may hemolyze faster than the patient's own inactivated, complement-coated erythrocytes. Every attempt should be made to keep the patients, particularly their extremities, warm. Splenectomy and corticosteroid therapy have helped in some cases. Treatment as for an underlying lymphoma has sometimes been successful.

Finally, patients with chronic immunohemolytic anemia of any type may suffer from folic acid deficiency and megaloblastosis. For this reason folic acid, 1 mg per day, should be prescribed. Many other therapeutic measures have been suggested but have proved to be of little benefit and will not be discussed.

Autoimmune Hemolytic Anemia in Association with Other Diseases

In a general hematology clinic, idiopathic autoimmune hemolytic anemia is relatively rare, but it does account for up to one-fourth of patients with overt hemolytic anemia. However, this number depends upon how one defines hemolytic anemia, since hemolysis of some degree occurs in association with many human diseases. Autoimmune hemolytic anemia usually accompanies malignant lymphomas, particularly lymphosarcomas, chronic lymphocytic leukemia, and systemic lupus erythematosus. It is sometimes associated with certain carcinomas (particularly ovarian), infectious mononucleosis, subacute bacterial endocarditis, inflammatory bowel diseases, infections, liver disease, and sarcoidosis. Most often the AIHA associated with these disease entities has the clinical features of the warm antibody type of idiopathic autoimmune hemolytic anemia.

Cold antibody-type autoimmune hemolytic anemia is most often found in association with lymphomas and other lymphoproliferative diseases such as chronic lymphocytic leukemia. Viral infections, particularly influenza, infectious mononucleosis, and acute *Mycoplasma* infections, cause high titer cold agglutinins and, occasionally, frank hemolytic anemia.

The pathogenesis of warm and cold antibody-type autoimmune hemolytic anemia in association with viral diseases or lymphoproliferative diseases is poorly understood. There is little evidence to enable us to choose between an abnormality in the patient's immune system and damage to the patient's blood group antigens. It is known in the case of the malignant lymphoproliferative diseases that the host's immune system is altered and abnormal. It is interesting that animal models for autoimmune hemolytic anemias often have lymphomas in association with autoimmune hemolytic anemia.

Coombs' Test-Positive Hemolytic Anemias Associated with Drug Ingestion

Four pathophysiologic mechanisms (see Table 5-2) account for most cases of drug-induced Coombs'-positive autoimmune hemolytic anemias.

Penicillin (and occasionally the cephalosphorin antibiotics such as cephalothin) provides the best example of the first pathophysiologic mechanism. Penicillin binds to red cell membranes both in vivo and in vitro. In this bound condition the drug acts as a hapten, and may cause a 7S, IgG-type, non-complement-fixing antibody to develop against it. In association with large doses of penicillin, or with small doses and in the presence of renal insufficiency, this antibody will react with erythrocytes coated with penicillin. This results in a positive DAT, and sometimes a frank hemolytic anemia. Thus there is a group of patients who have antipenicillin antibodies in their serum; a smaller group who, because of these antibodies, have positive DAT; and an even smaller group, usually those with high serum levels of penicillin, who develop frank hemolysis and anemia. Penicillin-coated red cells agglutinate in the presence of serum from these patients. A DAT performed with antiglobulin Coombs' reagent on red cells from these patients' cells will be positive, and testing done with an anticomplement Coombs' reagent will usually be negative.

Table 5-2 : Direct Antiglobulin Test-Positive (Coombs'-Positive) Hemolytic Anemias

Hemolytic Disease (DAT-positive)	Anti-γ-Globulin Coombs' Test	Anticomplement Coombs' Test	Antibody Specificity	Indirect Coombs' Test	Mechanism of Antibody Production
Autoimmune	Pos or Neg	Pos or Neg	Rh or none	Pos or neg	Defective immune system or altered red cells
Cold hemagglutinin	Neg	Pos	I or i	Pos	Defective immune system or altered red cells
Drug-induced					
Penicillin or Cephalin	Pos	Neg	Penicillin or cephalin	Pos with penicillin or cephalin	Hapten
Quinidine (innocent bystander)	Neg	Pos	Quinidine	Pos with quinidine	Hapten
Aldomet	Pos	Neg	Rh or none	Pos without Aldomet or neg	Altered red cells or defective immune system
Cephalin	Pos	Pos	None	Neg	Nonspecific binding due to alteration of red cell surface
Incompatible blood transfusion	Pos Transiently	Neg	One or several blood group antigens	Pos	Prior sensitization or natural isohemagglutinins

The second mechanism by which drugs induce Coombs'-test positive hemolytic anemias is most often encountered with the drug quinidine. Other drugs associated with this mechanism are stibophen, quinine, para-aminosalicylic acid, phenacetin, sulfonamides, chlorpromazine, and isoniazid. Quinidine complexes with an unknown macromolecular carrier and acts as a hapten. An IgM-type antibody directed against quinidine develops. The subsequent administration of quinidine results in an antigen–antibody reaction on or near the surface of erythrocytes. Complement is fixed to the red cell surface, but the antibody does not remain attached to the erythrocyte. The red cell is considered an *innocent bystander,* since its surface is being used as a site for a quinidine, not red cell, antigen–antibody reaction. As a result, the anticomplement direct Coombs' test is positive, and the anti-γ-globulin direct Coombs' test is negative. An indirect antiglobulin test will be positive only if the patient's serum contains quinidine or if quinidine has been added to the patient's serum prior to performing the test.

It is interesting that the antibody involved in quinidine-induced thrombocytopenia is a 7S IgG antibody rather than the IgM macroglobulin that is found in DAT-positive hemolytic anemia due to quinidine. Furthermore the antibodies associated with quinidine and quinine immunohemolytic anemias do not cross-react.

α-Methyldopa (Aldomet) is associated with the third pathophysiologic mechanism for drug-induced antibody-mediated hemolytic anemia. Up to one third of the patients receiving this drug may develop a positive reaction to the anti-γ-globulin direct Coombs' test. Usually this happens with a moderate dosage (2 gm per day) after 3 to 6 months of therapy. The disease closely resembles idiopathic, autoimmune, hemolytic anemia even to the point that Rh blood group specificity of the antibodies has been demonstrated. One small difference is that the anticomplement direct Coombs' test is rarely positive in the α-methyldopa-induced anemias. Of the patients who have positive direct Coombs' test results, usually fewer than one third actually hemolyze, and in only 3 percent does severe hemolysis develop. The presence of α-methyldopa is not required in order to obtain a positive indirect Coombs' test. L-Dopa, mefenamic acid, and chlordiazepoxide have also been described in association with this type of hemolytic anemia.

The final mechanism involved in producing positive DAT by drugs is not associated with an antigen–antibody reaction. Rather, cephalosporins such as cephalothin or cephaloridine, particularly in the presence of renal insufficiency or high serum levels, damage erythrocyte membranes; and, as a result, nonspecific uptake of serum proteins, including γ-globulin and complement, occurs.

The DAT is positive because of this coating of the red cell membrane, and the indirect antiglobulin test is positive in the presence of the cephalosporin.

Therapy of Drug-induced Coombs' Test-Positive Hemolytic Anemias

The hemolytic anemia associated with these drugs varies in severity; in many cases only the DAT is positive, but in a few, all the clinical findings associated with a moderate or severe hemolytic anemia are present. The only therapy required is discontinuation of the drugs. It may take several weeks or even months for the positive DAT result to disappear, but usually the hemolytic anemia ameliorates within days or weeks. Adrenal corticosteroids have been given in severe cases, although their benefit has not been proved. Sometimes they are used if an AIHA cannot be excluded from the differential diagnosis. Blood transfusions can usually be given safely once the drug has been eliminated from the patient's plasma, except in the case of α-methyldopa-induced hemolytic anemia, when it may be difficult to crossmatch the patient's blood, since his plasma contains antibodies against blood group antigens, especially the Rh group. Here crossmatching must be done, and in an emergency the blood that seems to be the least incompatible must be used. Usually the positive result to the antiglobulin test is the last manifestation of this type of immunohemolytic anemia to return to normal.

Incompatible Blood Transfusion Reactions

Transfusion reactions must be distinguished from autoimmune hemolytic anemia and immunohemolytic anemia secondary to drugs. These reactions are of two types. When a reaction due to ABO incompatibility occurs, it does not depend on prior sensitization, since individuals have in their plasma naturally occurring isoagglutinins. For example, a patient of blood group O has anti-A and anti-B in his plasma. If he is transfused with type A blood, a reaction occurs immediately between the A cells and the anti-A in his plasma. The donor A cells are immediately lysed, and the transiently positive DAT becomes negative.

In contrast, prior sensitization to blood group antigens in the Rh system, and in most other red cell antigen systems, is required before an antibody-mediated transfusion reaction to them can occur. The sequence of events usually goes as follows. A patient lacking an Rh blood group antigen, such as D, is given a transfusion with red cells carrying this D antigen. As a result the recipient develops anti-D antibodies within 2 to 3 weeks. If he is again transfused with red cells having D antigen on their surface, an antigen–antibody reaction results. Usually the D cells are not lysed immediately but rather are coated with immune, 7S, anti-D antibodies. These cells are then slowly destroyed in the reticuloendothelial system. Prior to destruction the DAT will reveal antibody coating. Since the cells giving the positive DAT are eliminated, however, the DAT ultimately becomes negative. The recipient continues to have in his plasma an anti-D antibody that can be demonstrated by the indirect Coombs' test. Thus, in this second type of transfusion reaction, the DAT may be positive for several days following transfusion, but it then becomes negative. Before transfusion the recipient has a negative indirect Coombs' test that becomes positive after sensitization. The antibody usually persists, so the indirect Coombs' test stays positive for weeks, months, or even indefinitely. In many cases the titer of antibody declines and the indirect Coombs' test becomes negative. However, an anamnestic rise in antibody can occur within a week, if subsequent transfusions of D cells are given.

Except for the days immediately following an incompatible blood transfusion, it is easy to separate transfusion reactions from autoimmune and drug-induced immunohemolytic anemia. The DAT remains positive in the latter two conditions but becomes negative following a hemolytic transfusion reaction.

Paroxysmal Cold Hemoglobinuria

Paroxysmal cold hemoglobinuria (PCH) is a rare disease associated with syphilis and occasionally with measles, mumps, chicken pox, and infectious mononucleosis. It may also occur in otherwise normal individuals. Both the idiopathic and the syphilitic forms are characterized by the presence of *Donath-Landsteiner antibody* in the patient's serum. This IgG, complement-fixing, 7S antibody is directed against the erythrocyte P antigen site. It does not react at $37°C$; but at $4°C$ it gives a positive result to DAT; and upon rewarming, complement lysis, not just agglutination, of the antibody-coated red cells occurs. Clinically, severe hemolysis and hemoglobinuria results from exposure to cold temperatures. The Donath-Landsteiner antibody must be distinguished from the usual cold agglutinins. The latter have anti-I specificity and do not usually cause hemolysis in vitro. In both CHAD and paroxysmal cold hemoglobinuria, the anticomplement Coombs' test is positive. The cold anti-γ-globulin Coombs' test is positive in PCH but usually not in CHAD. Therapy is not available for this disease; specifically, corticosteroids and splenectomy are not helpful. All that can be done is to protect the patient from cold in order to avoid acute hemolysis and hemoglobinuria.

APPROACH TO PATIENT WITH COOMBS' TEST-POSITIVE HEMOLYTIC ANEMIA

The diagnosis of Coombs' test–positive hemolytic anemia is made when a patient has documented hemolysis and positive results to direct or indirect antiglobulin tests performed with broad spectrum Coombs' reagent. In a few cases these tests are positive only at room temperature or below. Rarely, the Coombs' tests are negative because the titer of antibody is too low for detection

Approach to patient with Coombs' test-positive hemolytic anemia

I. History
  A. Blood transfusions
  B. Blood type
  C. Drug ingestion
  D. Hemoglobinuria
  E. Syphilis

II. Physical Examination
  A. Signs (lymphadenopathy, splenomegaly, etc.) associated with
    1. Chronic lymphocytic leukemia
    2. Malignant lymphoma
    3. Systemic lupus erythematosus

III. Laboratory Data
  A. Anticomplement direct Coombs' test
  B. Antiglobulin direct Coombs' test
  C. Antinuclear antibody and LE cell tests
  D. Blood smear (spherocytosis, polychromatophilia, lymphocytes characteristic of lymphoma or lymphocytic leukemia)
  E. Cold agglutinin titer
  F. Red cell typing and serum antibody screen (indirect Coombs' test)
  G. Reticulocyte count and production index
  H. Tests for hemolysis
  I. Other tests, when indicated
    1. Bone marrow
    2. Cold Coombs' tests
    3. Donath-Landsteiner antibody
    4. Lymph node biopsy
    5. Sensitive tests for complement and γ-globulin on red cells
    6. Test for specific antibodies to erythrocyte antigens
    7. Tests for syphilis

by routine methods. The diagnosis of antibody-mediated hemolytic anemia is then made on the basis of special immunologic tests that detect tiny amounts of γ-globulin or complement on red cells.

The cause of a Coombs' test–positive hemolytic anemia is usually determined by following the approach outlined in Table 5-2, page 137. A history of drug ingestion and transfusions; findings of symptoms and signs of lymphoma, lymphocytic leukemia, and systemic lupus erythromatosus; and the results of Coombs' tests and cold agglutinin titer, are most helpful in determining the etiology of the anemia.

Certain patterns of antiglobulin test reactions are helpful. A positive indirect Coombs' test (antibody screen) and negative DAT suggest sensitization to an erythrocytic antigen due to prior transfusion or pregnancy. This is particularly true if specificity of the antibody is limited to one or a few red cell antigens.

To distinguish between sensitization to erythrocyte antigens and autoimmunity, it is helpful to type the patient's red cells. If the antibody in his serum or on his cells corresponds to an antigen on his own cells, then by definition he has an autoimmune disease. On the other hand, if he lacks the red cell antigen, the conclusion must be that the antibody arose from prior sensitization to foreign red cells.

Positive anticomplement and negative anti-γ-globulin results are given to direct Coombs' tests by patients with chronic CHAD or quinidine-type drug-induced hemolysis and by some patients with autoimmune hemolytic anemia. Indirect Coombs' test results are positive in cases of drug-induced, antibody-mediated hemolysis only if the offending drug is present in the serum. α-Methyldopa-induced hemolytic anemias are an exception.

By using the patterns of reaction to antiglobulin testing shown in Table 5-2 it is possible to determine the etiology of a DAT-positive hemolytic anemia. In the few cases in which more than one diagnosis is possible, suspect drugs are eliminated and, if necessary, treatment with transfusions or adrenal corticosteroids is begun. With continued observation and testing, a definite etiologic diagnosis can usually be made.

CASE DEVELOPMENT PROBLEMS: COOMBS' TEST–POSITIVE HEMOLYTIC ANEMIA

Five case histories are presented here. In each case, the broad spectrum DAT is positive. On the basis of the information given in each case history, determine the best diagnosis(es).

Patient History No. 1

A 40-year-old woman with renal insufficiency was placed on continuous, intravenous, high dose penicillin therapy for an infection. After 3 weeks of therapy she was given 50 ml of red cells in a transfusion and immediately thereafter developed signs and symptoms of an acute hemolytic anemia.

Laboratory Data

Direct antiglobulin test	positive
Indirect antiglobulin test (antibody screen)	positive (penicillin was *not* added to the antiglobulin test reagents)
Antibody specificity	anti-c
Anti-γ-globulin direct Coombs' test	positive
Anticomplement direct Coombs' test	negative
Cold agglutinin titer	negative, undiluted

The differential diagnosis includes (1) hemolytic transfusion reaction due to previous sensitization to red cell c antigen, (2) penicillin-induced DAT-positive hemolytic anemia, and (3) autoimmune hemolytic anemia. The specificity of the antibody favors diagnosis 1, since the antibody involved in diagnosis 2 is directed against penicillin, not against erythrocyte antigens, and it is unusual to find such limited antibody specificity in diagnosis 3. The DAT may remain positive for several days after infusion of incompatible red cells, since these cells are coated with antibody prior to their destruction.

Patient History No. 2

A 60-year-old man with heart disease has been taking quinidine intermittently for years. One day after restarting quinidine therapy he developed a moderately severe hemolytic anemia. His urine was pale yellow. He has a past history of untreated syphilis and has recovered from a recent bout of influenza. He has never received blood transfusions.

Laboratory Data

Direct antiglobulin test	positive
Indirect antiglobulin test	positive, no hemolysis seen (quinidine was *not* added)
Antibody specificity	not done
Anti-γ-globulin direct Coombs' test	negative
Anticomplement direct Coombs' test	positive
Cold agglutinin titer	positive at 1:100,000 dilution

The differential diagnosis includes (1) cold hemagglutinin disease, (2) quinidine-induced immunohemolytic anemia, and (3) paroxysmal cold hemoglobinuria secondary to syphilis. The laboratory tests are completely consistent with diagnosis (1). There is no way to exclude diagnosis (2), however, if the cold agglutinins are presumed due to influenza; and quinidine was still present in his plasma. Diagnosis (3) is unlikely in the absence of hemoglobinuria. Furthermore the indirect antiglobulin test is usually negative with diagnosis (3); however, it is possible that the test was conducted at a low enough temperature for a Donath-Landsteiner antibody to fix complement and give a positive indirect antiglobulin test. Hemolysis should have been noted during indirect antiglobulin testing.

Patient History
No. 3

A 30-year-old woman developed high blood pressure during the third trimester of her second pregnancy and has been treated with α-methyldopa (Aldomet) since that time. At the time of her first delivery, 4 years ago, she had a hemolytic transfusion reaction.

Laboratory Data (4 months after second delivery)

Direct antiglobulin test	positive
Indirect antiglobulin test	positive (α-methyldopa *not* added)
Antibody specificity	multiple antigens of Rh blood group system
Anti-γ-globulin direct Coombs' test	negative
Anticomplement direct Coombs' test	positive
Cold agglutinin titer	negative, undiluted

The differential diagnosis includes (1) idiopathic autoimmune hemolytic anemia and (2) α-methyldopa-induced immunohemolytic anemia. All the data, with one exception, are compatible with both proposed diagnoses. Diagnosis (1) is more likely because it is very unusual for the anticomplement direct Coomb's test to be positive in α-methyldopa-induced hemolytic anemia. Although it is possible that some of the antibodies in the patient's serum are due to prior sensitization by pregnancy or transfusion, the positive DAT could not be related to the transfusions given 4 years previously.

Patient History
No. 4

A 55-year-old man with malignant lymphoma is being treated with large doses of the antibiotic cephalothin for an infection and has developed signs and symptoms of a mild hemolytic anemia. He has not received any blood transfusions.

Laboratory Data

Direct antiglobulin test	positive
Indirect antiglobulin test	negative (cephalothin *not* added)
Anti-γ-globulin direct Coombs' test	positive
Anticomplement direct Coombs' test	positive
Cold agglutinins	positive at 1:160 dilution

The differential diagnosis includes (1) autoimmune hemolytic anemia secondary to malignant lymphoma, (2) cephalothin-induced hemolytic anemia of nonimmune type, and (3) cold hemagglutinin disease. The findings are consistent with diagnosis (1). Low titer cold agglutinins are not frequently found in association with autoimmune hemolytic anemias of the warm antibody type. The indirect Coombs' (antiglobulin) test may be negative, if all the antibody is on the erythrocytes. Diagnosis (2) is also compatible with the laboratory data, although cephalothin therapy is rarely associated with frank hemolysis. Only by withdrawal of cephalothin therapy will it be possible to differentiate between diagnoses (1) and (2). The positive anti-γ-globulin direct Coomb's test and the low titer of cold agglutinins make diagnosis (3) very unlikely.

Patient History No. 5

Following a bout of infectious mononucleosis a 16-year-old girl has developed a very high reticulocyte count along with signs and symptoms of a hemolytic anemia. One year ago she received two transfusions as treatment for a bleeding duodenal ulcer.

Laboratory Data

Direct antiglobulin test	strongly positive
Indirect antiglobulin test	positive
Antibody specificity	anti-i
Anti-γ-globulin direct Coombs' test	negative
Anticomplement direct Coombs' test	positive
Cold agglutinin titer	positive at 1:10,000 dilution with fetal cells; negative with adult

The differential diagnosis includes (1) autoimmune hemolytic anemia secondary to infectious mononucleosis, (2) sensitization by prior transfusion, and (3) false positive DAT secondary to reticulocytosis. The clinical findings are most consistent with diagnosis (1). Anti-i antibodies, which react as cold agglutinins and fix complement, occasionally develop in patients with infectious mononucleosis. Unlike anti-I cold agglutinins, anti-i reacts with fetal cells, which have i, but not I, antigens on their membranes. A hemolytic transfusion reaction cannot account for the presently positive DAT. It is true that reticulocytes absorb transferrin to their surfaces, and if the Coombs' reagents contain antitransferrin antibodies, a positive result may be obtained. However, this reaction is usually weak, and most modern Coombs' reagents are free of antitransferrin antibody.

TOPICS FOR DISCUSSION: COOMBS' TEST-POSITIVE HEMOLYTIC ANEMIA

Production and standardization of Coomb's reagent

Significance of anti-γ-globulin and anticomplement Coombs' testing

Sensitive methods of detecting antibody and complement on red cells

Biochemistry of complement components and their function

Splenic and RES uptake of antibody and complement-coated red cells

Structure of immunoglobulins

Classification of DAT-positive hemolytic anemias

Pathogenesis of drug-induced immunohemolytic anemias

Therapy of immunohemolytic anemias

Animal models of immunohemolytic anemias

Donath-Landsteiner antibody

Cold antibody–mediated autoimmune hemolytic anemias

Immunohemolytic anemias secondary to lymphoma, lupus erythematosus, and lymphocytic leukemia

Pathogenesis of autoimmune hemolytic anemia
    Altered host immune system (proliferation of "forbidden clones" of antibody-producing cells)
    Altered red cell membrane

SELECTED REFERENCES

Bakemeier, R. F., and Leddy, J. P. Acquired Immune Hemolytic Disorders: Clinical Aspects and Laboratory Evaluation. In R. I. Weed (ed.), *Hematology for Internists.* Boston: Little, Brown, 1971.

Dacie, J. V. *Haemolytic Anaemias,* Part II, *The Auto-immune Anaemias* (2nd ed.). New York: Grune & Stratton, 1962.

Dacie, J. V., and Worlledge, S. M. Autoimmune hemolytic anemia. *Semin. Hematol.* 6:82, 1969.

Garratty, G., and Petz, L. D. Drug-induced immune hemolytic anemia. *Am. J. Med.* 58:398, 1975.

Griffin, J. P. Rapid screening for cold agglutinins in pneumonia. *Ann. Intern. Med.* 70:701, 1969.

Harris, J. W., and Kellermeyer, R. W. Acquired Hemolytic Disease Associated with Demonstrable Serum Factors. In J. W. Harris (ed.), *The Red Cell-Production Metabolism, Destruction: Normal and Abnormal.* Boston: Harvard University Press, 1970.

Jones, S. Autoimmune disorders and malignant lymphoma. *Cancer* 31:1092, 1973.

Mollison, P. L. The role of complement in antibody-mediated red-cell destruction. *Br. J. Haematol.* 18:249, 1970.

Rosse, W. F. Quantitative immunology of immune hemolytic anemia: I. The fixation of C_1 by autoimmune antibody and heterologous anti-IgG antibody. *J. Clin. Invest.* 50:727, 1971.

Rosse, W. F. Quantitative immunology of immune hemolytic anemia: II. The relationship of cell-bound antibody to hemolysis and the effect of treatment. *J. Clin. Invest.* 50:734, 1971.

Rosse, W. F. Hemolytic Anemia: II. The Immune Hemolytic Anemias. In C. E. Mengel, et al (eds.), *Hematology: Principles and Practice.* Chicago: Year Book, 1972.

Rosse, W. F. Correlation of in vivo and in vitro measurements of hemolysis in hemolytic anemia due to immune reactions. *Prog. Hematol.* 8:51, 1973.

Ruddy, S., Gigli, I., and Austen, K. F. The complement system of man. *N. Engl. J. Med.* 287:489; 545; 592; 642, 1972.

Sawitsky, A., and Ozaeta, P. B. Disease-associated autoimmune hemolytic anemia. *Bull. N.Y. Acad. Med.* 46:411, 1970.

Swisher, S. N. (ed.) Immune hemolytic anemias. *Semin. Hematol.* 13: 247, 1976.

Swisher, S. N. Erythrocyte Disorders — Anemias Due to Increased Erythrocyte Destruction Mediated by Antibodies. In W. J. Williams, E. Beutler, A. J. Erslev, and R. W. Rundles, (eds.), *Hematology* (2nd ed.). New York: McGraw-Hill, 1977.

Wintrobe, M. M., et al Immunohemolytic Anemias. In M. M. Wintrobe, et al (eds.), *Clinical Hematology* (7th ed.). Philadelphia: Lea & Febiger, 1974.

Worlledge, S. Immune drug-induced hemolytic anemias. *Semin. Hematol.* 10:327, 1973.

6 : Coombs' Test-Negative Hemolytic Anemias

Premature destruction of erythrocytes occurs in many human diseases. In the diseases described in Chapter 5, hemolysis was mediated by antibodies and complement. There are a great many hemolytic anemias in which antibody and complement are not involved, but which are caused by abnormal erythrocyte membranes, abnormal hemoglobins, deficient red cell enzyme activity, abnormal globin synthesis, hyperplasia of the reticuloendothelial system, traumatic disruption of the red cells, and other abnormalities. In fact hyperplasia of the reticuloendothelial system and decreased red cell life span occur in almost all diseases with an inflammatory component. For this reason we shall discuss only the important hematologic diseases, which result in increased destruction of erythrocytes. Rapid strides are being made in understanding the pathophysiology of these anemias, and it is not possible to summarize all that is known about them. The information relevant to their pathogenesis, diagnoses, and treatment presented here should enable the student to understand the results of laboratory investigation presented in monographs and books devoted to these diseases.

All the anemias listed here (p. 150) and discussed in this chapter have a hemolytic component and produce negative results in antiglobulin tests. Some are acquired, and others are inherited. In many the hemolytic component is quite prominent, but in others it is episodic or plays a relatively minor role. If a patient's anemia is characterized as hemolytic, and Coombs' test–negative, this group of diseases must be considered. We shall emphasize the differential characteristics that enable the hematologist to make a diagnosis.

Hereditary Spherocytosis
Clinical Findings

The typical patient with hereditary spherocytosis (HS) has a family history of spherocytosis, anemia, or jaundice that usually started in childhood. The patient himself is usually an infant with a hemolytic anemia characterized by the presence of many spherocytes in the peripheral blood. These spherocytes lyse more easily than is normal in mildly hypotonic saline solutions. The spleen is enlarged. These four findings — family history of anemia or jaundice, spherocytosis, splenomegaly, and increased osmotic fragility — characterize hereditary spherocytosis. The disease is inherited as an autosomal dominant. Jaundice secondary to in-

Coombs' test-negative hemolytic anemias

Hereditary spherocytosis
Hereditary elliptocytosis
Hemolytic anemia secondary to red cell enzyme deficiencies (congenital nonspherocytic hemolytic anemia)
Hemoglobinopathy
Thalassemia
Hypersplenism
Microangiopathic hemolytic anemia
Paroxysmal nocturnal hemoglobinuria
Hemolytic anemia secondary to toxins and infectious agents

direct bilirubinemia, skull x-rays revealing a tower skull as evidence of a hemolytic anemia with compensatory bone marrow hyperplasia, and normoblastic hyperplasia of the bone marrow are other features of this disease. Occasionally erythroid hyperplasia is severe enough to form tumors of extramedullary erythropoiesis.

The severity of HS varies greatly. Particularly in children, a *hemolytic crisis* with accelerated blood destruction may begin for no apparent reason. An *aplastic crisis* with reticulocytopenia and marrow erythroid aplasia may also occur in children, usually in association with infections or folic acid deficiency. A rapid fall in hematocrit should alert the physician to a hemolytic or aplastic crisis.

Patients with HS have all the laboratory evidence of a mild-to-severe hemolytic anemia. Except during hemolytic crises they do not have hemoglobinemia or hemoglobinuria. Examination of the peripheral blood smear shows large numbers of spherocytes (Plate 24). These cells have a small diameter and are hyperchromic or darker staining than normal. The normal erythrocyte's pale center is absent. Because of their spheroidal shape, which is due at least in part to loss of membrane area, they are more susceptible to osmotic stress as measured by the *osmotic fragility test* (see Figure 8). To perform this test, red cells are suspended in saline solutions of various tonicities. At lower tonicities water enters and swells the red cells, ultimately causing them to lyse. This normally occurs at a sodium chloride concentration of 0.55%. In patients with hereditary spherocytosis and in patients with other diseases in which large numbers of spherocytes are produced, lysis may begin at 0.70% sodium chloride concentration or even higher. This increased susceptibility to osmotic lysis is accentuated by prior incubation of the red cells for 24 hours at 37°C. Both normal subjects and HS patients will have increased osmotic fragility after incubation, but the effect is more marked for the patients with hereditary spherocytosis, whose cells may begin to lyse in 0.80% sodium chloride solution.

The *autohemolysis test,* during which red cells are incubated at 37°C for 48 hours in isotonic sodium chloride, is another stress test of the spherocyte. Because of their metabolic derangement, spherocytes from HS patients will lyse readily. Ten to fifty percent of HS erythrocytes lyse, compared to less than four percent of normals. Interestingly, the addition of glucose or ATP (adenosine triphosphate) to the incubation medium will decrease the extent of abnormal autohemolysis seen with red cells from HS patients.

Wintrobe indices are usually abnormal in clinically affected HS

Fig. 8 : Osmotic
fragility curves, pre-
incubation and post-
incubation, normal
and abnormal.

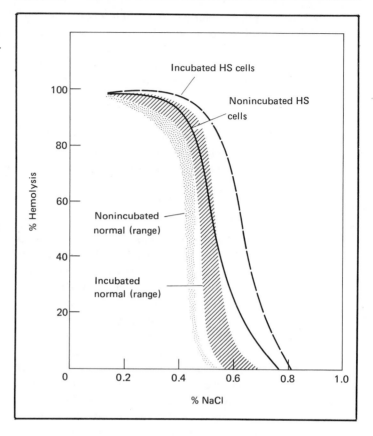

patients, MCV is low (83 ± 8.5 fl), and MCHC is characteristically high. HS is one of the few causes of an elevated MCHC. Adults with this disease usually come to the attention of a physician because of anemia, jaundice, bilirubin gallstones, splenomegaly, or high MCHC.

Pathogenesis of the Anemia in Hereditary Spherocytosis

The primary defect in the HS cell is unknown. However, investigators have agreed that certain abnormalities are characteristic. They also agree that the intrinsic cellular abnormality is not enough to cause the hemolytic anemia, but, rather, that there must be interaction of the HS cell with the reticuloendothelial system of the spleen. It is generally agreed that the following characteristics apply to the HS cell.

1. Increased glucose consumption, and presumably glycolytic rate, in the cell. If glucose is limited, there is a rapid decline in phosphate compounds such as ATP and 2,3-diphosphoglycerate (2, 3-DPG).

2. Increased passive influx of sodium into the cell. An ATP-dependent system is required to pump sodium out of the cell.
3. Reduction of total membrane lipid content.

The increased glycolytic rate has been attributed to the increased need for ATP production. Loss of membrane lipids may result from the increased membrane metabolic activity required for pumping sodium ions. However, coupling between membrane lipid metabolism and sodium pumping has not been demonstrated. Depletion of membrane lipids, in turn, can cause spherocytosis and loss of normal red cell deformability.

The *conditioning* role of the spleen in causing hemolysis is defined by the following observations.

1. HS cells have a decreased life span when transfused into normal people and in patients whose spleens are intact. Their survival is almost normal after splenectomy is performed on HS patients or normal subjects.
2. Normal red cells survive normally when transfused into non-splenectomized HS patients.

Thus there is an intrinsic defect in the red cell, but its expression depends upon the presence of a functioning spleen. It may be that the spheroidal, relatively less deformable shape of HS cells inhibits their ability to transverse the splenic sinusoids. As a result they are trapped in a glucose and oxygen-poor environment where the erythrocytes become more spherical and ultimately lyse after one or more passages through the spleen. The importance of the lack of cell deformability is emphasized by the fact that increasing the surface area of HS cells by the addition of excess membrane lipid does not alter their permeability to sodium but does permit a more discoid shape, an escape from splenic entrapment, and a longer survival.

Therapy

HS is one of the few hematologic diseases that can be cured, since splenectomy almost always returns red cell life span to normal or near-normal. It is recommended in all cases of diagnosed HS, for not only does it cure the anemia, it also reduces the potential for formation of bilirubin gallstones. Furthermore infection may convert mild or moderate hemolysis into a severe problem. Infection appears to turn off the normal bone marrow response to hemolysis and lead to the production of a severe, possibly life-threatening anemia. It may also increase splenic sequestration and destruction of erythrocytes. For these reasons diagnosis and immediate treatment of infections is mandatory. At the time of splenectomy an accessory spleen must be looked for, as hypertrophy of an accessory spleen occasionally causes recurrent hemolysis. In children, splenectomy is often delayed until after age 3 because of the increased incidence of overwhelming sepsis in patients below this age.

Folic acid should be prescribed, since this vitamin is often deficient in the presence of hemolysis and accelerated erythrocyte production. Occasionally folic acid treatment will result in an increase in hematocrit. Rarely, folic acid deficiency is severe enough to cause an aplastic crisis.

Hereditary Elliptocytosis (Hereditary Ovalocytosis)

Hereditary elliptocytosis (HE) is found in families afflicted with hereditary spherocytosis, to which it is closely related. HE is characterized by a family history of elliptocytosis, anemia, or jaundice and the presence of 25 percent, or usually more, elliptocytes in the peripheral blood. HE cells (Plate 25) are oval, with an axial ratio of less than 0.8. In the majority of cases hematocrit levels are near-normal. In 10 to 15 percent of HE patients erythrocyte destruction is substantially increased, leading to all the signs and symptoms of a true hemolytic anemia. Large numbers of elliptocytes and moderate poikilocytosis characterize the peripheral blood of these patients. HE cell metabolic abnormalities are similar to those of HS cells. The results of osmotic fragility and autohemolysis tests are abnormal. Splenomegaly, intermittent jaundice, bilirubin gallstones, and aplastic and hemolytic crises may all be present. Patients with severe hemolysis can be effectively treated with splenectomy.

It should be noted that elliptical cells also occur in thalassemia, iron deficiency, myelophthisic anemias, sickle cell disease, and megaloblastic anemia. Hereditary elliptocytosis is usually diagnosed in patients with mild or no hemolysis who have large numbers of elliptocytes in their peripheral blood for no apparent reason. Rarely is any extensive diagnostic testing or therapy indicated.

HEMOLYTIC ANEMIA SECONDARY TO ERYTHROCYTE ENZYME DEFICIENCY (CONGENITAL NONSPHEROCYTIC HEMOLYTIC ANEMIA)

Coombs' test–negative hemolytic anemia has been associated with at least ten red cell enzyme deficiencies. Of these, only two are of clinical significance. The rest occur rarely and will not be described here.

Glucose-6-Phosphate Dehydrogenase Deficiency

Deficiency of the enzyme glucose-6-phosphate dehydrogenase (G-6-PD) is by far the most common inherited erythrocyte enzyme deficiency. The gene for G-6-PD is sex-linked. According to the Lyon hypothesis X-inactivation is a random process, so more paternal- than maternal-derived, or vice-versa, X chromosomes may be inactivated. As a result individual female heterozygotes with one normal and one abnormal gene will have widely varying G-6-PD levels. Because of the X-linkage, male patients are more severely affected than females.

Also of significance is the fact that over 100 structural variants of this enzyme exist. The two most important have normal enzyme activity (+ sign indicates normal activity). Type B+ is the most common and is found in all populations. Type A+ is very prevalent among blacks. The enzymatic activity of both is normal, but there are differences in their electrophoretic mobility. Type A+ differs from type B+ by a single amino acid substitution. (A – sign following the variant type indicates that enzyme activity is deficient.) Among blacks the A– mutant is the type most commonly associated with enzyme deficiency. Ten percent of American black males carry this abnormality. Enzyme activity is reduced to 5 to 15 percent of normal, and when deficient patients ingest antimalarial or certain other drugs, episodic hemolysis results. Since the gene is sex-linked and some enzyme activity is associated with this variant, black females carrying only one abnormal X-linked gene may have normal or near-normal enzyme levels. Only a few female black patients have levels low enough to cause symptomatic hemolysis after ingestion of drugs. In white populations the most common variant is G-6-PD Mediterranean, but the frequency of this gene is extremely rare. Male patients who inherit this abnormality often have less than 1 percent of normal red cell enzyme activity.

Clinical Features

Unless specific enzyme or metabolic tests are undertaken, the red cells of affected individuals appear normal. There are no morphologic abnormalities nor, in most cases, evidence of hemolysis. However, when stressed by infections, drugs (see p. 156), or other agents, G-6-PD-deficient individuals may suddenly develop acute hemolytic anemia. Generally enzyme activity is one-fourth of normal before acute hemolysis will occur. Reticulocytosis, manifested by macrocytosis and polychromatophilia in the Wright-stained peripheral blood, is prominent 1 to 3 days after drug ingestion. Heinz bodies, or red cell inclusions of denatured hemoglobin, are found in peripheral blood erythrocytes. They are detected by phase microscopy, which depends on the differential refractive index of denatured as compared to normal hemoglobin, or by supravital staining with brilliant crystal violet or new methy-

Compounds associated with hemolysis in individuals with G-6-PD deficiency*

I. Analgesics and Antipyretics
   A. Acetanilid
   B. Aminopyrine
   C. Antipyrine
   D. Aspirin
   E. Phenacetin
II. Antimalarials
   A. Pamaquine
   B. Primaquine
   C. Quinacrine (Atabrin)
   D. Quinine
III. Nitrofurans
   A. Furadantin
   B. Furadin
IV. Sulfa Drugs
   A. Azulfidine
   B. Gantrisin
   C. Kynex
V. Sulfones
   A. Dapsone
   B. DDS
VI. Miscellaneous
   A. Chloramphenicol
   B. Dimercaptol (BAL)
   C. Fava beans
   D. Isoniazid
   E. Methylene blue
   F. Naphthalene (moth balls)
   G. Phenylhydrazine
   H. Probenecid (Benemid)
   I. Quinidine
   J. Vitamin K analogues

*Hemolysis has been observed in G-6-PD-deficient patients in association with viral or bacterial infections, diabetic ketoacidosis, acute or chronic hepatitis, and nephritis. This list may be reproduced for use by G-6-PD-deficient patients to help them avoid drugs to which they may be sensitive.

†Adapted from Wintrobe, M. M., et al. *Clinical Hematology,* 7th ed., p. 785. Philadelphia: Lea & Febiger, 1974.

lene blue are required to detect Heinz bodies. In the former method 1- to 2-μm refractile inclusions are found in unstained erythrocytes held in saline suspension. In supravital staining the blood is incubated with dye, and smears are prepared. Dark blue-staining inclusions appear in affected red cells. These Heinz bodies can be confused with the reticulocyte's ribonuclear protein network.

A number of enzyme assays are available that measure the rate of reduction of NADP to NADPH. Very sensitive tests that depend on detection of methemoglobin, an early product of hemoglobin oxidation, are used to find female carriers. Since young erythrocytes have higher G-6-PD enzyme activity than older cells, the G-6-PD enzyme level of moderately deficient patients may be near-normal, if assayed at the time of the acute hemolytic episode. Moderate deficiency should be suspected when a patient has reticulocytosis and normal or low G-6-PD levels, since normal individuals should have high G-6-PD levels in newly formed reticulocytes.

Several clinical syndromes are associated with hemolytic anemia due to G-6-PD deficiency. Black male patients with low G-6-PD levels develop severe hemolysis when treated with antimalarials. Such G-6-PD-deficient patients with active malaria have developed severe hemoglobinuria or *black water fever,* during treatment, as a result of acute hemolysis. Those with only moderately deficient G-6-PD levels who are given antimalarials prophylactically manifest a less severe, self-limited hemolysis that leads only to anemia and jaundice. The self-limited nature of this syndrome is due to the fact that young red cells have nearly normal G-6-PD levels and are therefore resistant to hemolysis. Even with continued dosing, the hemolytic anemia subsides. On the other hand white patients with severely deficient red cells of all ages (G-6-PD Mediterranean-type deficiency) often have severe hemolysis.

Patients with infectious hepatitis and G-6-PD deficiency may undergo an acute hemolytic episode that results in extremely high bilirubin levels. Certain G-6-PD-deficient patients with Mediterranean (not A–) phenotype develop acute hemolytic anemia upon ingestion of fava beans. Another factor besides G-6-PD deficiency is involved, since not all patients with similar enzyme deficiencies hemolyze after eating fava beans.

Rarely, G-6-PD deficiency has been associated with neonatal jaundice and confused with hemolytic anemia of the newborn. Patients with G-6-PD Mediterranean and other G-6-PD variants with markedly reduced activity may have a chronic, congenital, nonspherocytic, hemolytic anemia. Hemolysis is continuous and is exacerbated by infection or drugs. Usually the uncomplicated anemia is not very severe. Although these patients may have splenic enlargement, splenectomy usually does not ameliorate the anemia.

G-6-PD-deficient individuals are subject to episodic acute hemolysis and bilirubin gallstones, but there is no specific therapy other than blood transfusion. Splenectomy is of no use. G-6-PD-deficient patients should be given a list of drugs likely to cause acute hemolysis (see list). Severe hemolysis with hemoglobinemia and hemoglobinuria can result in shock and renal failure with a definite risk of death. This is particularly true of fava bean-sensitive patients and black males treated with antimalarials.

Screening tests should be performed on populations with a high frequency of gene carriers — blacks, Sardinians, Greeks, and Sephardic (oriental) Jews. The high frequency of the gene in areas where malaria has been prevalent has lead to the hypothesis that G-6-PD-deficient cells do not support parasites as well as normal cells. This theory remains to be proved.

Pathogenesis of Hemolysis Secondary to G-6-PD Deficiency

Glucose-6-phosphate dehydrogenase is a key enzyme in the hexose monophosphate pathway (HMP). The HMP is responsible for net production of NADPH from NADP. This cofactor, NADPH, is necessary to maintain glutathione in its reduced state (GSH). GSH helps prevent hemoglobin denaturation, maintains reduced sulfhydryl groups in the red cell cytoplasm and membrane, and prevents splitting of essential membrane disulfide bonds. Drugs that induce hemolysis in G-6-PD-deficient individuals generate forms of activated oxygen such as superoxide, hydroxyl radicals, and peroxide (see p. 172) which oxidize GSH. GSH in association with glutathione peroxidase is required to detoxify the hydrogen peroxide so generated. If the HMP is unable to function normally because of G-6-PD deficiency, exposure to increased amounts of activated forms of oxygen may result in damage to the red cell membrane or denaturation of hemoglobin. Heinz bodies are the end result of denaturation of hemoglobin. Once formed, these inclusions can be "pitted" out of erythrocytes by the spleen's reticuloendothelial cells, in some cases at the expense of cell integrity.

Drugs and other toxic agents vary in their ability to induce hemolysis, and the severity of enzyme deficiency varies greatly from person to person. These two factors probably account for the different clinical manifestations of G-6-PD deficiency. The explanation for individual sensitivity to oxidant stress lies in the nature of the enzyme defect. Glucose -6- phosphate dehydrogenase variants with decreased enzyme activity are due to structural abnormalities that either accelerate the enzyme's breakdown as the cell ages or cause reduced enzyme activity and unfavorable enzyme kinetics, e.g., a low affinity for NADP. At present there are no examples of G-6-PD deficiency due to abnormal regulatory genes that might reduce G-6-PD synthesis. Patients with G-6-PD variants having low activity and unfavorable kinetics are particularly sensitive to oxidant stress and may even hemolyze spontaneously (congenital nonspherocytic anemia).

Pyruvate Kinase Deficiency

Pyruvate kinase (PK) deficiency is the second most common erythrocyte enzyme deficiency. Rather than producing acute hemolysis in association with drug ingestion, it causes a chronic, congenital, nonspherocytic hemolytic anemia. Affected patients are sometimes confused with those suffering from hereditary spherocytosis. As we will see, there are definite biochemical and clinical differences between these diseases.

Clinical Features

The degree of anemia in affected individuals varies. Some patients may have splenomegaly and require frequent transfusions, while others have mild anemia and no overt clinical manifestations. Jaundice, bilirubin gallstones, and neonatal icterus are other possible clinical manifestations.

The peripheral blood may show evidence of reticulocytosis with polychromatophilic macrocytosis. Spherocytes are absent or rare. Irregularly contracted red cells or *burr cells* (Plate 26) may be prominent. The unincubated osmotic fragility is normal. The autohemolysis test gives abnormal results, which are poorly corrected by glucose but normalized by ATP (*type II autohemolysis test*). The relatively simple assay procedures available to detect PK deficiency will not be discussed here.

Splenectomy is sometimes of value, particularly in patients with large transfusion requirements. Aplastic and hemolytic crises can occur in association with infection. Folic acid supplementation should be given to prevent deficiency. In affected families, newborns must be observed carefully, so that jaundice and anemia can be treated as quickly as possible. The ultimate prognosis usually depends upon the severity of the hemolysis.

The diagnosis of pyruvate kinase deficiency is usually suspected in patients with a Coombs' test–negative hemolytic anemia who do not have large numbers of spherocytes in their peripheral blood but who have high reticulocyte counts. The finding of a family history (particularly in Amish populations) of anemia, abnormal type II autohemolysis, along with normal hemoglobin electrophoretic studies should suggest this diagnosis.

Pathogenesis of Erythrocyte PK Deficiency- Associated Hemolytic Anemia

Despite many investigations there is not total agreement as to the primary defect in PK deficiency. Some have argued that the detected PK enzyme deficiency is secondary to some other primary biochemical abnormality. Such an abnormality has not been demonstrated. It is also not entirely clear why cells from patients with PK deficiency are liable to premature destruction. The correlation between the degree of enzyme deficiency and the severity of the hemolysis is not particularly good. A generally accepted theory is that the hemolytic anemia is a result of the mature red cell's inability to produce its energy requirements, most of which depend upon anaerobic glycolysis. A deficiency of PK will limit the cell's ability to metabolize glucose and produce energy in the form of ATP by the following reaction:

$$\text{phosphoenolpyruvate} + \text{ADP} \xrightarrow{\text{PK}} \text{pyruvate} + \text{ATP}.$$

Reticulocytes are prominent in the peripheral blood, probably because they have an intact citric acid (Kreb's) cycle, which is an efficient energy source. Thus, in severely affected individuals, only the reticulocyte has the necessary metabolic machinery to maintain a viable red cell.

This enzyme deficiency as well as most others, except G-6-PD deficiency, is inherited as an autosomal recessive trait. The homozygotes have hemolytic anemia and splenomegaly, while the heterozygotes are clinically and hematologically normal. The latter's red cells often have half the normal PK activity. Abnormal PK activity can result either from a quantitative loss of activity or from the presence of an enzyme which is catalytically inefficient given the milieu of the red cell cytoplasm.

Hemolytic Anemia Due to Other Erythrocyte Enzyme Deficiencies

There are other, rarely encountered, red cell enzyme deficiencies associated with hemolytic anemia as well as some not associated with it. These rare disorders will not be discussed (see Selected References for relevant reviews) but should be suspected in patients who have a clinical picture similar to that of G-6-PD or PK deficiency, but have normal assays for these enzymes. The laboratory diagnosis of the rare erythrocyte enzyme disorders can only be made by specific assays.

HEMOGLOBIN-OPATHIES

Mutations in the DNA sequences controlling the synthesis of globin chains in hemoglobin result in either structurally abnormal hemoglobins or reduced globin chain synthesis or, sometimes, both. Generally the term *hemoglobinopathy* is used to signify a structurally abnormal hemoglobin with at least one amino acid substitution. *Thalassemia* refers to DNA mutations resulting in normally structured globins but with reduced or negligible synthetic rates. Structural abnormalities may cause premature red cell destruction; easily denatured hemoglobins; hemoglobins with abnormal oxygen affinity or altered solubility; and, in a few instances, reduced globin synthesis. The heme moiety of hemoglobin is synthesized normally and is structurally normal. As a result of abnormal globin synthesis, however, abnormalities in heme function may arise. In this chapter only the few clinically significant hemoglobinopathies are discussed, followed by a description of the thalassemias.

Structure and Function of Hemoglobin

The globin in hemoglobin consists of two pairs of identical polypeptide chains. In normal hemoglobin, so-called hemoglobin A, one pair of polypeptide chains is designated α^A and the other pair is called β^A. Normal hemoglobin A is therefore written as $\alpha_2^A\beta_2^A$. A normal hemoglobin present in low concentration is hemoglobin A_2. It is made up of two α^A-chains and two δ^{A2}-chains. The major hemoglobin found in the fetus, so-called fetal or F hemoglobin, contains α^A-chains and, in place of β-chains, γ^F chains. Hemoglobin F is written as $\alpha_2^A\gamma_2^F$. The α-, β-, δ-, and γ-chains differ in their amino acid sequences. The structure of β-, δ-, and γ-chains is similar, whereas the amino acid sequence of α-chains differs considerably from these. α-Chain genes in at least some individuals are carried on chromosome 2, and the β, γ, and δ structural genes are on a B group chromosome, either number 4 or number 5. It is possible that the γ and δ structural genes resulted from reduplication of an original β-like gene. Beta-, gamma-, and delta-chain genes are *alleles,* or genes that occupy the same locus on the B chromosome gene.

Both the α- and the β-chains contain helical and nonhelical regions. The helices are labeled with capital letters, and an amino acid can be located in a helix by giving the letter corresponding to the helix and a number corresponding to the location of the amino acid in that helix. It is also possible to give the location of the amino acid by the number corresponding to the distance from the N-terminal amino acid. The N-terminal amino acid is assigned the number 1, and each succeeding amino acid is given the next higher number until the C-terminal end is reached. For example, the β-chain substitution in sickle cell hemoglobin is at a glutamic acid residue 6 places from the N-terminal end or at helix A3. To each of the four polypeptides is joined a heme group. The heme iron is covalently bonded with a histadine at F8. When hemoglobin is oxygenated, the oxygen covalently binds with heme and with globin at histidine E7. Bonds also exist between heme and other parts of the hemoglobin molecule. Interchain amino acid contacts of functional significance have been specified as $\alpha_1\beta_1$ and $\alpha_1\beta_2$.

The process of oxygenation of a hemoglobin molecule results in changes in the tertiary and quaternary structure of hemoglobin but leaves the primary amino acid and secondary helical structures unchanged. The tertiary structure, or the folding of the individual polypeptide chains, changes slightly with oxygenation, whereas the quaternary structure, or the manner in which the four polypeptide chains are joined to form a single molecule, changes significantly and accounts for the sigmoidal shape of the hemoglobin-oxygen dissociation curve. This change in oxygen affinity during oxygenation is called *heme-heme interaction*. The sequence of molecular changes on oxygenation occurs in the following manner: Oxygen is added first to an α-chain, then to a second α-chain, and finally to the two β-chains. After the second or third oxygen is added, the quaternary structure changes considerably. 2,3-DPG, which had stabilized the deoxygenated form of hemoglobin, is now expelled from the molecule. Movement occurs at the $\alpha_1\beta_1$ and $\alpha_1\beta_2$ contact points, particularly the $\alpha_1\beta_2$. Once the change from the deoxygenated to the oxygenated configuration is underway, oxygen affinity is greatly increased (accounting for the steep rise in the oxygen dissociation curve of hemoglobin), and oxygen is added to the hemes of the remaining β-chain or chains.

Details of the *"respiration of hemoglobin"* obviously have been omitted. Study of the structure–function relationships of the hemoglobin molecule are interesting and important but will not be discussed further except as they relate to the pathogenesis of hemoglobin disorders.

Hemoglobin Nomenclature

Hemoglobins were first assigned a letter of the alphabet on the basis of their electrophoretic mobility. When the letters of the alphabet were used up, subsequent hemoglobins were named after the geographic location in which they were described. If the hemoglobin had characteristics of one of the letter hemoglobins, the geographic designation was used as a subscript, for example, hemoglobin $J_{Capetown}$. If the hemoglobin had been characterized as to the amino acid substitution, this was designated by a superscript after the globin chain involved: for example, hemoglobin S, $\alpha_2\beta_2^{(6\ Glu\rightarrow Val)}$. This means that there is a substitution 6 amino acids from the N-terminal end of the β-chain: glutamic acid is no longer present and valine has been substituted for it.

Pathogenesis of Hemoglobinopathies

Several different genetic mechanisms account for abnormal hemoglobin production:

1. Substitution of a single DNA nucleotide for another (*point mutation*). The hemoglobin product of this mutated DNA gene has a substitution of one amino acid for another. Almost al-

ways, only one of the three bases coding for the amino acid is changed.

2. Point mutation in a "stop" codon. Extra amino acid residues are added to the normal hemoglobin chain.

3. Crossovers between chromosomal pairs, resulting in gene deletions or fusion of genes. Hemoglobins made up partially of β-chains and partially of δ-chains may result from the latter.

4. "Frameshifts" in which a single DNA nucleotide is added or deleted. Codons further on in the chain will, therefore, be altered, usually in a nonsensical manner. These nonsense mutations can be tolerated only if the amino acids involved are at the end of a chain. The location of an amino acid substitution will often determine the functional abnormality and the clinical findings. At least five different locations for substitutions have been described:

   a. Substitution at the surface of the hemoglobin molecule (for example, hemoglobin S). This results in a molecule with reduced solubility, and in stacking of hemoglobin chains to cause shape abnormalities and hemolytic anemia.

   b. Substitution in the internal nonpolar residues. This results in hemoglobin instability and in some cases hemolytic anemia (for example, hemoglobin$_{Köln}$).

   c. Substitution of tyrosine for histidine near the heme iron. The ionic bond between heme and tyrosine stabilizes the heme iron in the ferric state and leads to methemoglobinemia and cyanosis (for example, hemoglobin M).

4. Substitution at an $\alpha_1\beta_2$ contact point. This impairs heme–heme interaction and results in increased oxygen affinity and erythrocytosis (for example, hemoglobin$_{Chesapeake}$).

5. Substitutions at an $\alpha_1\beta_2$ contact point and near the heme moiety. Decreased oxygen affinity and cyanosis result (for example, hemoglobin$_{Kansas}$).

Hemoglobin S

By far the most important hemoglobinopathies are those related to the presence of sickle hemoglobin (HbS). This hemoglobin is present in approximately 10 percent of blacks. Depending upon many factors, which we will discuss, its presence may result in severe disease causing early death or in a clinically benign condition of importance only when the individual is stressed. Before detailing the clinical manifestations of the diseases related to sickle hemoglobin we shall discuss the pathogenesis of the anemia and the thrombotic tendency associated with it.

Pathophysiology of Sickle Hemoglobin

Sickle hemoglobin results from replacement of the sixth amino acid from the N-terminal end of the β-chain, glutamic acid, by valine. This substitution occurs because of the substitution in messenger RNA of uridine for adenine in the second nucleotide of the glutamic acid codon (adenine for thymidine in the DNA codon). As a result of the replacement of the hydrophilic amino acid, glutamic acid, by the hydrophobic amino acid, valine, cyclization of the N-terminal end of the β-chain of sickle hemoglobin takes place after deoxygenation. This is a valine–valine cyclization between the valine residues at the 1 and the 6 positions. The resulting structure interlocks with an adjacent normal or abnormal hemoglobin molecule in an oxygenated or deoxygenated state. This leads to the formation of hemoglobin monofilaments which associate to form hemoglobin rods. Each rod is formed from six monomolecular strands of hemoglobin S twisted into a spiral. These rods align to form parallel fibrobundles, or *tactoids,* which deform the cell into an elongated, rigid, sickle-shaped form.

It should be emphasized that two events must occur in order that monofilaments be formed: (1) the substitution of glutamic acid by valine and the formation of hydrophobic valine–valine bonds and (2) the deoxygenation of HbS to cause a configuration change in the hemoglobin which allows interlocking between the valine-valine ring structure and adjacent hemoglobin molecules. Once shape changes have occurred in the red cells, viscosity of the whole blood increases and deformability of the sickled cell decreases. As a result of both these factors, sickled red cells flow poorly through small arterioles and may actually act as a plug. The interference with arteriolar blood flow results in infarction and death of tissues supplied by these arterioles.

The mildly sickled cell may revert to normal on exposure to oxygen, while the filamentous form becomes irreversibly sickled. These abnormal forms contain small Heinz bodies or denatured hemoglobin, rendering them susceptible to fragmentation, loss of membrane, and hemolysis. They may be sequestered in the reticuloendothelial system, particularly in the liver, thereby causing hemolysis.

Several clinical manifestations result from thrombosis: chronic leg ulcers, particularly around the ankles; bone infarction with severe pain; and splenic infarction causing autosplenectomy and hyposplenism. Damage to the heart, liver, central nervous system, and lung may also result from infarction of these vital tissues. The hemoconcentration, anoxia, and low pH associated with the renal medulla makes it quite susceptible to sickling and infarctions. For this reason, hematuria and an inability to concentrate urine normally are found in patients with sickle hemoglobin.

The hemolytic anemia is often complicated by infections that decrease the rate of erythropoiesis, so that compensation for chronic hemolysis does not occur. Characteristic skull, vertebral, and long bone abnormalities are the result of chronic hemolysis and erythroid hyperplasia. Deficiency of folic acid, due to increased utilization, may lead to megaloblastic anemia. Probably related to bone infarctions are an increased incidence of salmonella osteomyelitis and a "hand–foot" syndrome characterized by painful swelling of hands or feet, seen primarily in children.

Hemoglobin S
Clinical Syndromes

Four important clinical syndromes are associated with sickle hemoglobins. In order to understand these syndromes, it is necessary to review the inheritance of sickle hemoglobin and the factors that moderate the formation of sickle cells.

Hemoglobins A, S, and the β-chain variant, C; a gene that results in the continued production of hemoglobin F after infancy (hereditary persistence of fetal hemoglobin); and the thalassemia gene are alleles of the β-chain locus. In every individual there are two non-sex-linked gene loci for β-chains, one from each parent. Both alleles are expressed, and therefore hemoglobins are inherited as *autosomal codominants.*

The presence of hemoglobin A and F in cells with hemoglobin S will modify the severity of the sickling. This is particularly important in patients who are heterozygous for hemoglobin S and have hereditary persistence of hemoglobin F, for in these individuals the presence of hemoglobin F prevents sickling despite the presence of 50 percent or more hemoglobin S. Similarly, patients with sickle cell trait with 50% A in each red cell (HbSA) have a benign clinical course.

Sickle Cell Trait (HbSA). Patients with *sickle cell trait* are not anemic, do not hemolyze, and are asymptomatic. They may have difficulty in concentrating urine and occasionally develop hematuria. If rendered hypoxic during anesthesia or while flying in an unpressurized aircraft, they may develop splenic infarctions.

Sickle Cell Anemia (HbSS). Patients with *sickle cell anemia* have the most severe clinical manifestations of sickle hemoglobin. They are moderately to severely anemic from birth. They may have splenomegaly in early childhood, but with repeated thromboses resulting in autosplenectomy, their spleens become impalpable. Because of the increased turnover of red cells due to hemolysis they develop bilirubin gallstones. Leg ulcers, bony abnormalities (aseptic necrosis), priapism, maternal and fetal morbidity and mortality, congestive heart failure, pulmonary infarctions, and neurologic defects including convulsions and paralysis often make their lives miserable. In most populations these patients usually do not live beyond the second decade of life. HbSS patients have painful crises usually occurring spontaneously or in association with infection. The pain is severe in the bones, joints, and back, and may be so severe in the abdomen as to suggest an abdominal catastrophe. The white blood cell count and temperature are elevated. The crisis may last for several hours or for days with gradual subsidence of pain.

Sickle Cell-β-Thalassemia (HbS-thal). If a patient inherits two abnormal alleles, one for S hemoglobin and one for thalassemia, one of two different syndromes may result. In one, there may be 90 percent or more S hemoglobin and complete suppression of hemoglobin A synthesis. In the other, β-chain synthesis is not completely suppressed, and there may be 25 to 35 percent hemoglobin A. Because of the presence of hemoglobin A, the clinical course is much milder than when complete suppression of normal β-chain synthesis occurs. The pathogenesis of these two forms of *sickle cell-thalassemia* will be discussed later in this chapter under Thalassemias. Suffice it to say that patients with sickle cell-thalassemia have an extremely variable clinical picture ranging from all the manifestations of sickle cell anemia to a more benign disease resembling that of sickle cell trait. The spleen may be enlarged. The severity of the disease seems to be correlated with the concentration of HbS present in the erythrocytes.

Sickle Cell-Hemoglobin C (HbSC) Disease. Individuals with *sickle cell-hemoglobin C disease* carry two abnormal β-alleles, hemoglobin S and hemoglobin C. These patients are sometimes severely affected but generally less so than with HbSS disease; and this disorder is more likely to be compatible with long life. It includes many of the symptoms and signs described for HbSS disease. Unlike sickle cell anemia it may cause splenomegaly in adults, and there are numerous reports of pregnancies with complications to the baby and mother. The patients may also be predisposed to hemorrhages in the fundus of the eye. Corkscrew-shaped conjunctival capillaries are characteristically seen in this and other sickle hemoglobin syndromes.

Differential Diagnosis of the Sickle Hemoglobin Syndromes

In all sickle hemoglobin syndromes, sickling (Plate 27) of red blood cells may be demonstrated by sealing blood under a cover slip and adding 2% sodium metabisulfite. This agent chemically deoxygenates hemoglobin and makes the sickle cells assume their characteristic appearance under a microscope.

Sickle hemoglobin has a characteristic mobility when electrophoresed on paper, cellulose acetate, or agarose gel. However, the rare hemoglobin D has the same electrophoretic mobility. It may be separated from hemoglobin S by acid-agar electrophoresis at pH 6 or by the decreased solubility of hemoglobin S as compared to hemoglobin D. Irreversibly sickled cells are seen on Wright-stained peripheral blood smears from patients with HbSS disease and HbS-thalassemia. They may occasionally be present in HbSC disease but are not seen in smears from patients with sickle cell trait. Target cells (Plate II) and poikilocytes are seen in the peripheral blood of all patients with hemoglobin S syndromes (except HbSA). Bone marrow is characterized by active erythropoiesis; and investigation of the blood shows evidence of hemolytic anemia.

All hemoglobins that sickle are not necessarily hemoglobin S. It is known that hemoglobin C_{Harlem}, and hemoglobin $C_{Georgetown}$, and the α-chain variant, hemoglobin I, sickle when deoxygenated. High concentrations of hemoglobin $_{Bart's}$ (γ_4) also sickle.

The clinical picture, hematocrit, hemoglobin electrophoresis, assay for hemoglobin F, and presence or absence of individual HbF-containing cells will usually enable us to distinguish between HbS syndromes. In a few cases special research techniques or a thorough study of the family may be required. Sickle cell trait (HbSA) is characterized by a normal hematocrit and blood smear. The sickle cell test is positive, and hemoglobin electrophoresis reveals almost equal quantities of HbA and S. Sickle cell anemia (HbSS) is associated with anemia and severe clinical abnormalities, including painful crises. Hemoglobin electrophoresis reveals almost all hemoglobin S, and the assay for fetal hemoglobin shows only small quantities. The diagnosis is secure if hemoglobin A is recognized on hemoglobin electrophoresis. The only other diagnostic possibilities would be hemoglobin SD disease or the presence of another hemoglobin with the electrophoretic mobility of HbS. These can be distinguished by family studies, hemoglobin electrophoresis on acid-agar gel, or differential solubility studies. It is sometimes difficult to distinguish sickle cell anemia from sickle cell–thalassemia, particularly when hemoglobin A production is completely suppressed in the sickle cell-thalassemia patient. Sickle cell–thalassemia with complete suppression of hemoglobin A synthesis may also be suspected if the patient has marked hypochromia, microcytosis, and decreased red cell mean corpuscular volume. Family studies may help, but in some cases the differential diagnosis requires analysis of the in vivo synthesis of hemoglobin chains by the patient's reticulocytes. Thalassemics will have marked depression of either α- or β-chain production.

Patients with hemoglobin S and hereditary persistence of fetal hemoglobin are characterized by the distribution of fetal hemoglobin among all the red cells. When the Kleihauer technique is used, the presence of hemoglobin F is detected by acid elution of hemoglobin A from dried red cells. The remaining cytoplasmic hemoglobin F is stained pink; and under a microscope, hemoglobin F–containing cells are readily counted. Patients with sickle cell–thalassemia may have high hemoglobin F values, but the fetal hemoglobin will be seen in only a relatively small number of cells (heterogenous distribution). Patients with hemoglobin S and hereditary persistence of hemoglobin F will have varying quantities of hemoglobin F in many cells (homogenous distribution).

Therapy for
Sickle Hemo-
globin Syndromes

Patients with mild HbS syndromes require no therapy. Usually patients who require treatment have high concentrations of sickle hemoglobin and no ameliorating hemoglobins. Frequent, painful crises are the major problem with these patients, and at present there is no therapy that will prevent or consistently ameliorate these symptoms. Recently attempts have been made to use high concentrations of urea in vivo to stop valine–valine cyclization and thereby prevent sickling. Although this treatment method is still controversial, the bulk of the evidence indicates that it is not of value. Risk is associated with the high concentrations of infused urea, which result in severe dehydration unless plasma volume is meticulously monitored and replaced.

Carbamyl phosphate and cyanate are drugs that carbamylate, that is, add $H_2N\text{-}C\diagup^{0}$-groups to the free N-terminal end of β-chains, thereby preventing hemoglobin molecules from stacking in helical arrangements and forming sickle cells. They also cause a shift to the left of the oxygen dissociation curve (Figure 1); and as a result of the increased oxygen affinity, less deoxygenated hemoglobin is present at a given partial pressure of oxygen. This, too, would tend to impair sickling under hypoxic conditions. Studies in which carbamylation is carried out in vitro on blood removed from patients and then reinfused indicate that red cell life span can be prolonged. Although this might be of some benefit, it is more important to find a therapy that will prevent or ameliorate painful crises. Initial studies of oral sodium cyanate therapy seem to indicate that any benefit gained is slight and certainly difficult to measure; furthermore, neurotoxicity and weight loss have been detected with chronic use.

Certainly hydration of the patient and administration of oxygen carry little risk and may be of some benefit in ameliorating painful crises. However, alkalization, anticoagulants, dextran, carbon monoxide, nitrites, phenothiazines, vasodilators, defibrination, and most of the other treatments proposed for sickle cell crisis have been proved unsuccessful. In certain high risk patients, particularly those pregnant or about to undergo major surgery, partial exchange transfusion with normal blood can be performed in an attempt to minimize complications. Enough of the patient's blood is removed and replaced by normal blood to obtain a final hematocrit of between 0.30 and 0.35 with at least 50 percent hemoglobin A. This treatment has been used for symptomatic crises as well as in anticipation of complications of delivery or surgery. The fear of transmitting hepatitis with the blood transfusions has prevented its widespread adoption, as has the lack of controlled studies to demonstrate its effectiveness. Perhaps with the use of frozen blood, which is essentially free of hepatitis virus, large scale trials can be performed. Chronic maintenance of patient hemoglobin A levels at 50 percent in all patients with sickle cell disease would sorely tax our blood supplies and transfusion facilities, so that at present this unproved therapy should be limited to severely affected or high risk patients.

Androgens increase red cell mass by increasing erythropoietin to supranormal levels. Unfortunately sickle hemoglobin concentration increases and, in children, this leads to an increase in painful crises. Anemic adults might benefit from this therapy, since they do not develop an increased frequency of attacks.

A recent report suggesting inhibition of sickling in vitro by amino acids, homoserine, asparagine, and glutamine will stimulate the search for nontoxic drug therapy of sickle cell anemia. In the meantime conventional therapy for painful crises now consists of hydration, narcotics, and careful studies to detect and treat infection.

Despite therapy most patients with sickle cell anemia will die at an early age; some will survive to adulthood, and a few will live out a normal life span. Some patients with clinically mild sickle cell anemia but with high concentrations of HbS are double heterozygotes. They have genes for HbS and for another disorder: for example, thalassemia (α- or β-chain variety), $Hb_{Memphis}$ (α23 Glu$\rightarrow$Gln), $HbD_{Los Angeles}$, or hereditary persistence of F. Interaction between sickle hemoglobin and hemoglobins A,F,D, and Memphis tends to reduce a patient's sickling tendency. The mild nature of the disease in specific populations is unexplained. In certain Jamaican and Saudi Arabian populations unknown factors cause elevated intraerythrocyte HbF concentrations.

Since a cure has not been found and the life of most patients with hemoglobin SS disease is miserable, painful, and short, the role of genetic counseling must be considered. It is possible with mass screening programs to find individuals carrying the sickle cell genes and, theoretically, with the use of premarital counseling, to inform potential parents of the possibility of having a severely affected infant. Whether mass screening for sickle cell trait should be undertaken at all is still questioned, since premarital genetic counseling may have only a small effect on the number of births of severely affected infants. It has also become possible in medical centers to detect the presence of an affected child in utero. Abortion is then possible. It is clear that, if screening techniques were put into widespread use, employment, social acceptance, and insurability would all be affected by the detection of the sickle cell gene.

Hemoglobin C Syndromes

Since hemoglobin C (HbC) is probably the second most common hemoglobinopathy (2 to 3 percent gene frequency in black populations), four important hemoglobin C syndromes will be discussed. HbC molecules are caused by substitution of lysine for glutamic acid in the sixth position from the N-terminal end of the β-hemoglobin chain (same location as the substitution in HbS).

Hemoglobin C Trait (HbCA)

Hemoglobin C trait is the most commonly encountered syndrome. Patients are asymptomatic and not anemic. The peripheral blood smear shows increased numbers of target cells (Plate II); and hemoglobin electrophoresis reveals about 40 percent hemoglobin C migrating faster than HbS but slower than HbA. Splenomegaly is usually not present.

Hemoglobin C Disease (HbCC)

Hemoglobin C disease is characterized by a mild hemolytic anemia associated with splenomegaly and by a peripheral blood smear showing many target cells and some microspherocytes. Hemoglobin C crystals may appear after slow drying of a peripheral blood smear and may account for the marked targeting, with puddling and then crystallization of hemoglobin in the center of these cells. Symptomatically these patients can have acute episodes of hemolysis when stressed, particularly by infections. In some cases they have gallstones. Since the prognosis is good, little is required in the way of therapy.

Hemoglobin SC Disease (HbSC)

Hemoglobin SC disease is of intermediate severity between hemoglobin SS disease and hemoglobin CC disease. It is associated with bone, joint, or abdominal pains, pulmonary infarctions, hematuria, aseptic necrosis of the femoral head, splenomegaly, splenic infarctions, osteomyelitis, maternal or fetal mortality, and fundal hemorrhages. Anemia, targeting, hemoglobin crystals, and occasional sickle forms are seen in the peripheral blood. Mild hemolysis is often present. Equal amounts of hemoglobin S and C and normal or slightly elevated hemoglobin F are found. In general the prognosis is good and no specific therapy is required except good oxygenation during delivery or operations. Occasional patients with severe symptoms may require partial exchange transfusion prophylactically or as therapy for painful occlusive crises. As in hemoglobin CC disease, massive enlargement of the spleen may require splenectomy.

Hemoglobin C-β-Thalassemia (HbC-Thal)

HbC-thalassemia resembles HbCC disease clinically, but the concentration of HbC is greater than 50% and HbA is usually detectable. Occasionally, if HbA is absent, family studies are needed to distinguish HbC-thalassemia from HbCC. Since the disorder is usually symptomless, no therapy is required.

Hemoglobinopathies Associated with Cyanosis

Cyanosis can be caused by increased levels of deoxyhemoglobin (> 5 gm per deciliter) or by the presence of abnormal hemoglobins. Methemoglobin is a form of hemoglobin in which the iron moiety of heme is maintained in the ferric (Fe^{+++}) rather than the ferrous (Fe^{++}) state. As a result, reversible oxygenation of the iron moiety cannot take place. Methemoglobinemia occurs if the enzyme systems of the red cell are unable, because of inherited defects or overwhelming oxidant stress, to maintain iron in the ferrous state. Toxic methemoglobinemia due to drugs has been reported with amyl nitrite (coronary artery vasodilator); acetanilid and phenacetin (analgesics); prilocaine (local anesthetic); dapsone; and sulfonamide (sulfa antibiotic); menadione (vitamin K analogues); and naphthalene (moth balls). G-6-PD deficiency will enhance methemoglobin production.

Abnormal hemoglobins with light absorption spectra different from normal methemoglobin arise from amino acid substitutions in the microenvironment surrounding the heme group. These *M hemoglobins* have substitutions in their α- or β-chains that fix the heme iron in a ferric state. The cyanotic or brownish color of affected persons' skin is secondary to the abnormal light absorption properties of the HbM hemes. They are detected by special electrophoretic techniques or by their spectroscopic characteristics. Still other abnormal hemoglobins cause cyanosis because of their abnormally low affinity for oxygen (see p. 173).

Patients with cyanosis or a purplish, brownish, or slate gray appearance to their skin since birth should be given a battery of tests: assay of the methemoglobin reduction enzyme systems, spectroscopic measurement of deoxyhemoglobin and methemoglobin concentrations, evaluation of oxygen affinity, and test for electrophoretically abnormal or unstable hemoglobins; and should be asked about exposure to cyanosis-producing drugs.

The cyanide moiety (CN) binds to heme and prevents normal oxygenation. Furthermore, normal respiration of the hemoglobin molecule is disturbed even if only one of the four heme groups is bound to CN. As a result of this abnormal heme–heme interaction, the oxygen dissociation curve becomes markedly abnormal and oxygen loading is markedly decreased at any given oxygen concentration. Death from cyanide poisoning actually results from the binding of CN to cytochrome oxidase, which inhibits a key enzyme in cellular respiration and causes cytotoxic hypoxia. In the presence of methemoglobin, the formation of the cytochrome-CN complex is minimal. Therefore nitrites are administered to cyanide victims in order to convert hemoglobin to methemoglobin.

Cherry red cyanosis caused by carbon monoxide poisoning is due to the bright red color of carboxyhemoglobin (carbomonoxyhemoglobin). The affinity of CO for heme is 218 times that of oxygen, but CO can be quickly dissociated from carboxyhemoglobin through oxygen therapy. Carboxyhemoglobin cannot carry oxygen, and anoxic death will result from prolonged exposure to high concentrations of this odorless, colorless gas.

Hemoglobinopathies Associated with Unstable Hemoglobins (Heinz Body Hemolytic Anemia)

Unstable, readily denaturable hemoglobins are the result of amino acid substitutions in areas critical to oxygen binding, at sites in the interior of the molecule, in helical regions, and at contacts between chains. Because the substitution often affects heme function, unstable hemoglobins may have increased or decreased oxygen affinity. These unstable hemoglobins are detected by the presence of a hemoglobin fraction that precipitates on incubation at $50°C$ or in buffered isopropanol at $37°C$; by an abnormal electrophoretic band; or by the appearance of Heinz bodies, cytoplasmic inclusions made of hemoglobin subunits, in blood smears. These Heinz bodies can be visualized with phase microscopy or supravital staining, particularly after splenectomy. Hemolytic anemia of varying severity is found in patients with unstable hemoglobins, and a hemolytic crisis may follow use of sulfa drugs.

Hemoglobin$_{Köln}$ is probably the most commonly encountered example of an unstable hemoglobin. The anemia associated with it may be mild or severe and is usually improved by splenectomy. Hemoglobin$_{Zürich}$ is found only after exposure to sulfa drugs and is associated with Heinz body formation.

The sequence of events in the denaturation of unstable hemoglobins involves oxidation of heme iron, separation of unlike hemoglobin chains, formation of hemichromes (subunits with heme attached), heme-globin dissociation, and finally Heinz body formation. In some cases heme has been found in the Heinz bodies. Liberated heme is catabolized to dark brown dipyrroles (mesobilifuscin), which are excreted in the urine.

Normally in oxyhemoglobin there is polarization of the electron shared by the heme iron and bound oxygen. This shared electron is returned to the heme iron when oxygen is released from hemoglobin, and the iron therefore retains its ferrous (Fe^{++}) state. The return of the electron to iron is prevented if water enters the pocket in which heme sits. As a result superoxide (O_2^-) radicals (activated oxygen) are released. Methemoglobin production increases greatly if an amino acid substitution allows distortion of the heme pocket, increased entry of water or other small anions, increased production of superoxide, and oxidation of hemoglobin to methemoglobin. These changes also lead to denaturation and Heinz body formation.

Besides their appearance in unstable hemoglobins, Heinz bodies may be found in the blood or bone marrow of patients with thalassemia, HbH disease, G-6-PD deficiency, or after ingestion of phenylhydrazine, phenacetin, naphthalene, nitrofurantoin, sulfasalazine, sulfa drugs, dapsone, and other oxidant drugs.

Hemoglobinopathies Associated with Abnormal Oxygen Affinity

Increased oxygen affinity (decreased P_{50}) is found not only with unstable hemoglobins such as Köln, Zürich, and Gun Hill but also with stable hemoglobins like Yakima, Rainer, and Bethesda. Tissue anoxia due to impaired release of oxygen initially stimulates erythropoietin production, sometimes resulting in erythrocytosis. Whether erythrocytosis develops depends on the concentration of abnormal hemoglobin, its stability, and the nature of the mutation. Many of these hemoglobins have a defect at $\alpha_1\beta_2$ contact points or at the carboxy-terminal end of the β-chain. These defects impair hemoglobin oxygenation, heme–heme interaction, or binding of 2,3-DPG to deoxyhemoglobin.

Decreased oxygen affinity (increased P_{50}) is found with the unstable hemoglobins Torino, Seattle, and others and with the stable hemoglobin Kansas. Either cyanosis due to increased concentration of deoxyhemoglobin or a lowered hematocrit without physiologic anemia may result from the decreased binding of oxygen to hemoglobin. The amino acid substitutions are near the heme group or the $\alpha_1\beta_2$ contact point.

THALASSEMIAS

The normal adult carries three types of hemoglobin, A (96–98 percent), F (2–3 percent), and A_2 (2–3 percent). Two types of hemoglobin F exist, one whose γ-chains have glycine in position 136, the other with alanine in this position. After birth the γ-loci are switched off, and β- and δ-loci are fully activated. The α-chains combine with β- and δ-chains to produce hemoglobin A and A_2, respectively. Most structural hemoglobin variants, such as sickle cell hemoglobin, arise from a single amino acid substitution in the globin peptide chains. Such changes in structure may lead to hemoglobins that sickle, that are unstable, or that have abnormal oxygen affinities. The site of amino acid substitution will determine the functional abnormality.

Less commonly, structural mutations that arise from genetic

mechanisms, such as *unequal crossing over*, lead to decreased synthesis of globin peptide chains, for example in Hb_{Lepore}. The *thalassemia* genes represent a type of genetic defect that leads to the decreased synthesis of globin chains. No structurally abnormal hemoglobin can be identified; but presumably a genetic defect leads, in an unknown way, to decreased chemical amounts of hemoglobin messenger RNA (mRNA) for one or more chains of hemoglobin. The reduction in amount of mRNA may result from decreased intranuclear synthesis, defective processing or transport, or increased degradation.

While the loci for the α- and β-chain genes are probably on separate chromosomes, genes for β- and δ-chains are closely linked. There is evidence for more than one gene locus for γ-chains and in some populations for α-chains as well. There appears to be only one β-chain structural locus in man. Double heterozygotes with two β-chain mutations, that is, patients who have inherited a structural variant in each of their β-chain loci, produce no hemoglobin A. The β-thalassemia gene is either allelic or closely linked to the β structural gene. A gene that allows continued synthesis of γ-chains and hemoglobin F in adult life also appears to be allelic to the β-chain loci. Thus an individual can inherit genes for only two of the following: β-chain structural mutants, β-thalassemia, or hereditary persistence of fetal hemoglobin.

β-Thalassemia Syndromes

Four clinical types of β-thalassemia are recognized (see Table 6-1).

Thalassemia Major. The most severe type is *β-thalassemia major.* This disease is usually recognized during the first years of life. Small size, poor weight gain, progressive severe anemia (4–6 gm per deciliter), jaundice, chronic leg ulcers, mongoloid facies — flattened nose and wide-apart eyes with bossing of the skull, hypertrophy of the upper maxillae, and prominent malar eminences characterize affected children. X-rays of the skull show dilation of the space between the tables of bone with a series of radiating striations, giving a *hair-on-end appearance.* The long bones are thin, and fractures are not uncommon. These patients do not develop normally physically and may not be normal mentally. Sexual development is delayed and may not appear at all. Hepatosplenomegaly, with massive enlargement of the spleen, is common. Infections of the bones, gallbladder (gallstones are common), and sinuses occur less commonly. Examination of the bone marrow shows erythroid hyperplasia, and in many patients there are megaloblastic changes because of folate deficiency. Some patients die as a result of infections or iron deposition in tissues, such as the myocardium, leading to organ failure. The iron overload is probably due to transfusions and possibly to increased iron absorption.

Table 6-1 : Classification of Thalassemia Syndromes

Genotype	Clinical	Hemoglobin Pattern (%)		
		HbA	HbA$_2$	HbF
$\delta\beta$ $\delta\beta$	Normal	96–98	2–3	2–3
$\delta\beta$ $\delta^{thal^?}\beta$	δ-Thal. minima (silent thal. gene)	N1	Dec.	N1
$\delta\beta$ $\delta\beta^{thal^?}$	β-Thal. minima	N1	N1	N1
$\delta\beta$ $\delta\beta^{thal^+}$	β-Thal. minor (thal. trait)	Slt. dec.	Inc.	N1
$\delta\beta$ $\delta\beta^{thal^0}$	β-Thal. minor (thal. trait)	Slt. dec.	Inc.	Slt. inc.
$\delta\beta$ $(\delta\beta)^{thal^0}$	$(\delta\beta)$-Thal. minor [$(\delta\beta)$-Thal. trait]	Dec.	N1	5–20
$\delta\beta^{thal^0}$ $\delta\beta^{thal^?}$	Thal. intermedia	Dec.	Slt. inc.	6–12
$\delta\beta^{thal^0}$ $(\delta\beta)^{thal^0}$	$(\delta\beta)$-Thal. intermedia	0 or mkd. dec.	Dec.	60–99
$(\delta\beta)^{thal^0}$ $(\delta\beta)^{thal^0}$	$(\delta\beta)$-Thal. intermedia (High F-thalassemia)	0	0	100
$\delta\beta^{thal^+}$ $\delta\beta^{thal^+}$	Thal. major (classic Cooley's anemia)	Mkd. dec.	N1 or Slt. inc.	20–80
$\delta\beta^{thal^0}$ $\delta\beta^{thal^0}$	Thal. major	0	N1 or Slt. inc.	95

N1 = Normal; Slt. inc. = Slight increase; Mkd. dec. = marked decrease.

Thalassemia Intermedia. The second clinical type is *thalassemia intermedia,* with which patients have similar abnormalities to thalassemia major in their hemoglobin patterns but suffer only a moderate degree of anemia and require intermittent or no transfusions. They may live with chronic disease lasting into childhood or may survive into adult life.

Thalassemia Trait. The third type is *thalassemia trait,* in which there is little in the way of symptoms, and the diagnosis is made on the basis of family studies or on examination of the peripheral blood, which shows marked abnormalities in the face of mild or no anemia.

Thalassemia Minima. Thalassemia minima, a fourth type, is undetectable clinically, but its presence is determined by genetic studies of the patient's family.

Anemia in β-Thalassemia

Anemia in β-thalassemia is a result of (1) decreased synthesis of the β-globin chains of hemoglobin and (2) precipitation and subsequent removal of excess α-globin chains which in turn leads to hemolysis.* Hypochromia, microcytosis, fragmented forms, inclusion bodies, and evidence of hemolysis are found in blood from severely affected thalassemic patients (see Plates 28 and 29).

The hypochromia is a result of decreased cellular content of hemoglobin, a major defect in thalassemia. The bone marrow is hyperplastic and produces large numbers of poorly hemoglobinized cells. Because of an increased number of cell divisions, microcytosis predominates. Further complicating the production abnormality is excessive ineffective erythrocytosis and rapid destruction of newly formed erythrocytes in the peripheral blood. Intramedullary and extramedullary red cell destruction appears to be the result of an attempt of the reticuloendothelial cells to remove Heinz bodies — intracellular inclusions made up of excess, denatured α-chains from erythrocytes. This occurs particularly in the spleen, where *pitting* from red cells occurs. The splenic reticuloendothelial cells may first deform cells into teardrop shapes while plucking out the inclusions. Further injury leads to increased permeability of the red cell and formation of fragmented forms. Triangular forms, target cells, tiny microcytes, teardrop forms, and other shape abnormalities are commonly seen. Macrocytes, basophilic stippling, polychromatophils, and nucleated red cells are also present. Supravital staining or phase microscopy reveals reticulocytosis and Heinz inclusion bodies. The latter are most numerous after splenectomy and in patients with severe anemia. Red cell osmotic fragility is decreased, presumably because of a decreased content of hemoglobin that leaves more space for water absorption.

The anemia stimulates bone marrows to maximum activity, resulting in expansion of the bone marrow cavity and the skeletal abnormalities previously described. Besides erythroid hyperplasia there may be defective hemoglobinization and periodic acid–Schiff (PAS)–staining material in normoblasts. Iron is abundant, and small numbers of ringed sideroblasts may be found.

In milder forms of thalassemia, microcytosis and hypochromia are the only peripheral blood findings. In thalassemia minima, these abnormalities are minimal or absent.

Clinical Severity and Hemoglobin Constitution of β- and δ-Thalassemias

On the basis of the clinical findings, peripheral blood smear, and hemoglobin pattern, it is usually possible to predict the genotype of the β- or δ-thalassemia. In δ-thalassemia there is a defective synthesis of the δ-chain. In some forms of thalassemia defective

*Hemolysis may also be due to increased amounts of activated oxygen forms (superoxide), which attack the cell membrane. Hypochromia facilitates the oxidation of the membrane by reducing the amount of hemoglobin available for buffering protection. The excess α-chains act like unstable hemoglobulins that allow water to enter the heme pocket, thereby produc-

synthesis of both β- and δ-chains occurs, and this is referred to as $(\delta\beta)$-*thalassemia.* The deficit of either β- or δ-chain synthesis may be either partial or total. In Table 6-1 a zero superscript following "thal" (thal^0) indicates that no β-chain or δ-chain is produced, and a plus (thal$^+$) indicates reduced, but not absent, synthesis of the β- or δ-chain. A close study of this table will allow some logical sense to be made out of the confusing clinical pictures and hemoglobin patterns presented by various thalassemic patients. In clinical practice it is necessary only to determine whether the patient's anemia is severe enough to require blood transfusion, for if it is not, the patient is heterozygous for the thalassemia gene, and no therapy is required.

It is possible for the β^{thal^0} and the β^{thal^+} genes to interact with a sickle mutation. Patients with $\beta^S\beta^{thal^0}$ genes have almost all sickle hemoglobin and no HbA, whereas patients with $\beta^S\beta^{thal^+}$ genes have some HbA present. The amount of sickle hemoglobin determines the clinical severity of the disease, so that a patient with sickle gene and β^{thal^0} will be clinically indistinguishable from one with homozygous sickle cell disease.

The milder manifestations of thalassemia intermedia are the result of interaction of β^{thal^+}, β^{thal^0}, and $(\delta\beta)^{thal^0}$ genes with $(\delta\beta)^{thal^0}$ β^{thal^0}, and thalassemia minima genes or with structural hemoglobin mutants or Hb$_{Lepore}$ genes. In general, clinical severity has a direct correlation with the degree of the α–β-chain imbalance and the presence of Heinz bodies in erythrocytes.

Hemoglobin Lepore (Hb$_{Lepore}$) Syndromes

As a result of a structural defect in hemoglobin, a thalassemia-like picture can be produced in patients who carry genes for Hb$_{Lepore}$. This hemoglobin results from an unequal crossover between the closely linked β- and δ-chain gene loci. It has the electrophoretic mobility of hemoglobin S, a δ-chain sequence at one end, and a β-chain sequence at the other. Patients with two Hb$_{Lepore}$ genes synthesize hemoglobin at a reduced rate, presumably because they lack a normal β-chain gene. The clinical findings resemble those of thalassemia major.

Hereditary Persistence of Fetal Hemoglobin (HPFH)

Hereditary persistence of fetal hemoglobin can be looked upon as a form of β-thalassemia in which there is total compensation for the lack of β-chain synthesis by persistent δ-chain production. The gene for this abnormality behaves as an allele for the β-chain locus. In the usual classic form of β-thalassemia, HbF levels may be elevated, but HbF is confined to only a small population of cells. In HPFH, on the other hand, some HbF is found in most or

ing methemoglobin and superoxide. In thalassemia, inclusion body formation is important, but evidence is accumulating that indicates a significant role for direct oxidation of cell membranes in hemolysis.

all cells. HbF distribution is tested for by incubation of a peripheral blood smear with citric acid–phosphate buffer (pH 3.2), which elutes hemoglobin A and leaves behind HbF. This Kleihauer-Betke or acid elution stain thus detects cells that contain fetal hemoglobin. If the gene for HPFH interacts with a gene for sickle cell, a syndrome results in which the sickle cell hemoglobin concentration is high, but the clinical symptoms are mild, because the hemoglobin F in each cell ameliorates sickling. The HPFH gene is revealed by the homogeneous distribution of the fetal hemoglobin in patients with high HbF and normal hemoglobin levels. This gene may also interact with thalassemia genes and structural hemoglobin mutations.

α-Thalassemia

There is now evidence that in at least some populations four gene loci (two closely linked genes on each chromosome) exist for synthesis of hemoglobin α-chains. Thalassemia-like mutations may affect one or all four of these gene loci. Different clinical pictures result, depending on the number of gene loci affected. All the evidence that supports the theory of four gene loci for the α-chain will not be reviewed here. Populations of African origin appear to have chromosomes possessing only one α-chain locus, whereas white populations may have two.

The four main α-thalassemic syndromes in order of increasing severity are α-thal$_2$ trait, α-thal$_1$ trait, hemoglobin H disease, and hemoglobin$_{Bart's}$ (γ_4) hydrops fetalis. Patients with α-thal$_2$ trait are clinically normal and have normal hematologic findings except for reduced MCV and MCH. These patients have a thalassemic defect in one of the four α-chain loci. The α-thal$_1$ trait is characterized by two abnormal loci both on the same chromosome. In this case the patient is clinically normal, but there are mild hematologic abnormalities (anemia, low MCV and MCH, and hypochromia) compatible with thalassemia trait. Hemoglobin H disease results from three abnormal α-chain loci. It is clinically characterized by the clinical picture of thalassemia intermedia and by variable amounts of hemoglobin H, a β-chain tetramer. The most severe form of α-thalassemia occurs only in anemic, edematous, stillborn infants whose hemoglobin composition is almost all hemoglobin$_{Bart's}$. These patients have four thalassemic α-chain loci and therefore can produce in the fetal state only γ-chains, which polymerize to form Hb$_{Bart's}$. Interestingly, the amount of Bart's hemoglobin in a fetus or newborn has a direct correlation with the number of thalassemic α-chain loci, so that 1 to 2 percent is found in fetuses carrying α-thal$_2$ trait, 5 to 6 percent in α-thal$_1$, 25 percent in HbH disease, and greater than 80 percent in hydrops fetalis.

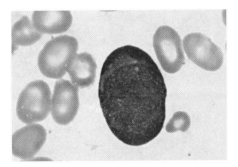

1 : Pronormoblast (Erythroblast)

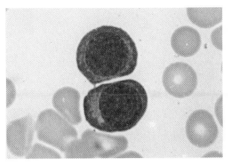

2 : Basophilic normoblast

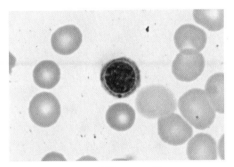

3 : Polychromatophilic normoblast

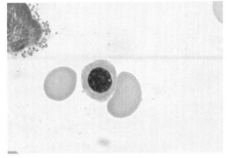

4 : Orthochromatic normoblast

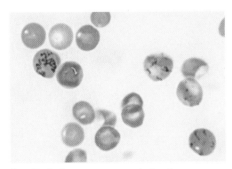

5 : Reticulocytes — supra vital stain

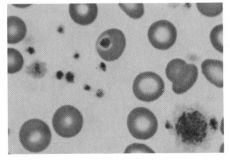

6 : Platelets

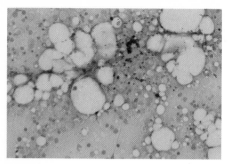

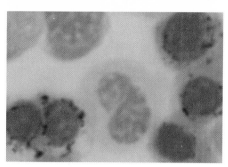

7 : Normal smear – iron stain, marrow, extra-cellular iron

8 : Ringed sideroblast

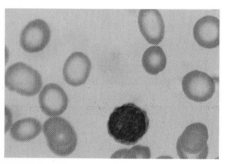

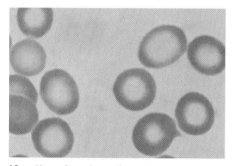

9 : Microcytosis

10 : Hypochromic erythrocytes

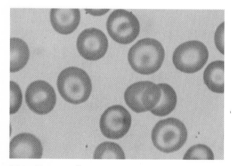

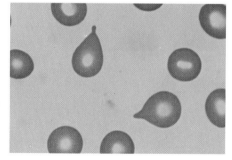

11 : Target cells

12 : Teardrop cells

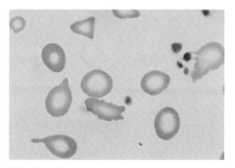

13 : Poikilocytes

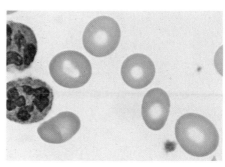

14 : Dimorphic red cells

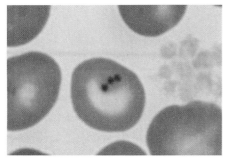

15 : Pappenheimer bodies – iron stain

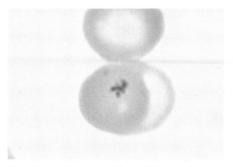

16 : Pappenheimer bodies – Wright stain

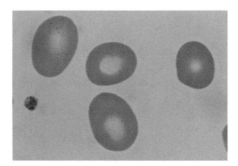

17 : Macroovalocytes

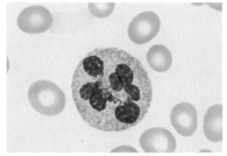

18 : Hypersegmented poly

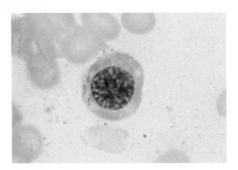

19 : Megaloblast

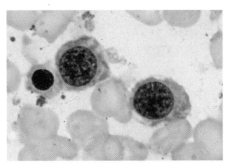

20 : Megaloblast

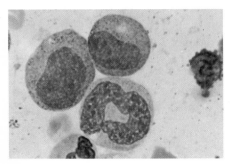

21 : Giant myeloid forms

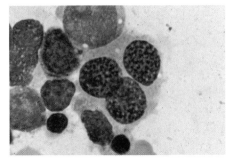

22 : Erythroleukemia — gigantoblast

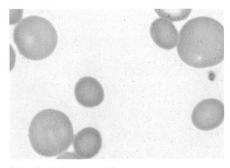

23 : Polychromatophils

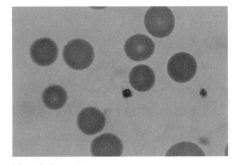

24 : Spherocytes

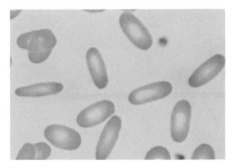

25 : Ovalocytes

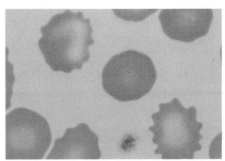

26 : Burr cells

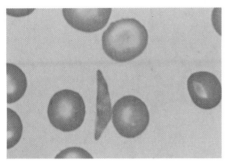

27 : Sickle cell

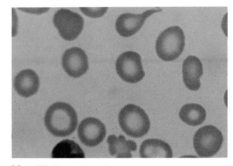

28 : Thalassemia minor

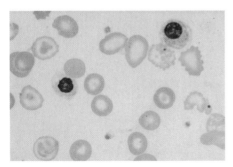

29 : Thalassemia major

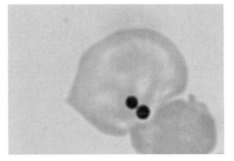

30 : Howell-Jolly bodies

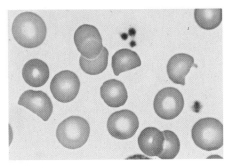

31 : Helmet cells

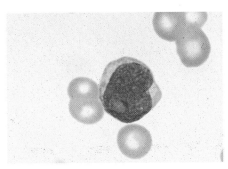

32 : Myeloblast

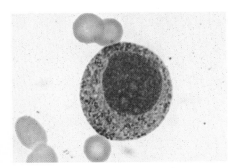

33 : Promyelocyte

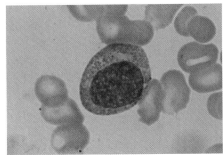

34 : Myelocyte

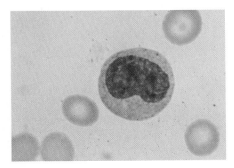

35 : Metamyelocyte

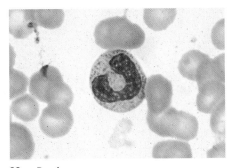

36 : Band

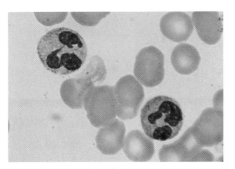

37 : Neutrophil (poly)

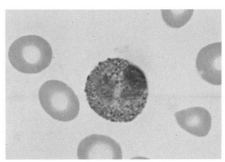

38 : Eosinophil

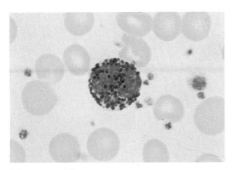

39 : Basophil

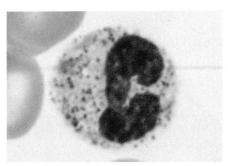

40 : Döhle body

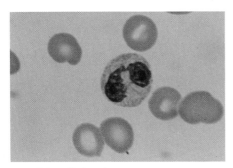

41 : Pelger-Huët – heterozygous

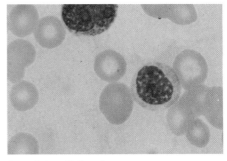

42 : Pelger-Huët – homozygous

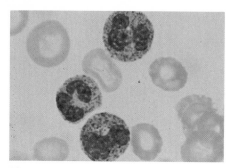

43 : Toxic granulations

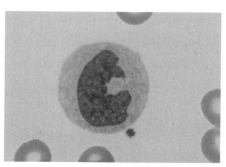

44 : Monocyte

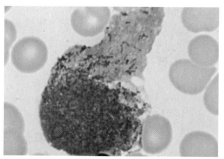

45 : Reticuloendothelial cell (macrophage)

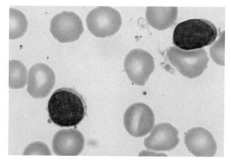

46 : Lymphocytes, small

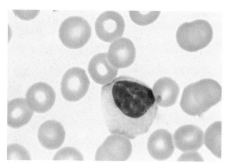

47 : Lymphocyte, large

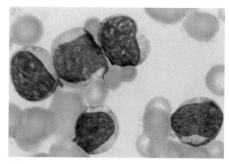

48 : Acute lymphocytic leukemia (lymphoblasts)

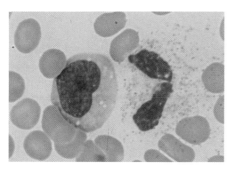

49 : Atypical lymphocyte – vacuolated

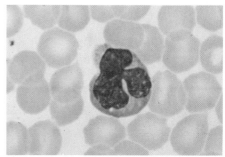

50 : Atypical lymphocyte – monocytoid nucleus

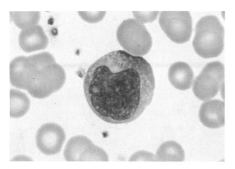

51 : Atypical lymphocyte – nucleoli

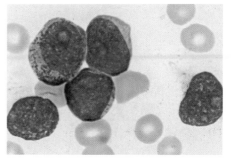

52 : Acute granulocytic leukemia (blast, promyelocyte)

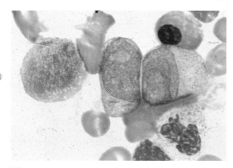

53 : Auer rods

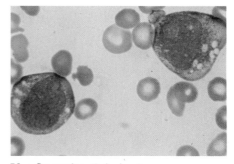

54 : Promyelocytic leukemia

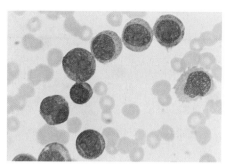

55 : Acute myelomonocytic leukemia

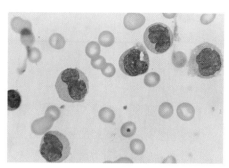

56 : Acute monocytic leukemia

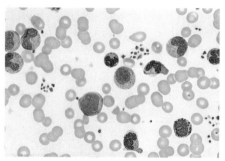

57 : Chronic granulocytic leukemia

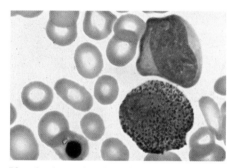

58 : Leukoerythroblastosis

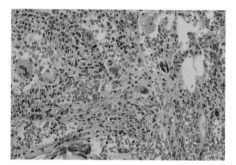

59 : Marrow fibrosis, biopsy, H&E

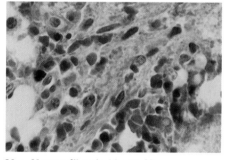

60 : Marrow fibrosis, biopsy, Masson trichrome stain

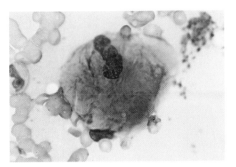

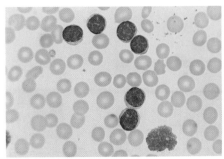

61 : Gaucher disease

62 : Chronic lymphocytic leukemia

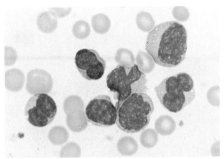

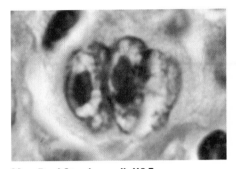

63 : Chronic lymphosarcoma cell leukemia

64 : Reed-Sternberg cell, H&E

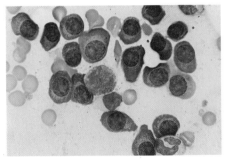

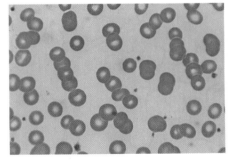

65 : Plasma cells and plasmablasts (multiple myeloma)

66 : Rouleaux

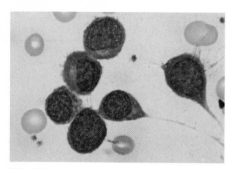

67 : Plymphocytes

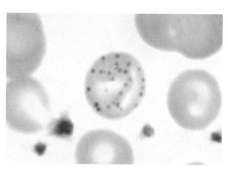

68 : Coarsely stippled red cell

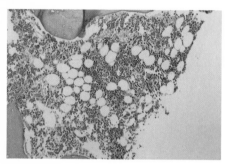

69 : Normal marrow biopsy

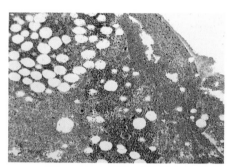

70 : Normal clot section, H&E 45×

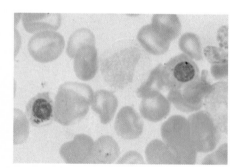

71 : Normal smear — iron stain, normal marrow, intracellular iron

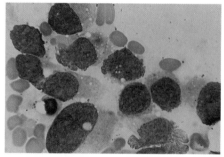

72 : Tumor cells

An interesting α-chain structural mutant is hemoglobin$_{Constant Spring}$ (HbCS). This hemoglobin is characterized by an α-chain elongated at the C-terminal end by 31 amino acid residues. It arises from mutation of the terminating codon of the normal α-gene. This gene is similar to Lepore hemoglobin in that it has a thalassemia-like effect causing reduced synthesis of the α-CS chain. Double heterozygosity for α-thalassemia trait (two affected α-chain loci) and HbCS results in a picture similar to that of hemoglobin H disease but with a small percentage of HbCS also present. If there were only two gene loci for α-chains, then double heterozygotes for HbCS and α-thalassemia should have a hemoglobin composition consisting of only hemoglobin$_{Bart's}$ (γ_4) and HbCS. Furthermore HbCS has not been found in any Hb$_{Bart's,}$ hydropic, stillborn infant. If there were only two gene loci, homozygosity for HbCS should prevent HbA production and result in hydrops fetalis with HbCS and Hb$_{Bart's}$. As long as no such hydropic infants with HbCS are found, the four gene loci model (duplication of the human α-chain locus) is most likely correct, at least for some populations.

HbH (β_4) is electrophoretically fast, unstable, and thermolabile and has an oxygen affinity ten times normal (no heme–heme interaction). Anemia results from Heinz body formation in marrow and peripheral blood erythrocytes. These inclusion bodies can be demonstrated, particularly after splenectomy, by incubation of red cells with brilliant cresyl blue for 20 minutes. This dye oxidizes free thiols in the HbH molecules, thereby causing HbH to precipitate. Presumably, newly produced erythrocytes contain soluble HbH, which precipitates during the cell's life, and the Heinz body formed is pitted from the cell by the spleen. The increased oxygen affinity of HbH further complicates the anemia by preventing normal release of oxygen to tissues. Luckily the majority of the hemoglobin present in patients with HbH disease is HbA. Microcytosis, hypochromia, target cells, stippling, and small poikilocytes are found on examination of peripheral blood smears.

Treatment of Thalassemia

Transfusion remains the mainstay of treatment for patients with thalassemia major or Cooley's anemia. There is debate as to whether the hemoglobin should be kept at 5 to 6 gm per deciliter or whether transfusions should be given up to a normal hemoglobin level. The lower level has the advantage of requiring fewer transfusions and therefore producing less of an iron load. There is no evidence, however, that the increased iron load of a normal hemoglobin level does any more harm than a lower hematocrit. Patients maintained with high hematocrits develop more normally, grow faster, exhibit fewer complications, and have less trouble with skeletal deformities, hepatosplenomegaly, and cardiac failure. However, despite frequent transfusions these patients do not survive beyond the second decade of life. In some young patients splenectomy may decrease the transfusion requirement, but there is an increased incidence of severe infections following this operation.

Transfusions necessarily lead to an increased load of iron. Iron-chelating agents such as desferrioxamine or diethylenetriamine pentaacetate (DTPA) may be given parenterally to chelate iron and cause its excretion in the urine. Complications of chelating therapy include a falling off of the daily iron excretion rate, despite continued therapy; allergic reactions; and pain from daily intramuscular injections. Thus far, the initial promise of iron-chelating agents has not been fulfilled, but new methods of administration that avoid these complications are being developed. It is important to find means for reducing iron load, since a common cause of death in young patients with thalassemia major is cardiac failure due to hemachromatosis. Certainly iron therapy given as a result of an erroneous diagnosis of iron deficiency anemia should be stopped. Folic acid (1 mg per day) is recommended because of the degree of ineffective erythropoiesis in thalassemia major. In general, transfusion and folic acid therapy are needed only for patients with thalassemia major. Genetic counseling may help prevent the birth of homozygous β-thalassemic children.

Diagnosis of Thalassemia

The diagnosis of thalassemia major is usually made from a family history of the thalassemia gene, skeletal and facial abnormalities at birth, and the presence of a severe microcytic and hypochromic anemia (Plate 29) with evidence of ineffective erythropoiesis. Confirmation comes from measuring hemoglobin A_2 and hemoglobin F levels (Table 6-1). Hemoglobin A_2 is generally determined by starch block electrophoresis or DEAE column chromatography. Hemoglobin F is measured by addition of potassium hydroxide to a hemoglobin solution. In this method denatured HbA is precipitated by ammonium sulfate and removed by filtration. The alkali-resistant HbF remains in the supernatant. The proportion of alkali-resistant hemoglobin F is expressed as a percentage of the total hemoglobin present. Normal hemoglobin A_2 and F levels are 0 to 2 percent.

In some cases family studies will be necessary to determine a thalassemic patient's genotype; rare, in other instances, special chain separation procedures are required to confirm the diagnosis of thalassemia, as follows: Reticulocytes from a patient are incubated with radiolabeled amino acids, and the newly synthesized hemoglobin purified. After separation of the hemoglobin chains, it is possible to measure by assaying radioactivity the amount of nascent α- and β-chains. In β-thalassemic patients the ratio of β-chain production to α-chain production is reduced 50 percent in the heterozygote and considerably more in the homozygote. In α-thalassemics increased β-chain-to-α-chain ratios are found. These techniques can actually be performed on small amounts of blood from newborn infants in order to make the diagnosis of thalassemia at birth.

In the adult the diagnosis of thalassemia intermedia or minor is usually suspected in patients of Mediterranean ancestry with hypochromic anemia. Examination of their peripheral blood (Plate 28) shows microcytosis, hypochromia, target cells, and poikilocytosis. These patients usually have a normal or near-normal hematocrit in the case of thalassemia minor and may be mildly anemic in the case of thalassemia intermedia. The discrepancy between the severe abnormalities of shape and the mild or nonexistent anemia should suggest the diagnosis. An unusual β-thalassemia gene has been described in association with severe anemia, although only one β-chain locus is abnormal. The severity of the anemia may be due to an unusual propensity to form inclusion bodies of precipitated α-chains.

Some thalassemic patients come to attention because of their extremely low MCV — 75 femtoliters or less by the Coulter counter. Iron deficiency may cause MCV values this low, but normally an MCV of 75 fl or less means severe anemia. The following calculation serves as a rule of thumb: $MCV(fl)/PCV(L/L) \times 0.1$. A value of less than 13 suggests the diagnosis of thalassemia rather than iron deficiency anemia.

α-Thalassemia heterozygotes are rarely detected, except when unexplained microcytosis or low HbA_2 is discovered. Of course, in certain Greek, Southeast Asian, and Chinese populations, hemoglobin H disease may be suspected and supravital staining for the characteristic erythrocyte inclusions performed. $Hb_{Bart's}$ disease should be suspected in Oriental women with a history of repeated hydropic stillbirths.

HYPER-SPLENISM

The syndrome of hypersplenism is characterized by

1. Splenomegaly
2. Anemia, leukopenia, thrombocytopenia, or any combination of these cytopenias
3. Hyperplasia of bone marrow precursors
4. Correction of the peripheral blood cytopenias by removal of the spleen

Mechanisms of
Hypersplenism

The spleen is thought to affect peripheral blood counts by three possible mechanisms

Production of a substance in the spleen which decreases marrow production
Destruction of blood elements within the spleen
Trapping or sequestration of blood elements in the organ

The evidence for the production of toxins by the spleen is fragmentary. Antibodies may be produced in the spleen — for example, against platelets. The collection of lymphocytes and plasma cells around the arterioles feeding into the spleen may serve as a source of antibody production. This white pulp is known to proliferate after intravascular injection of antigens. A few cases of anemia associated with a hypoplastic bone marrow have been reported to improve after splenectomy.

The spleen plays a role in the destruction of abnormal red cells, such as those found in immunohemolytic anemia, hereditary spherocytosis, and elliptocytosis, spur cell anemia of liver disease, and Heinz body hemolytic anemia. In the case of red cells coated with antibodies or complement, the reticuloendothelial cells of the spleen and monocytes in the peripheral blood remove parts of the red cell membrane, reducing the membrane to volume ratio. This results in a spheroidal shape and loss of ability of red cells to deform. As a result cells in various stages of losing membrane may be trapped in the sinusoids of the spleen. Here they are exposed to further stress (conditioning), hypoglycemia, and decreased pH. Even if the cell initially escapes the spleen, its susceptibility to later entrapment because of decreased deformability is increased. Finally the cell becomes irreversibly trapped and destroyed in the spleen.

In hereditary spherocytosis, perhaps as a result of a membrane lipid or protein defect, the influx of sodium is increased and the capacity for the cell to extrude sodium is exceeded. Because of intracellular osmotic pressure, water may enter the cell and cause swelling and the formation of macrospherocytes. Deformability is reduced by the decrease in membrane surface-to-volume ratio. Microspherocytosis also occurs, perhaps as a result of membrane loss due to action of monocytes or reticuloendothelial cells. These cells are trapped, conditioned and lysed in the spleen.

In the spur cell anemia of severe liver disease, there is an increased serum cholesterol and an increased uptake of cholesterol into the cell membrane. This results in an abnormal cell with scalloped borders called a *burr* or *spur cell*. Because of loss of deformability, the cell is trapped and "conditioned" in the spleen in a manner similar to what happens in hereditary spherocytosis. This leads to even more severe poikilocytosis, production of cells with long and irregular spicules, and finally hemolysis.

In Heinz body hemolytic anemias the affected erythrocytes flow through arterioles first into the white pulp, then through the red pulp into sinusoids lined by cords of spleen cells. Since these are narrow passages, red cells may be trapped, especially if their deformability is reduced. The reticuloendothelial cells lining these passages have been observed to pit out Heinz bodies, sometimes resulting in production of deformed cells with membrane projections and loss of membrane surface area. Continued pitting, deformation, and conditioning results in cell lysis.

Removal of the spleen in patients with HS cures the anemia by preventing the conditioning process. Splenectomy also may improve red cell survival in immunohemolytic anemias, Heinz body anemia, and thalassemia. In Heinz body hemolytic anemia and thalassemia, splenectomized patient's erythrocytes contain large numbers of inclusion bodies because the pitting function of the spleen has been eliminated.

Etiology and Effects of Splenomegaly

Any disease that causes an enlarged spleen either by infiltration of abnormal cells or by stimulation of the reticuloendothelial cells can result in the syndrome of hypersplenism. In some cases a vicious cycle is set up by which hemolysis leads to reticuloendothelial cell hyperplasia, which in turn leads to further damage, entrapment, and lysis of red cells in the spleen. For this reason certain chronic hemolytic anemias such as thalassemia, pyruvate kinase deficiency, and unstable hemoglobin variants may be helped by splenectomy (see p. 184).

The pathogenesis of the thrombocytopenia (decreased platelets) appears to be different from the anemia. Recent evidence strongly suggests that platelet lysis rarely occurs in an enlarged spleen but that, rather, a large percentage of a patient's platelets are trapped or sequestered without destruction in splenic pools. These platelets may be available to the patient following stress such as hemorrhage. Because of this, what appears to be a dangerously low peripheral blood platelet count may not lead to serious bleeding.

There is evidence that an enlarged spleen may in some way increase peripheral plasma volume. This leads to hemodilution and an apparently low peripheral blood hematocrit. Removal of the spleen has sometimes increased the hematocrit, primarily by reduction of plasma volume rather than by increase in red cell mass.

Leukopenia and granulocytopenia secondary to splenomegaly have not been well studied. There may well be enlarged splenic

Causes of hypersplenism in adults

Chronic, congenital hemolytic anemias, e.g., hereditary spherocytosis,
  hemoglobinopathies, and erythrocyte enzyme deficiencies
Chronic infections such as tuberculosis, subacute bacterial endocarditis,
  infectious mononucleosis, and infectious hepatitis
Chronic lymphocytic leukemia
Chronic myelocytic leukemia and agnogenic myeloid metaplasia
Cirrhosis of the liver with portal hypertension and congestive
  splenomegaly
Idiopathic or primary splenomegaly
Lipid storage diseases, e.g., Gaucher's disease
Malignant lymphomas
Polycythemia vera
Rheumatoid arthritis and Felty's syndrome
Sarcoidosis
Thalassemia

pools of leukocytes in certain leukemias and other diseases associated with splenomegaly. It is not entirely clear whether actual destruction of leukocytes occurs in enlarged spleens.

Diagnosis and Treatment of Hypersplenism

Diagnosis of hypersplenism is usually easy, once splenomegaly and cytopenias are discovered. To confirm the diagnosis, a bone marrow aspiration should be performed to demonstrate hyperplasia of the blood elements involved. Bone marrow examination is also done to diagnose leukemia, lymphoma, or other infiltrative diseases of the marrow. Of course, a complete physical examination and history review of the patient's history should be done to detect any underlying illness. In some cases, treatment of the underlying disease is all that is required to reduce the spleen size to normal and cure the hypersplenism. In patients with hereditary spherocytosis, thalassemia, hemoglobinopathies, Heinz body hemolytic anemias, pyruvate kinase deficiency, lymphomas, and leukemias, removal of the spleen may be required. The treatment of Coombs' test–positive hemolytic anemia, idiopathic thrombocytopenic purpura, and aplastic anemia may also include splenectomy. Adults usually tolerate splenectomy well. Perioperative mortality is related to the age and underlying disease. Very large spleens are difficult to remove technically and predispose the patients to infections such as subdiaphragmatic abscesses.

In young patients, particularly those under 5 and to some degree in patients up to age 30, there appears to be an increased risk of infections with overwhelming sepsis. Some pediatricians recommend prophylactic antibiotic treatment for patients under 5 who have a splenectomy performed. Close observation and early treatment of infection in older children and adults is certainly required.

Except in the case of chronic myelocytic leukemia, splenic irradiation is usually of little benefit to patients with enlarged spleens, although occasionally patients with lymphoma and leukemia are successfully treated.

Hyposplenism

The removal of the splenic function by surgery, by infarction of its arterial supply, or by autoinfarctions as occurs in sickle cell anemia and some myelocytic leukemias may result in a syndrome called *hyposplenism.* Children with congenital heart disease and other diseases can lose the trapping function of the spleen, although the spleen size is normal. Congenital agenesis of the spleen is another rare cause of hyposplenism. Patients with hyposplenism have changes in their peripheral blood that help confirm the diagnosis (see p. 186). Howell-Jolly bodies (Plate 30) are processed DNA and appear as large, dark-staining, single or double

Peripheral blood changes in patients with hyposplenism*

Variable eosinophilia and basophilia
Transient erythrocytosis
Howell-Jolly bodies
Increased inclusion bodies in Heinz body hemolytic anemias and
 thalassemias
Chronic monocytosis and lymphocytosis
Acute neutrophilia
Pappenheimer bodies (siderocytes)
Increased platelet count (transitory or permanent)
Increased poikilocytosis, particularly target, burr, and fragmented cells
Nucleated red cells
Increased reticulocyte count and polychromatophilia
Elevated white cell counts
Immature white cells

*Except for Howell-Jolly bodies, which are consistently present, these changes may appear transiently or not at all in some patients with decreased or absent splenic function.

inclusion bodies in erythrocytes from patients with hyposplenism. Probably these inclusions are produced all the time, but in the absence of the spleen's pitting function, they are detected in the peripheral blood. Pappenheimer bodies (Plates 15 and 16), small dark inclusions usually appearing in clusters of three or more, are also prominent in erythrocytes (siderocytes) from patients with hyposplenism. They are smaller than Howell-Jolly bodies and have ragged, rather than smooth, surfaces. These inclusion bodies stain with Prussian blue for hemosiderin. They are also present in iron-loading anemias. Occasionally the misshapen red cells seen following splenectomy lead to a mistaken diagnosis of microangiopathic hemolytic anemia, but hyposplenism should be suspected if the hematocrit is normal or near-normal.

MICROANGIO-PATHIC HEMOLYTIC ANEMIA

A Coombs' test–negative hemolytic anemia characterized by the presence of abnormal, fragmented erythrocytes in the peripheral blood smear is called a *microangiopathic hemolytic anemia*. Helmet cells (Plate 31), triangular cells, burr or spur cells (Plate 26) with membrane scalloping or projections, and tiny fragments of cells are prominent. The helmet, burr, and triangular cells are called *schistocytes* or *irregularly contracted cells* and are diagnostic for microangiopathic hemolytic anemias. Often associated with these cells are microspherocytes, nucleated red cells, polychromatophilia, and other peripheral blood findings characteristic of hemolytic anemia. The anemia may be mild or severe, and the reticulocyte count is usually elevated.

Etiology of Microangiopathic Hemolytic Anemia

Defective aortic valve prostheses are probably the most common cause of fragmented erythrocytes. Calcified and stenotic aortic, and in some rare cases mitral, valve abnormalities can also cause fragmented cells. If hemolysis is happening at a significant rate, hemoglobinemia, hemoglobinuria, and hemosidinuria will arise. The loss of iron through the kidneys may be severe enough to produce iron deficiency anemia. Therefore, in cases of Coombs' test–negative hemolytic anemia and iron deficiency, a defective cardiac valve should be suspected. Jet streams of blood flowing through any part of the heart, particularly when they impinge upon nonendothelialized surfaces, lead to red cell fragmentation. The hemolysis appears to be due to mechanical breakdown of the red cell membranes, which are unable to withstand the sheer stress forces. Mechanical trauma from marching or jogging in nonprotecting shoes (march hemoglobinuria) can also lead to erythrocyte fragmentation and hemolysis.

Abnormalities of the vascular endothelium, particularly the arterioles, account for many cases of microangiopathic hemolytic anemia. Some investigators believe that red cell flow through

Causes of fragmented erythrocytes

I. Traumatic Causes
   A. Cardiac prostheses (defective valves, jet streams)
   B. Cardiac valvular diseases (calcific, stenotic, jet streams)
   C. March hemoglobinuria
II. Vascular Abnormalities
   A. Arteriovenous shunts
   B. Carcinomatosis
   C. Malignant hypertension
   D. Renal failure, renal cortical necrosis, glomerulonephritis
   E. Thrombotic thrombocytopenic purpura (hemolytic-uremic syndrome)
   F. Toxemia of pregnancy
   G. Vasculitis (periarteritis nodosa and systemic lupus erythematosus)
III. Intravascular Coagulation
   A. Disseminated
      1. Abruptio placentae
      2. Septicemia
   B. Local
      1. Cavernous hemangioma
      2. Purpura fulminans
      3. Renal hemograft rejection

damaged vascular endothelium causes the fragmentation. Others suggest that fibrin deposits in these small vessels capture red cells as a result of folding of the erythrocytes over fibrin strands. If sufficient force is supplied by the bloodstream, the erythrocyte membrane may be torn by the fibrin strand. The membrane tears reseal, and the erythrocyte fragments continue to circulate in the peripheral blood.

A very rare but frequently fatal microangiopathic hemolytic anemia is known as *thrombotic thrombocytopenic purpura* (TTP). It is characterized by (1) Coombs' test-negative hemolytic anemia with many fragmented forms in the peripheral blood; (2) thrombocytopenic purpura (low platelet count and cutaneous hemorrhages), sometimes with serious bleeding; (3) fever; (4) neurologic and psychiatric abnormalities including convulsions, coma, paralysis, and hallucinations; and (5) renal failure. Microthrombi are found in many small blood vessels, along with evidence of vasculitis. The diagnosis is made on the basis of the clinical findings and biopsy of lymph node, bone marrow, kidney, or other organs containing small blood vessels. Treatment is usually unsuccessful, but improvement or spontaneous remission has been associated with large doses of adrenal corticosteroids and splenectomy. Heparin, dextran, and renal dialysis have also been tried, usually with poor results. Recently drugs known to interfere with platelet function, aspirin and Persantin, have been employed with success in a small number of patients.

Probably closely related to TTP is a similar disease seen in children, the *hemolytic-uremic syndrome,* and systemic lupus erythematosus, a disease caused by a vasculitis of unknown etiology.

Disseminated intravascular coagulation (DIC) refers to a syndrome caused by inappropriate intravascular activation of the coagulation process. This results in the laying down of fibrin, which leads to fragmentation of red cells. Although the mechanism by which DIC produces microangiopathic erythrocytes is not agreed upon, this diagnosis should be suspected in the face of microangiopathic red cell changes and evidence for activation of the coagulation cascade. Typically platelets and soluble coagulation factors consumed during clotting are reduced as a result of the intravascular clotting. The treatment for this form of microangiopathic hemolytic anemia is removal of the cause for DIC, replacement of coagulation factors, or in severe cases administration of the anticoagulant, heparin.

Severe poikilocytosis can sometimes be mistaken for microangiopathic erythrocytes. For example, in patients with severe megaloblastic or iron deficiency anemias, thalassemia, thermal burns, and hyposplenism, the red cells may be so abnormally shaped as to suggest microangiopathic blood.

Therapy for microangiopathic hemolytic anemia is treatment of the underlying disease. For example, replacement of defective cardiac valve prostheses may be required.

PAROXYSMAL NOCTURNAL HEMOGLOBINURIA

Paroxysmal nocturnal hemoglobinuria (PNH) is a rare disease that merits discussion only because of the pathophysiologic mechanisms associated with its clinical presentation. A membrane abnormality of some or all PNH red blood cells makes them susceptible to the hemolytic action of complement. Associated with this sensitivity to complement lysis are numerous clinical and biochemical abnormalities.

Clinical Findings in PNH

Affected patients are characterized by bouts of hemoglobinuria, usually worse at night. It is known that patients who reverse their sleep habits reverse their pattern of hemoglobinuria. Other factors such as infections, inoculations, and vaccinations may precipitate hemolytic crises. Because of hemolysis and loss of hemoglobin iron through the kidneys, PNH patients become iron-deficient. Treatment with transfusions or iron often results in a severe hemolytic episode. It is suspected that iron allows deficient bone marrows to produce more abnormal red cells, which are sensitive to complement lysis. In some patients, the degree of hemolysis is not enough to produce hemoglobinuria.

The disease often unfolds over a period of years, some patients developing pancytopenia and marrow aplasia. Some investigators feel that the abnormal erythrocytes peculiar to PNH result from defective stem cells. The same defect in stem cells may cause the marrow aplasia. Interestingly, complement-sensitive erythrocytes may also be found in patients with leukemia, marrow aplasia due to drugs or idiopathic causes, and in some other, apparently unrelated, diseases.

Commonly seen in PNH patients are thrombotic and embolic phenomenon. Hepatic, portal, cerebral vein, and other venous thromboses have been known to occur. Abdominal and back pain without any apparent etiology may be due to small venous thromboses.

Laboratory Abnormalities in PNH

Biochemically the disease is characterized by the ability of acidified normal serum to lyse PNH cells (Ham test). Fresh normal serum is acidified with hydrochloric acid to a pH of 6.7, and the cells to be tested are incubated with it for 30 minutes at $37^\circ C$. Using appropriate controls the amount of lysis is determined. PNH, but not normal cells, will lyse under these conditions. The serum used in these tests may be taken from any normal individual, although serums do vary in their ability to cause lysis. This is the same test that may be positive in hereditary dyserythropoietic anemia. In the case of PNH no antibody against red cell antigens has been demonstrated in active serums. It is believed that the test depends on activation of complement in the serum to cause lysis of sensitive erythrocytes. Another procedure that activates complement is called the *sucrose lysis* or *sugar water test*. Cells and small amounts of serum are suspended in isotonic sucrose. Because of the reduced ionic strength, complement is activated and sensitive cells are lysed. Weak false-positive reactions are sometimes seen. This procedure serves as an excellent screening test for PNH, but a positive acidified serum lysis test is required for confirmation.

Although an antibody has not been shown to be required for lysis, a serum protein, properdin, has been implicated in the initiation of complement lysis. Probably the same membrane defect that predisposes to complement lysis also causes an absence of the membrane enzyme acetylcholine esterase. No detectable clinical problem is associated with low or absent enzyme levels. Occasionally assay for this enzyme is needed to confirm the diagnosis of PNH.

In the past, electron micrographs were thought to show abnormal pits in the membrane surfaces of these cells. More recent studies show no specific abnormality in the membrane. It is interesting that normal red cells can be made to resemble PNH cells functionally by treatment with certain sulfhydryl compounds. Treated cells become sensitive to complement lysis. It may be that PNH cells have fewer thiol groups on their surface, since these chemicals artificially reduce available thiol groups by production of mixed disulfides.

Another biochemical abnormality is the absence of the enzyme leukocyte alkaline phosphatase. This enzyme is detected by incubating methanol-fixed white cells with an organic phosphate at alkaline pH. In the presence of alkaline phosphatase the phosphate group is removed and the organic substrate precipitates in the cytoplasm, yielding a distinctive blue or brown color. Typically, in chronic myelocytic leukemia and in PNH, the leukocyte alkaline phosphatase score is low or zero. Interestingly, some patients with PNH have developed acute myelocytic leukemia.

It is possible that the hemolysis and intravascular release of red cell stroma, a thromboplastic substance, causes a hypercoagulable state and the thrombotic complications of PNH.

Treatment of PNH   There is no known treatment for this disease. Transfusions must be given very carefully, as washed packed red cells, since transfusion has been known to precipitate hemolytic and thrombotic crises. Iron therapy is often required but, as previously noted, may result in more hemolysis from the production of complement-sensitive red cells. Androgens, corticosteroids, and splenectomy have had varying degrees of success in this difficult-to-treat disease. Anticoagulant therapy with heparin, coumadin, or dextran has not been particularly successful. Usually the moderately to severely affected patients survive for a period of years, often suffering pain and discomfort from the complications of the disease. More mildly affected patients survive with little in the way of clinical problems and may ultimately improve. Protection from infection and prompt treatment of infections is important for patients with marrow aplasia. Bleeding complications from thrombocytopenia may require emergency treatment with platelet transfusions.

MISCELLANEOUS CAUSES OF COOMBS' TEST-NEGATIVE HEMOLYTIC ANEMIA

As noted earlier in this section, Coombs' test–negative hemolytic anemia may be a part of many, if not all, diseases that affect man. We will briefly discuss unusual causes of this type of hemolytic anemia.

Patients with severe hypophosphatemia and reduction in high energy phosphate compounds may hemolyze. This problem has been encountered in association with acute pancreatitis. Patients with a blood type Rh_{null} have a decreased red cell life span. This may be due to a membrane abnormality associated with the absence of Rh blood groups. In premature infants, a vitamin E deficiency syndrome is sometimes associated with hemolytic anemia. Vitamin E normally protects membranes from oxidation by activated oxygen. Patients with high copper levels due to contamination of hemodialysis fluids have hemolytic anemias. Interestingly, patients with Wilson's disease, an inherited disease associated with high serum copper levels, also suffer from hemolytic anemia. It is thought that hemolysis is due to increased oxidative stress on erythrocytes. About one-third of patients with Gilbert's syndrome, an inherited disease associated with high levels of unconjugated bilirubin in an otherwise asymptomatic patient, have an unexplained hemolytic anemia. These obscure causes of Coombs' test–negative hemolytic anemia should not be considered until the more common causes have been ruled out.

APPROACH TO PATIENT WITH COOMBS' TEST-NEGATIVE HEMOLYTIC ANEMIA

On the basis of the patient's history, physical examination, and blood smear, in particular the red cell morphology, a Coombs' test–negative hemolytic anemia can usually be assigned to one of eight categories. These are listed in Table 6-2 along with their associated erythrocyte abnormalities. Confirmatory tests are then performed to define the diagnosis further. For example, a finding of many target cells in a hematologically normal patient with

Approach to patient with Coombs' test-negative hemolytic anemia

I. History
   A. Burns
   B. Cardiac valvular disease or prostheses
   C. Drugs
   D. Family history of anemia, jaundice, splenomegaly, or spherocytosis
   E. Infections, e.g., *Clostridium welchii,* malaria
   F. Hemoglobinuria
   G. Liver disease
II. Physical Examination
   A. Jaundice
   B. Signs of secondary diseases associated with Coombs' test-negative hemolytic anemia
   C. Skeletal and facial abnormalities of congenital hemolytic anemias
   D. Splenomegaly
III. Laboratory Data
   A. Complete blood counts, including WBC, WBC differential, platelet estimation, and Wintrobe indices
   B. Hemoglobin electrophoresis (blacks)
   C. Red cell morphology
   D. Reticulocyte count
   E. Sickle cell preparation (blacks)
   F. Tests for hemolytic anemia as previously outlined in Table 4–1
IV. Tests to be Considered after Initial Evaluation
   A. Determination of P_{50}
   B. Erythrocyte enzyme assays
   C. Family studies
   D. Ham or sugar water test
   E. Heinz body preparation
   F. Hemoglobin A_2 and hemoglobin F assays, HbF cellular distribution
   G. Hemoglobin heat stability or isopropanol tests
   H. Osmotic fragility and autohemolysis
   I. X-rays of skull, hands, and long bones

Table 6-2 : Red Cell Morphologic Abnormalities Associated
with Coombs' Test–Negative Hemolytic Anemias

Anemia	Red Cell Morphologic Abnormalities
Hereditary spherocytosis	Many spherocytes, polychromatophilia
Hereditary elliptocytosis	Many elliptocytes, poikilocytosis
Congenital nonspherocytic anemias	No abnormalities, except possibly burr cells
Hemoglobinopathies	Sickle cells, target cells, and hemoglobin crystals
Thalassemia	Poikilocytosis with target and teardrop cells, hypochromia, microcytosis, and stippling
Hypersplenism	Mild spherocytosis and poly-chromatophilia
Microangiopathic hemolytic anemia	Helmet cells, triangular cells, burr cells, or other fragmented forms
Paroxysmal nocturnal hemoglobinuria	Poikilocytosis, polychromato-philia, and hypochromia

splenomegaly suggests the presence of a hemoglobinopathy. Hemoglobin electrophoresis may confirm the diagnosis of HbC disease.

Indiscriminate laboratory screening without an adequate history, physical examination, or study of the peripheral blood smear is wasteful not only of laboratory resources but also of patients' money. Remember that Coombs' test–negative hemolytic anemias can be secondary to any inflammatory or malignant disease, but a secondary anemia can be diagnosed only after primary hematologic causes have been evaluated and dismissed.

CASE DEVELOPMENT PROBLEMS: COOMBS' TEST-NEGATIVE HEMOLYTIC ANEMIA

Each of the following patients has a Coombs' test–negative hemolytic anemia. Indicate the mechanism(s) for the pathogenesis of the hemolytic anemia in each case.

1. A 35-year-old woman has toxemia of pregnancy and a blood smear showing marked anisocytosis and poikilocytosis with burr cells, triangular forms, and helmet cells.

This patient probably has a microangiopathic hemolytic anemia secondary to toxemia of pregnancy. Some investigators believe that toxemia of pregnancy is due to a vasculitis leading to fragmentation of red cells, which are sequestered and lysed in the reticuloendothelial system of the spleen.

2. A 24-year-old male has anemia and hemoglobinuria. He may have paroxysmal nocturnal hemoglobinuria. Patients with this disease produce red cells that are inordinately sensitive to complement lysis. In many cases complement is activated at night while the patient is asleep, leading to lysis of red cells, free hemoglobin in the serum and urine, and loss of iron. An aplastic bone marrow sometimes complicates the iron deficiency and hemolytic anemia.

3. An 18-year-old boy has a normal hemoglobin, many spherocytes in his peripheral blood, and Howell-Jolly bodies in his red cells.

This patient may have been born with congenital spherocytosis. A splenectomy was done to cure his disease, but this left him with spherocytes in his peripheral blood and Howell-Jolly bodies in his red cells. The latter are remnants of DNA that are seen when the spleen has been removed.

4. A 25-year-old black male patient developed signs, symptoms, and laboratory data diagnostic of a recent acute hemolytic anemia following ingestion of primaquine, but his radiochromium 51 red cell survival is now normal.

This patient almost certainly has glucose-6-phosphate dehydrogenase deficiency. An acute hemolytic crisis was touched off as a result of primaquine ingestion, presumably for the treatment of malaria. In blacks, older cells are destroyed, but younger ones with adequate G-6-PD levels are not lysed. If the red cell survival test is done, even a few days after the acute hemolytic episode, the red cells that are still viable will be young and have a normal survival time. Therefore a normal red cell survival time as determined by radiochromium does not exclude a recent hemolytic episode.

5. A 1-year-old black infant has a hematocrit of 0.25 (25%) and shows no HbS on hemoglobin electrophoresis. One parent has 70 percent hemoglobin S, 10 percent hemoglobin F, and 20 percent hemoglobin A. The other parent has a normal hematocrit and a peripheral blood smear showing target cells, hypochromia, and stippled red cells.

This infant's hemolytic anemia is due to thalassemia major. The parent with sickle cell hemoglobin has sickle cell–thalassemia. When the sickle cell trait interacts with the thalassemia trait, the amount of sickle hemoglobin present is greater than 50 percent. The other parent has thalassemia trait, since he has the typical morphologic changes and a normal hematocrit. One of every four children of this parentage will have thalassemia major with severe anemia in infancy.

6. A 35-year-old white woman takes extremely large amounts of phenacetin for her headaches. Her G-6-PD red cell activity is assayed and found to be elevated.

This Coombs' test–negative hemolytic anemia is due to phenacetin-induced hemolysis. Glucose-6-phosphate dehydrogenase deficiency need not be present for lysis to develop, if erythrocytes are exposed to a high enough concentration of this drug. On the other hand G-6-PD deficiency in whites is associated with hemolytic anemia after exposure to phenacetin. The elevated G-6-PD activity effectively rules out the Mediterranean type of deficiency.

7. A 45-year-old man has an artificial aortic valve and presents with high fever and blood cultures indicating an infection of his valve prosthesis.

This patient's Coombs' test–negative hemolytic anemia could be due to two causes. First, the infected and probably defective artificial valve could be causing fragmentation of red cells and a microangiopathic hemolytic anemia. Alternatively a bacterial infection and associated reticuloendothelial cell hyperplasia could be shortening red cell life span.

8. A 29-year old male alcoholic of Italian extraction presents with jaundice (yellow skin) and an enlarged spleen. Physical examination shows no enlargement of the lymph nodes nor of the liver.

a. What initial laboratory tests would you order?

Hematocrit, Wintrobe indices, white blood cell count, blood smear for morphology and platelet estimation, reticulocyte count, Coombs' tests and fractionated bilirubin levels.

The following laboratory data were obtained:

Hematocrit	0.30 (30%)
White blood count	$3.0 \times 10^9/L$
Blood smear:	hypochromia (MCHC low), target and teardrop cells, stippled red cells, and polychromatophilia
Reticulocyte count	8 percent
Direct Coombs' test:	negative
Bilirubin, direct and indirect	elevated

b. What is your differential diagnosis?

On the basis of information obtained thus far, this patient has a Coombs'-negative hemolytic anemia and a hypochromic anemia. The hemolysis may be due to hypersplenism, hemo-globinopathy, PNH, or thalassemia. The hypochromia may be due to iron deficiency, the anemia of chronic disease, or an iron-loading anemia such as thalassemia or lead poisoning.

c. Would a bone marrow examination be helpful? Why?

It might confirm the diagnosis of hypersplenism, if hyperplasia of the red cells, white cells, and megakaryocytes was seen. Fur-thermore iron stores could be evaluated and ringed sideroblasts searched for. On the other hand there is enough evidence to make the diagnosis of hypersplenism without a bone marrow examination, and a serum iron and total iron-binding capacity might give enough information about iron stores. It would not help in diagnosing a hemoglobinopathy, PNH, nor thalassemia (unless inclusion bodies were found by phase microscopy). A bone marrow examination was performed and serum iron and total iron-binding capacity determined. The bone marrow showed hyperplasia of all three blood cell lines and normal iron stores without ringed sideroblasts. The serum iron was 120 mg per deciliter, and total iron-binding capacity was 290 mg per deciliter.

d. What is the differential diagnosis now, and how would you confirm a suspected diagnosis?

The diagnosis of hypersplenism seems secure. Liver function tests or liver biopsy should be considered to determine whether the patient's alcoholism has led to cirrhosis, portal hyperten-sion, and splenomegaly. A hemoglobinopathy such as hemo-globin C disease might also explain the patient's splenomegaly, but whites seldom have HbC disease. Hemoglobin electrophore-sis would determine this. On the basis of the blood smear alone, thalassemia still must be considered. Determination of hemo-globin A_2 and F levels, along with family studies, is needed to confirm or eliminate this diagnosis. A urine lead level would tell whether the stippled red cells are related to an increased body lead load. PNH is unlikely, since hemoglobinuria, bleed-ing, thrombosis, and iron deficiency are not present.

TOPICS FOR DISCUSSION: COOMBS' TEST-NEGATIVE HEMOLYTIC ANEMIA

Primary defect in hereditary spherocytosis

Relationship of congenital elliptocytosis to congenital spherocy-tosis

Red cell membrane sodium and potassium pumps

Methemoglobins

Structure and function relationships in G-6-PD variants

Abnormalities of glutathione and related enzymes in hemolytic anemia

Primary defect in pyruvate kinase deficiency

Normal hemoglobin structure and function

Hemoglobin structure and the unstable hemoglobinopathies

Hemoglobins with abnormal oxygen affinity

Mild thalassemia syndromes

Mild sickle cell syndromes

Hemoglobin F in thalassemia, sickle cell disease, and other hemoglobinopathies

Treatment of sickle cell disease

Treatment of thalassemia

Molecular basis for thalassemia

Molecular basis for sickle cell disease

Screening methods for thalassemia and sickle cell disease

Genetic counseling in the hemoglobinopathies and thalassemia

Structure and function of spleen

Pathophysiology of hypersplenism

Effect of splenomegaly on hematologic diseases

Splenectomy in congenital enzyme deficiencies

Indications for and complications of splenectomy

Hyposplenism

Role of vascular endothelium and fibrin in microangiopathic hemolytic anemias

Natural history of and etiology of paroxysmal nocturnal hemoglobinuria

Complement lysis in paroxysmal nocturnal hemoglobinuria and Coombs' test–positive hemolytic anemias

SELECTED REFERENCES

General Considerations

Dacie, J. V. *Haemolytic Anemias,* Part I, The Congenital Anaemias, (2nd ed.). New York: Grune & Stratton, 1960.

Dacie, J. V. *The Haemolytic Anaemias,* Part 3, Drug-induced Haemolytic Anaemias, Paroxysmal Nocturnal Haemoglobinuria, Haemolytic Disease of the Newborn. (2nd ed.). New York: Grune & Stratton, 1967.

Dacie, J. V. *The Haemolytic Anaemias,* Part 3, Secondary or Symptomatic Haemolytic Anaemias, (2nd ed.). New York: Grune & Stratton, 1967.

Harris, J. W., and Kellermeyer, R. W. Red Cell Destruction and the Hemolytic Disorders. In J. W. Harris (ed.), *The Red Cell-Production, Metabolism, Destruction: Normal and Abnormal.* Boston: Harvard University Press, 1970.

Jaffe, E. R. Oxidative hemolysis, or "what made the red cell break?." *N. Engl. J. Med.* 286:165, 1972.

Mengel, C. E., Kann, H. E., and Carolla, R. L. Hemolytic Anemia: I. General Considerations, Enzymatic and Membrane Abnormalities, and Nonimmune Acquired Disorders. In C. E. Mengel, et al (eds.), *Hematology: Principles and Practice.* Chicago: Year Book, 1972.

Shohet, S. B. Hemolysis and changes in erythrocyte membrane lipids. *N. Engl. J. Med.* 286:557; 638, 1972.

Weed, R. I. Disease States Resulting from Abnormalities in Hemoglobin Synthesis. In R. I. Weed (ed.), *Hematology for Internists.* Boston: Little, Brown, 1971.

Hereditary
Spherocytosis

Cooper, R. A., and Jandl, J. Erythrocyte Disorders — Anemias Due to Increased Destruction of Erythrocytes With Abnormal Shape and Normal Hemoglobin (Membrane Defects?). In W. J. Williams, E. Beutler, A. J. Erslev, and R. W. Rundles (eds.), *Hematology* (2nd ed.). New York: McGraw-Hill, 1977.

Valentine, W. N. The molecular lesion of hereditary spherocytosis (HS): A continuing enigma. *Blood* 49:241, 1977.

Wintrobe, M. M., et al Hereditary Spherocytosis and Other Hemolytic Anemias Associated with Abnormalities of the Red Cell Membrane. In M. M. Wintrobe, et al (eds.), *Clinical Hematology* (7th ed.). Philadelphia: Lea & Febiger, 1974.

Young, L. E. Hereditary Spherocytosis. In R. I. Weed (ed.), *Hematology for Internists.* Boston: Little, Brown, 1971.

Erythrocyte Enzyme
Deficiencies — Con-
genital Non-
Spherocytic
Hemolytic Anemias

Beutler, E. *Red Cell Metabolism: A Manual of Biochemical Methods* (2nd ed.). New York: Grune & Stratton, 1975.

Beutler, E. Glucose 6-Phosphate Dehydrogenase Deficiency. In W. J. Williams, E. Beutler, A. J. Erslev, and R. W. Rundles (eds.), *Hematology* (2nd ed.). New York: McGraw-Hill, 1977.

Carrell, R. W., Winterbourn, C. C., and Rachmilewitz, E. A. Activated oxygen and haemolysis. *Br. J. Haematol.* 30:259, 1975.

Desforges, J. Genetic implications of G-6-PD deficiency. *N. Engl. J. Med.* 294:1438, 1976.

Miwa, S., Nakashima, K., Ariyoshi, K., Oda, S., and Tanaka, T. Four new pyruvate kinase (PK) variants and a classical PK deficiency. *Br. J. Haematol.* 29:157, 1975.

Valentine, W. Pyruvate Kinase Deficiency; Deficiency of Other Enzymes Leading to Anemia. In W. J. Williams, E. Beutler, A. J. Erslev, and R. W. Rundles (eds.), *Hematology* (2nd ed.). New York: McGraw-Hill, 1977.

Wintrobe, M. M., et al Glucose-6-Phosphate Dehydrogenase Deficiency and Related Deficiencies Involving the Pentose Phosphate Pathway and Glutathione Metabolism. In M. M. Wintrobe, et al (eds.), *Clinical Hematology* (7th ed.). Philadelphia: Lea & Febiger, 1974.

Wintrobe, M. M., et al Hereditary Hemolytic Anemias Associated Mainly with Abnormalities in the Glycolytic Metabolic Pathway of Enythrocytes.

In M. M. Wintrobe, et al (eds.), *Clinical Hematology* (7th ed.). Philadelphia: Lea & Febiger, 1974.

Hemoglobinopathies   Bertles, J. F. Hemoglobin interaction and molecular basis of sickling. *Arch. Intern. Med.* 133:538, 1974.

Bradley, T. B., and Ranney, H. M. Acquired disorders of hemoglobin. *Prog. Hematol.* 8:77, 1973.

Brewer, G. J. A view of the current status of antisickling therapy. *Am. J. Hematol.* 1:121, 1976.

Bromberg, P., et al Hemolytic Anemia III; Hemoglobin and Its Abnormalities. In C. E. Mengel, et al (eds.), *Hematology: Principles and Practice.* Chicago: Year Book, 1972.

Bunn, F. H., Forget, B. G., and Ranney, H. M. *Hemoglobinopathies.* Philadelphia: W. B. Saunders, 1977.

Charache, S. The treatment of sickle cell anemia. *Arch. Intern. Med.* 133:698, 1974.

Gordon-Smith, E. C. and White, J. M. Oxidative haemolysis and Heinz body haemolytic anaemia. *Br. J. Haematol.* 26:513, 1974.

Huntsman, R. G., and Lehmann, H. Treatment of sickle-cell disease. *Br. J. Haematol.* 28:437, 1974.

LaCelle, P. L. The Heinz Body Disorders. In R. I. Weed, (ed.), *Hematology for Internists.* Boston: Little, Brown, 1971.

Lehmann, H., et al Erythrocyte Disorders — Anemias Related to Abnormal Globulin. In W. J. Williams, E. Beutler, A. J. Erslev, and R. W. Rundles (eds.), *Hematology* (2nd ed.). New York: McGraw-Hill, 1977.

McCurdy, P., et al Hemoglobin S-G (S-D) syndrome. *Am. J. Med.* 57:665, 1974.

Miller, D. R., and Lichtman, M. A. Clinical Implications of Altered Affinity of Hemoglobin for Oxygen. In R. I. Weed (ed.), *Hematology for Internists.* Boston: Little, Brown, 1971.

Murayama, M. Molecular mechanism of red cell sickling science. *Science* 153:145, 1966.

Powars, D. R. Natural history of sickle cell disease — the first ten years. *Semin. Hematol.* 12:267, 1975.

Ranney, H. M. (ed.). Hemoglobinopathies. *Semin. Hematol.* 11:383, 1974.

Ranney, H. M., and Nagel, R. L. Drug-induced oxidative denaturation of hemoglobin. *Semin. Hematol.* 10:269, 1973.

Smith, R. P., and Olson, M. V. Drug-induced methemoglobinemia. *Semin. Hematol.* 10:253, 1973.

Steinberg, M. H., Dreiling, B. J., Morrison, F. S., and Necheles, T. Mild sickle cell disease. Clinical and laboratory studies. *J.A.M.A.* 224:317, 1973.

Weatherall, D. J. (ed.) Haemoglobin: Structure, function and synthesis. *Br. Med. Bull.* 32:193, 1976.

Wintrobe, M. M., et al The Hemoglobinopathies: Structural Abnormalities in Globin; General Principles, Unstable Hemoglobin Disease; Hemoglobinopathies S,C,D,E, and O, and Associated Diseases. In M. M. Wintrobe et al (eds.), *Clinical Hematology* (7th ed.). Philadelphia: Lea & Febiger, 1974.

Thalassemia

Benz, E. J., Jr., and Forget, B. G. Molecular genetics of the thalassemia syndromes. *Prog. Hematol.* 9:107, 1975.

Forget, B. G., and Kan, Y. W. Thalassemia and the Genetics of Hemoglobin. In D. G. Nathan and F. A. Oski (eds.), *Hematology of Infancy and Childhood*. Philadelphia: W. B. Saunders, 1975.

Orkin, S. H., and Nathan, D. C. The thalassemias. *N. Engl. J. Med.* 295: 710, 1976.

Pearson, H. A., and O'Brien, R. T. The management of thalassemia major. *Semin. Hematol.* 12:255, 1975.

Wasi, P. Is the human globin α-chain locus duplicated? *Br. J. Haematol.* 24:267, 1973.

Weatherall, D. J. The Thalassemias. In W. J. Williams, E. Beutler, A. J. Erslev, and R. W. Rundles (eds.), *Hematology* (2nd ed.). New York: McGraw-Hill, 1977.

Weatherall, D. J., and Clegg, J. B. *Thalassaemia Syndromes* (2nd ed.). Oxford, Engl.: Blackwell, 1972.

Weatherall, D. J., and Clegg, J. B. Hereditary persistence of fetal haemoglobin. *Br. J. Haematol.* 29:191, 1975.

Spleen and Hypersplenism

Aster, R. H. Platelet sequestration studies in man. *Br. J. Haematol.* 22: 259, 1972.

Crosby, W. H. Hypersplenism. In W. J. Williams, E. Beutler, A. J. Erslev, and R. W. Rundles (eds.), *Hematology* (2nd ed.). New York: McGraw-Hill, 1977.

Diamond, L. K. The concept of functional asplenia. *N. Engl. J. Med.* 281:958, 1969.

Jacob, H. S. Hypersplenism: Mechanisms and management. *Br. J. Haematol.* 27:1, 1974.

Spencer, R. P., and Pearson, H. A. The spleen as a hematological organ. *Semin. Nucl. Med.* 5:95, 1975.

Weed, R. I. Determinants of Erythrocyte Survival in Hemolytic States: Indications for Splenectomy. In R. I. Weed (ed.), *Hematology for Internists*. Boston: Little, Brown, 1971.

Weiss, L. A scanning electron microscopic study of the spleen. *Blood* 43:665, 1974.

Wintrobe, M. M., et al The Reticuloendothelial (Mononuclear Phagocyte) System and the Spleen; Disorders Primarily Involving the Spleen. In M. M. Wintrobe, et al (eds.), *Clinical Hematology* (7th ed.). Philadelphia: Lea & Febiger, 1974.

Microangiopathic Hemolytic Anemia

Brain, M. C. Microangiopathic hemolytic anemia. *Annu. Rev. Med.* 21: 133, 1970.

Marsh, G. W., and Lewis, S. M. Cardiac haemolytic anemia. *Semin. Hematol.* 6:133, 1969.

Wintrobe, M. M., et al The Red Cell Fragmentation Syndromes. In M. M. Wintrobe, et al (eds.), *Clinical Hematology* (7th ed.). Philadelphia: Lea & Febiger, 1974.

Paroxysmal

Rosse, W. F. Paroxysmal Nocturnal Hemoglobinuria. In W. J. Williams, E. Beutler, A. J. Erslev, and R. W. Rundles (eds.), *Hematology* (2nd ed.). New York: McGraw-Hill, 1977.

202

Paroxysmal Nocturnal Hemoglobinurias

Wintrobe, M. M., et al Paroxysmal Nocturnal Hemoglobinuria (PNH). In M. M. Wintrobe, et al (eds.), *Clinical Hematology* (7th ed.). Philadelphia: Lea & Febiger, 1974.

Miscellaneous Coombs' Test Negative Hemolytic Anemias

Beutler, E. Erythrocyte Disorders: Anemias Related to Erythrocyte Damage Mediated by Chemicals. In W. J. Williams, E. Beutler, A. J. Erslev, and R. W. Rundles (eds.), *Hematology* (2nd ed.). New York: McGraw-Hill, 1977.

Davidson, R. J. L. Phenacetin-induced haemolytic anaemia. *J. Clin. Pathol.* 24:537, 1971.

Deiss, A., Lee, G. R., and Cartwright, G. E. Hemolytic anemia in Wilson's disease. *Ann. Intern. Med.* 73:413, 1970.

Jacob, H. S., and Amsden, T. Acute hemolytic anemia with rigid red cells in hypophosphatemia. *N. Engl. J. Med.* 285:1446, 1971.

Manzler, A. D., and Schreiner, A. W. Copper induced acute hemolytic anemia. A new complication of hemodialysis. *Ann. Intern. Med.* 73:409, 1970.

Mayer, K., and Ley, A. B. Hemolysis of red cells due to sulfone. *Ann. Intern. Med.* 72:711, 1970.

Ritchie, J. H., Fish, M. B., McMasters, V., and Grossman, M. Edema in hemolytic anemia in premature infants. *N. Engl. J. Med.* 279:1185, 1968.

Rosse, W. F. Erythrocyte Disorders — Anemias Related to Mechanical Damage to Erythrocytes. In W. J. Williams, E. Beutler, A. J. Erslev, and R. W. Rundles (eds.), *Hematology* (2nd ed.). New York: McGraw-Hill, 1977.

Sturgeon, P. Hematological observations on the anemia associated with blood type Rh_{null}. *Blood* 36:310, 1970.

7 : Aplastic Anemia, Blood Banking, and Secondary Anemias

APLASTIC ANEMIA

Anemia secondary to a reduction in bone marrow cellularity, particularly of erythroid elements, is called *aplastic anemia.* Patients with aplastic anemia usually are *pancytopenic* — that is, all three major blood elements, red cells, white cells, and platelets are reduced or absent in them. In some patients the bone marrow is totally devoid of erythroid, myeloid (white cell), and platelet precursors. In others the cellularity is only reduced, or there are focal areas of acellular marrow intermixed with areas of normal cellularity or even hypercellularity. Unfortunately the term *aplastic anemia* is sometimes used synonymously with pancytopenia. For example, pancytopenia and a hypercellular bone marrow is referred to as *aplastic anemia with hypercellular bone marrow.* For the purposes of this discussion patients diagnosed as having aplastic anemia have reduced or absent bone marrow precursor cells. The terms *aplasia, aplastic,* and *hypoactive* refer to bone marrows that have little or no cellularity and *hyperplasia, hyperplastic,* and *hyperactive* refer to increased marrow cellularity. Hyperplasia or hypoplasia of one of the three major blood elements is called *erythroid, myeloid,* or *megakaryocytic hyperplasia* or *hypoplasia.* Biopsy specimens or clot sections should be used to confirm the diagnosis of hyper- or hypocellularity of one or more marrow cell lines.

Bone Marrow Stem Cell Physiology

Continued production of blood cells by the bone marrow depends on the presence of *stem cells,* which have two important characteristics: (1) the potential to divide (proliferate) and ultimately mature (differentiate) into functional cells, such as hemoglobin-containing erythrocytes, and (2) the unique ability to divide and produce cells identical to themselves. Without the latter characteristic the bone marrow would quickly become deficient in the precursor cells necessary for continued proliferation and maturation of marrow cells.

Data from various experiments suggest that stem cells vary in their potential for producing various cell lines. This implies that as stem cells differentiate, they lose certain potentialities. Until recently stem cells were a physiologic concept, but now certain lymphocytoid cells are suspected of being *pluripotential* or of limited potential, *committed stem cells.* A simplified diagram of the relationships between various types of stem cells and their corresponding mature cell lines is shown in Figure 9.

The evidence for a stem cell with the potential to produce erythroid, myeloid, and megakaryocytic stem cell lines is derived from at least two sources. Marrow cells injected into lethally irradiated mice produce splenic colonies, each derived from a single cell, as determined by cytogenic studies. Each colony may contain erythrocytes, neutrophils (mature white cells), or megakaryocytes. The single cell producing such colonies is called a *colony-forming unit* (CFU). Other evidence comes from study of patients with chronic myelocytic leukemia (CML), whose erythroid, neutrophilic, and megakaryocytic cell lines contain an abnormal chromosome (Philadelphia) but whose lymphoid line is devoid of this abnormality.

The evidence for the existence of committed stem cells is reviewed in Chapters 1 (Anemia) and 8 (Leukocytes). Figure 9 represents one viewpoint derived from many complicated and difficult-to-interpret experiments.

Etiology of Aplastic Anemia

Aplastic anemia may be the result of injury to stem cells, so that these unique cells cannot reproduce themselves, and failure of one or more marrow cell lines results. The cellularity of the bone marrow is reduced, leading to anemia, neutropenia, or thrombocytopenia. Drugs, x-irradiation, viruses, or congenital defects could cause injury to stem cells.

Injury to the bone marrow's microcirculation might also cause aplastic anemia. Evidence supporting this theory comes from studies of animals whose bone marrows have been irradiated. For example, in one study a radioactive beam was used to produce a pencil-thin aplasia in the bone marrow of mice. Active hematopoiesis was present outside the irradiated area but did not recur within the exposed area, presumably because of destruction of the microcirculation necessary to support marrow growth. Similarly, after local irradiation of marrow there is prompt initial aplasia resulting from damaged differentiated elements and stem cells. This is followed by recovery, presumably by migration of normal stem cells from nonirradiated areas. However, 2 to 4 weeks later aplasia in the irradiated area recurs secondary to death of the more slowly proliferating and less radiation-sensitive cells responsible for maintenance of the marrow's microcirculation. One ultrastructural study of marrow microcirculation in patients with aplastic marrows, however, revealed no differences from normal.

A small group of patients has been described who have aplasia of

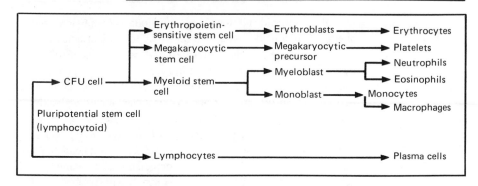

Fig. 9 : Simplified diagram of stem and mature cell interrelationships. [Adapted from Wintrobe, M. M., et al (eds.), Clinical Hematology, 7th ed. p. 52. Philadelphia: Lea & Febiger, 1974.]

only the erythroid cell line. These individuals are characterized by anemia, reticulocytopenia, and severe hypoplasia or aplasia of the marrow erythroid cells. This *pure red cell aplasia (PRCA)* has been seen in association with tumors of the thymus gland; drugs, such as chloramphenicol, sulfa drugs, benzene, and diphenylhydantoin (Dilantin); and various malignancies, including leukemia. Immunologic abnormalities have been postulated as the cause of idiopathic and thymoma-associated PRCA. Cytotoxic IgG autoantibodies directed against erythroblasts and, in one case, an antibody to erythropoietin have been detected in some patients with acquired PRCA.

Preleukemia, hypogammaglobulinemia, paroxysmal nocturnal hemoglobinuria, carcinomas, and viral infections, including hepatitis and infectious mononucleosis, have all been associated with aplastic anemia, but the pathogenesis of the stem cell injury is unknown.

Diagnosis of Aplastic Anemia

The clinical diagnosis of aplastic anemia is usually based on the presence of an insidiously developing anemia or other cytopenia(s) along with a hypocellular bone marrow. Examination of a marrow biopsy specimen shows large areas of acellular stroma and fat with clusters of lymphocytes, reticulum cells, and plasma cells. The reticulocyte count is usually low. Serum iron is increased, and transferrin saturation may be 50 percent or greater. Ferrokinetic studies reveal slow disappearance of iron from plasma, decreased uptake of radioiron by the marrow, and decreased incorporation of iron into circulating erythrocytes.

The anemia is usually normochromic and normocytic; however, there may be macrocytosis despite normal vitamin B_{12} and folic acid levels. Fetal hemoglobin levels may be elevated, particularly in children, for whom elevated levels (> 0.4 gm per deciliter) are associated with a better prognosis. Erythropoietin levels are high.

Splenomegaly is present only occasionally. In patients with cytopenia(s) and splenomegaly, causes of hypersplenism such as leukemia, lymphoma, or miliary tuberculosis should be suspected. As these diseases usually do not present with hypoplasia of the marrow, bone marrow examination should eliminate any confusion with aplastic anemia.

Radioactive tracers that localize in normally functioning marrow have been used to demonstrate functional marrow aplasia and to define its severity. In normal marrow, normoblasts take up radioactive iron (^{59}Fe). Its uptake can be measured by use of an Anger γ-ray camera. A photograph from this camera anatomically locates normally functioning marrow sites in ribs, skull, vertebrae, and proximal long bones. Scintillation counters can also be used as probes over bone marrow, liver, and spleen to measure the radio-activity at these sites: they detect uptake of injected radioiron by normal marrow cells or, in aplastic anemia, by the liver. Indium III chloride, a lower energy γ-emitter than ^{59}Fe, is also taken up in normally active marrows by either erythroid or reticuloendo-thelial cells, and scintillation scanners can be used to locate ^{111}In activity. Indium III chloride and radioiron studies of patients with aplastic anemia show decreased radioactivity in bones normally containing functioning marrow.

Drug-Induced Aplastic Anemia

The following drugs (p. 208) are known to cause marrow aplasia (and drugs chemically related to those listed are also often asso-ciated with the disease). Although the evidence is not strong, it is thought that those drugs cause marrow hypoplasia by injury to bone marrow stem cells. The mechanism and nature of the injury are unknown. Congenitally determined host susceptibil-ity to stem cell injury may explain the relative rarity of aplastic anemia in association with these frequently prescribed drugs.

Chloramphenicol, a once widely used antibiotic, suppresses mar-row function in two ways. It causes idiosyncratic aplastic anemia in certain rare individuals who, if they ingest even small amounts of the drug, present weeks or months later with a usually fatal, severe, aplastic anemia, presumably due to irreparable stem cell damage. Study of affected identical twins suggests that a genetic factor is necessary for the development of this idiosyncratic reac-tion. Chloramphenicol also causes marrow suppression in patients taking large cumulative doses of the drug. Typically, after taking 2 gm per day for three weeks, patients develop reticulocytopenia, increased serum iron and transferrin saturation, and ultimately anemia, sometimes followed by neutropenia or thrombocytopenia.

Examination of the bone marrow immediately separates idio-syncratic aplastic anemia from dose-related marrow suppression. When the bone marrow is suppressed, instead of being aplastic it has markedly increased cellularity. Typically there is vacuolization in the nucleus and cytoplasm of early erythroid precursors and often similar vacuoles in myeloid and other marrow cells. In-creased iron stores and ringed sideroblasts may also be seen. Un-like the outcome in idiosyncratic aplasia, all the clinical and bone marrow findings of dose-related suppression are reversed once chloramphenicol therapy has been stopped. Seldom if ever does the patient go on to develop fatal aplastic anemia. There are in-dividual differences in susceptibility to chloramphenicol's ability to suppress marrow function. The rate or extent of the drug's detoxification may partially account for these differences. It has been proposed that abnormalities of mitochondrial protein syn-thesis and mitochondrial ultrastructure, which have been seen

Drugs associated with marrow hypoplasia

   I. Anticonvulsants
- A. Diphenylhydantoin (Dilantin)
- B. Methylphenylethylhydantoin (Mesantoin)
- C. Trimethadione (Tridione)

  II. Antimicrobials
- A. Arsenicals
- B. Chloramphenicol
- C. Quinacrine
- D. Sulfa drugs

 III. Antithyroid Drugs
- A. Carbimazole
- B. Tapazole

 IV. Benzene

  V. Cytotoxic Drugs used in Cancer Chemotherapy

 VI. Colchicine

VII. Hair Dyes

VIII. Hypoglycemic Agents
- A. Chlordiazepoxide (Librium)
- B. Tolbutamide (Orinase)

 IX. Insecticides
- A. DDT
- B. Parathion

  X. Phenylbutazone

 XI. Sulfa Drugs

and described, are the physiologic basis for chloramphenicol's toxicity in marrow.

X-Irradiation-Associated Aplastic Anemia

The aplastic anemia associated with irradiation is probably due to damage to stem cells. With higher doses of radiation, damage also occurs to the vascular microcirculation and stroma of the bone marrow, which are needed to support cellular proliferation. Destruction of these support structures means that the bone marrow eventually cannot be repopulated by the patient's own stem cells or exogenously supplied bone marrow. In some cases of radiation damage the patient dies from complete aplasia; in others sublethal damage to stem cells leads to chronic bone marrow hypoplasia with varying degrees of pancytopenia. Chromosomal abnormalities may be detected even years after radiation exposure. The clinical picture of aplastic anemia secondary to radiation is similar to that of idiopathic aplastic anemia.

Congenital Aplastic Anemia (Fanconi's Anemia)

Fanconi's anemia is an aplastic anemia seen in children and is associated with a familial history of bone marrow hypoplasia. This anemia is often accompanied by multiple congenital abnormalities, such as brown skin pigmentation, hypoplasia of the kidney and spleen, absent thumb or radius, microcephaly, and mental and sexual retardation. Multiple chromosomal abnormalities may be detected in the bone marrow. There is a high incidence of leukemia.

The *Blackfan-Diamond syndrome* or *congenital hypoplastic anemia* affects children in the first two years of life and is characterized by pure red cell aplasia. Usually there is no history of congenital anemia in preceding generations, and major birth defects are absent. Marrows are cellular but devoid of erythroid precursors, and the patients do not have thymomas. The syndrome is usually responsive to treatment with adrenal corticosteroids. Recently an inhibitor of erythropoiesis has been detected in the serum of these patients. It is thought that this inhibitor may block erythropoietin-sensitive stem cell receptor sites, causing decreased responsiveness to the hormone. Finally, cell culture techniques indicate that some patients with the Blackfan-Diamond syndrome have mononuclear leukocytes (lymphocytes) that inhibit erythroid stem cells from normal subjects.

Other Aplastic Anemias

As previously mentioned the diagnosis *aplastic anemia with hypercellular bone marrow* is probably a misnomer. Pancytopenia and hyperplastic bone marrows fall into a heterogenous group of hematologic disorders. Perhaps some are the result of deficient vitamin-like substances, since a few patients respond to Valentine's liver extract. In other cases removal of the spleen induces a remission. When there are ringed sideroblasts in the bone marrow, the diagnosis is *acquired sideroblastic anemia.* A few patients, particularly those exposed to benzene, go on to develop acute leukemia.

Therapy of Aplastic Anemia

Transfusion

Transfusions serve mainly to support patients until they spontaneously recover or respond to androgens or adrenal corticosteroids. Packed red cells are used to maintain the hematocrit at 0.25 (25%) to 0.30 (30%), which will usually keep the patient symptom-free. In cases of severe thrombocytopenia (less than 15–20 $\times$ 10^9 cells per liter), platelets obtained from one (a *single*) donor by plateletphoresis are valuable for preventing or treating hemorrhage. Thrombocytopenic patients with infections or markedly prolonged bleeding times are more likely to bleed. Use of a single donor and continuous flow centrifugation avoids exposure of the patient to many platelet antigens; fewer antibodies are produced, and it is possible to maintain supplies of platelets for a longer period of time. Histocompatibility (see Tissue Typing for Marrow Transplantation) between donor and recipient will further reduce the chance of sensitization of the patient to donor platelets. Once sensitization occurs, fever and a suboptimal rise in platelet count complicates platelet transfusion therapy.

It is possible to collect granulocytes by continuous centrifugation or by use of nylon filters that concentrate leukocytes. Infusion of 5 $\times$ 10^{10} or more white cells daily is required to raise the granulocyte count to about 1,000 per cubic millimeter. A donor with a high white cell count — for example, a patient with chronic myelocytic leukemia or a normal person pretreated with corticosteroids — is used to supply granulocyte transfusions for treatment of life-threatening infections.

Antibiotics

Prophylactic treatment of aplastic anemia patients with antibiotics is not recommended. Instead, complete bacteriologic evaluation should be undertaken whenever one of these patients presents with fever; and infection, if present, must be vigorously treated. Bowel sterilization with nonabsorbable antibiotics has been tried in an effort to prevent infectious complications but no dramatic benefits have been reported from it. Similarly, complete bacteriologic isolation of patients has not prolonged their survival and has reduced important interpersonal contacts between family, physician, and patient. Face masks, careful washing of hands, and avoidance of infected individuals, rather than total isolation, should be tried. It is possible that further development of laminar flow rooms (Chapter 8, p. 261) and *life islands* will decrease the incidence of infectious complications.

Adrenal
Corticosteroids

Except as therapy for the Blackfan-Diamond syndrome, adrenal corticosteroids have played little role in the induction or maintenance of remissions from aplastic anemia. Steroids may reduce vascular fragility and prevent hemorrhage due to low platelets. Balanced against this undocumented benefit are the side effects of corticosteroids, including Cushing's syndrome, duodenal ulcers, and enhanced susceptibility to infections. Except possibly for the treatment of severe thrombocytopenia, steroids are not recommended.

Splenectomy

Some patients have reduced transfusion requirements following splenectomy. The rare patient has gone into complete remission, suggesting that the spleen had been producing a humoral factor which caused bone marrow suppression. In patients with severe thrombocytopenia and massive transfusion requirements splenectomy may be of benefit.

Androgens

Androgens appear to induce remission in some cases of aplastic anemia. Granulocytopenia and thrombocytopenia are often ameliorated as well. Patients with hypocellularity of the bone marrow rather than complete aplasia are more likely to respond. Androgens are probably effective because of their ability to raise erythropoietin levels to supernormal heights. They may also increase responsiveness of erythroid precursors to erythropoietin. Oxymetholone, 100 mg a day by mouth, or intramuscular injections of testosterone enanthate, 200 mg per week, have been recommended. Some of the observed benefits may be due to the ability of these agents to reduce plasma volume and thereby increase the hematocrit without any substantial effect on red cell mass. In general a therapeutic trial should be carried out for 2 to 3 months before one considers abandoning it in the absence of a response. Side effects include masculinization in the female, increased libido, liver function abnormalities, and fluid retention. In general the judicious use of transfusion therapy combined with androgens has led to long-term survival for patients with aplastic anemia — in some cases, to complete or partial remission.

Bone Marrow
Transplantation

Recent reports suggest that it is feasible to infuse bone marrow from an identical twin or from an individual with similar tissue antigens into a patient with aplastic anemia. The marrow donor is usually a sibling (results with identical twins are best) matched with the patient for the major human histocompatibility loci (Human Leukocyte Antigen, or HLA) and by mixed leukocyte culture (MLC) tests. To prevent rejection of the bone marrow, patients are pretreated with immunosuppressive drugs such as cyclophosphamide and, after grafting, may be given other drugs, such as methotrexate to prevent a graft-versus-host (GVH) reaction. The GVH reaction is characterized by fever, rash, diarrhea, and liver dysfunction, and in severe cases it is usually fatal. Single donor, and if possible HLA-matched, platelet transfusions and frozen, washed, red cells are used before and after grafting to decrease exposure to foreign tissue antigens. The complications of aspirating large amounts of marrow from various bones have been few, although the process is time-consuming and physically taxing for donor and surgeons. Besides GVH disease, cytomegalic virus infection, probably causing interstitial pneumonia, and other infectious agents complicate the clinical course of the graft recipient. As more experience is obtained and it becomes possible to suppress immunologic response without drastically altering the host's resistance to infection, bone marrow transplantation will become the treatment of choice for severe aplastic anemia.

Tissue Typing for Marrow Transplantation

The HLA system plays a major but not yet completely defined role in human allograft responses. HLA antigens are inherited independently of major antigenic systems such as blood groups and platelet antigens. Platelets do carry HLA antigens, but red cells do not. The HLA region in human chromosomes has at least two loci* (A and B) that are inherited together, that is, very closely *linked*. As diagrammed in Figure 10 one set of loci is inherited from each parent. Therefore, only one of every four children is likely to be HLA-identical. It is also clear that children seldom have the same phenotype as their parents. Phenotypes are detected by immunologic reaction with typing sera obtained from individuals sensitized to tissue antigens by pregnancy or prior transfusion.

Besides HLA compatibility, blood group compatibility between donor and recipient is usually required. Graft rejection or graft-versus-host reactions can occur as a result of differences between non-HLA loci that are undetected by current techniques.

Mixed lymphocyte or leukocyte culture (MLC) tests are also performed prior to grafting. These tests determine whether histocompatibility exists and, if not, whether the recipient's lymphocytes can "turn on" and produce cytotoxic antibodies in response to incompatibility. *Stimulating cells,* irradiated, killed, donor lymphocytes, are mixed in tissue cultures with *responding cells,* living, recipient lymphocytes. If the responding, recipient's cells recognize a stimulating, donor cell antigen(s) as foreign, the responding cell will incorporate increased amounts of radiolabeled

*A description of the true complexity of the HLA system is given in Bach, F. H., and van Rood, J. J., The major histocompatibility complex — genetics and biology, *New England Journal of Medicine* 295:806–812, 872–878, 927–936, 1976.

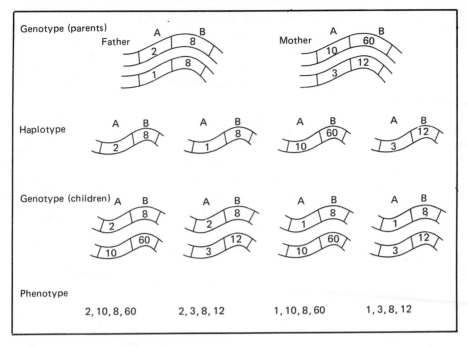

Fig. 10 : Inheritance of HL-A subtypes.

thymidine into DNA. An increase in thymidine incorporation indicates nonhistocompatibility and the possibility of a graft-versus-host reaction. The MLC genetic locus is closely linked to the HLA loci, so that HLA-compatible individuals are usually MLC-compatible unless the rare event, crossing over, has occurred.

Approach to Patient with Aplastic Anemia

The history and bone marrow examination are most important in the study of a patient with suspected aplastic anemia. An anemia characterized by a low reticulocyte count and production index along with (an)other cytopenia(s) is often due to marrow aplasia, particularly if splenomegaly is not present. Examination of the peripheral blood and bone marrow confirms the destruction of hematopoietic elements and effectively rules out megaloblastic, myelophthisic, and hypersplenic anemias. Drug, x-ray, and occupational exposures most frequently define the cause for marrow damage, although often no etiologic agent is uncovered.

Case Development Problems: Aplastic Anemia

A 22-year-old woman with a history of chronic urinary tract infections since childhood presents with acute pyelonephritis (kidney infection) due to an organism that is sensitive only to chloramphenicol. She is treated with this drug in a moderately high dosage. At the end of the second week of treatment her hematocrit has fallen from a normal level to 0.25 (25%) and her white blood count is 2.8×10^9 per liter with 30 percent neutrophils; her platelet count is 20×10^9 per liter. She has taken no other drugs and has not been exposed to x-irradiation. Her physical examination is entirely normal. Peripheral blood smear shows reduced platelets and granulocytes but no immature white cells.

1. What laboratory tests would you do, and what would be the most likely results of these tests?

   The most likely cause for the pancytopenia is the dose-related, reversible, bone marrow suppression caused by chloramphenicol. The reticulocyte count would be low, serum iron level elevated, and total iron-binding capacity near saturated. Bone marrow examination usually reveals a hypercellular marrow with vacuolated erythroid and possibly granulocyte precursors.

With cessation of antibiotic therapy her blood counts return to normal. Three months later, however, because of symptoms of an upper respiratory tract infection, she medicates herself with leftover chloramphenicol tablets. Six months after that she is again found to be pancytopenic, with a hematocrit of 0.20 (20%) and a white blood count of 1.0×10^9 per liter with less than 10 percent neutrophils. Her platelet count is 20.0×10^9 per liter. Upon examination the bone marrow is found to be completely aplastic

Approach to patient with aplastic anemia

I. History
   A. Drugs, toxins, other marrow-suppressive agents
   B. Hepatitis
   C. Occupational history, exposure to solvents, pesticides, dyes, etc.
   D. X-irradiation
II. Physical Examination
   A. Bleeding manifestations
   B. Infection
   C. Lymphadenopathy
   D. Splenomegaly
III. Laboratory Tests
   A. Blood counts and peripheral blood smear
   B. Bone marrow examination
   C. Chest x-ray (thymoma)
   D. Hemoglobin F
   E. Reticulocyte count (and production index)
   F. Sugar water or Ham test

with only lymphocytes, plasma cells, and reticulum cells visible, except for a very few erythroid and myeloid precursors.

2. What abnormalities would you expect in the physical examination, serum iron level, total iron-binding capacity, reticulocyte count, erythropoietin level, and radioiron kinetics?

Her physical examination would show evidence of bleeding, including petechiae and purpura, and possible mild splenic enlargement. Serum iron would be high and total iron-binding capacity saturated. The reticulocyte count would be very low, perhaps down to 0.1 percent. Radioiron kinetics would show prolonged plasma iron clearance, failure of radioactive iron to appear in peripheral blood erythrocytes, and a near-normal red cell life span. Marrow scanning would show little or no uptake in marrow-bearing areas such as the pelvis, vertebrae, and ribs. Some uptake would be seen in the spleen, where islands of myeloid metaplasia might be responsible for erythropoietic activity. Her erythropoietin level would be very high.

The diagnosis is aplastic anemia secondary to an idiosyncratic reaction to chloramphenicol. Because of the low platelet count and evidence of bleeding into the skin and mucous membranes, platelet transfusions are requested.

3. Who would be the optimal donor(s) for these platelets, and if they are unavailable, what other donor(s) should be used?

The optimal donor for platelets is an HLA-identical donor, most likely a sibling of the patient. Platelets from such a donor are likely to produce a good recovery and allow chronic administration for months or longer. If platelets are used from random donors, antibodies will develop against multiple platelet antigens: in time infusion of platelets will yield little rise in the platelet count; and after weeks or months there may be febrile reactions without any platelet rise. If an HLA-identical donor is not available, platelets may be obtained from a single donor by plasmaphoresis, using a cell separator. In this way the recipient is exposed to platelet antigens from only one individual. If he becomes sensitized to the platelets from one donor, then another can be used. The use of plateletphoresis from one individual at a time makes it possible to prolong the period during which platelet transfusions can be given to a patient with chronic aplastic anemia.

The patient's ABO blood type and Rh type are determined. Her blood is cross-matched with several donors, and because of her anemia she receives several units of packed red cells over a period of weeks. Following the last transfusion she develops fever and abdominal pain, and is found to be excreting red urine.

4. What tests would you order, and what results would you expect?

The patient is probably having a hemolytic transfusion reaction. The first step in the investigation of transfusion reactions is to look for evidence of hemolysis. A sample of the patient's plasma, perhaps from a microhematocrit tube, and a urine sample should be tested with benzadine tablets for the presence of blood. In hemolytic transfusion reactions, both specimens react positively. Serum haptoglobins should be low and the methemalbumin test positive. The direct Coombs' test may give positive results during the first day or so following the administration of the incompatible blood; the indirect Coombs' test should be positive.

Testing documented the presence of a hemolytic transfusion reaction. The patient's indirect Coombs' test results were positive.

5. How would you obtain blood for further transfusions?

The first step is to find out which antibody caused this transfusion reaction. By reacting the serum with a panel of red cells carrying known antigens, the specificity of the antibody can be determined. If, for example, the patient has a Kell antibody, then we would expect her serum to react with all cells in the panel having Kell antigen and not with Kell-negative cells. Once the specificity of the antibody is determined, then red cells lacking this antigen can safely be transfused into this patient. Antibody production by aplastic anemia patients can sometimes be prevented by completely typing the patient's red cells and avoiding transfusion with red cells containing antigens that her own cells lack.

6. Besides supportive transfusion with red cells, platelets, and perhaps granulocytes, and treatment of infections with antibiotics, what other therapy can be offered?

A trial of androgen therapy is useful, particularly if some normal erythroid, myeloid, or megakaryocytic elements are present. Complete aplasia carries a very grave prognosis. Usually a reticulocyte response appears first, followed by improvement in white cell and platelet counts. It is unusual for complete remission to occur. If a patient fails to respond and gives no sign of remission, marrow transplantation from an identical twin or an HLA-matched sibling should be seriously considered. Early transplantation has been suggested for complete marrow aplasia and hepatitis-associated aplastic anemia.

BLOOD BANKING

ABO Blood Groups The human erythrocyte carries on its cell wall many antigenic substances. The most important antigen system represented is the ABO. Almost all human red cells can be placed in one of four major blood groups, A, B, AB, and O. Red cell type is identified by cell reaction with typing sera. Human red cells that react with anti-A typing serum and not anti-B typing serum are type A. Conversely, cells that react with anti-B typing serum and not with anti-A are type B. Patients who react with both sera belong to type AB, and those who react with neither are type O. Anti-A typing serum contains 17S macroglobulin antibodies to type A antigen, which because of their large size directly agglutinate type A red cells. These agglutinating antibodies are found naturally in patients whose erythrocytes are type B. Patients whose red cells contain type B antigen have in their serum naturally occurring, agglutinating antibodies directed against type A cells. Serum from type AB individuals contain no such agglutinating antibodies; and humans whose red cells react with neither anti-A nor anti-B have serum that contains both anti-A and anti-B. These data are summarized in Table 7–1.

If red cells of known type A or B are available, it is possible to identify the patient's naturally occurring serum antibodies. This *back-typing* is often done to confirm the red cell type. For example, if typing serum indicates that a patient's red cells contain group A, then his serum should agglutinate known group B red cells. If this reaction does not occur, then the original typing is suspect.

The ABO blood group system is most important, because the transfusion of group A red cells into a patient who has anti-A antibody will result in an antigen–antibody reaction the consequences of which can be catastrophic. The patient becomes hypotensive, and renal failure develops secondary to hypotension and other effects of the antigen–antibody reaction. For this reason patients must be transfused with blood that is *ABO-compatible*. Type O cells are compatible with recipient plasma of any ABO type. Patients with type AB erythrocytes have no anti-A or anti-B in their serum and therefore can receive cells from donors with any of the four major ABO blood types without fear of reaction. For these reasons type O individuals are referred to as *universal donors* and type AB as *universal recipients*. They are universal donors or recipients only in regard to the ABO system,

Table 7-1 : ABO Blood Group System

| Cell Type | Typing Sera Reaction | | Serum Antibody |
	Anti-A	Anti-B	
A	+	−	Anti-B
B	−	+	Anti-A
AB	+	+	None
O	−	−	Anti-A, Anti-B

since hemolytic transfusion reactions due to other red cell antigen (or antibody) incompatibility can occur.

The anti-A and anti-B antibodies found normally in human serum are large enough and have enough binding sites so that they can span the distance between corresponding antigenic groups on two red cells. This allows direct agglutination of erythrocytes in vivo; and no other reagents are required in vitro to detect the binding of antibody to red cell antigens. As we will see, this is usually not the case with other blood group systems. In other systems, the antibodies occur only after an antigenic stimulus; and smaller (7S) antibodies are produced that do not directly agglutinate cells with corresponding antigens. The addition of protein or the use of Coombs' reagent may be needed to facilitate agglutination. The mechanisms by which protein facilitates agglutination are not entirely known. There is some evidence that it affects the normal negative charge on red cells, causing a decreased repulsion among erythrocytes. Coombs' reagent contains anti-γ-globulin, which reacts with 7S antibodies attached to red cell antigens. This results in the formation of a matrix between red cells and antibodies and allows agglutination to occur. Probably the major reason for the lack of direct agglutination with most 7S antibodies is that they are too small to span the distance between antigenic groups on different erythrocytes.

The ABO blood groups are inherited. Each individual inherits two genes for expression of blood type, one derived from his father and one from his mother. There are three alleles, A,B, and O, for each of the two genetic loci. A and B are said to be dominant. Thus, a patient who has blood group A may have one or two A genes. If he has only one, the other is O. It is only through family studies that the genotype of an individual can be conclusively determined. Table 7-2 gives a few examples of the possible inheritance of ABO blood types.

Many other blood group systems are known and are still being discovered. These usually are revealed when serum from a patient fails to react in any previously known pattern with a panel of human red cells. Studies are rapidly done to show that its antibodies differ from all other known antibodies. In many cases other antisera are found that can be used to define antigens that are alleles within the newly discovered system. The second most important blood group system, *Rh* or *Rhesus,* was discovered in this manner.

Rh System

As in the ABO system two parental genes determine the antigens of the Rh system on each human red cell. Each gene is more complex, however, because it is expressed on three linked loci. There are many alleles for each of these loci, but we will discuss only the clinically important ones. The loci are referred to as *C, D,* and *E.* C and c are the two important alleles found at the *C* locus. D and d are found at the *D* locus, and E and e at the *E* locus. The alleles in each of the loci on the same chromosome are inherited together. The antigens denoted by the capital letters are said to be dominant. An example of a genotype is *D c e/D C e.* The gene to the left of the slash is contributed by one parent, and that to the right by the other. The phenotype would be DCe. Phenotypes are determined in the laboratory by reacting cells with typing sera, anti-C, anti-c, anti-D, anti-E, and anti-e. Anti-d serum has never been found or made, so the *dd* genotype is inferred if reaction with anti-D is negative. In the example here the phenotype of the *C* locus is C, (the dominant allele) even though only one C allele is present. Only when there are two c's present will the phenotype be c. The phenotype of the *E* locus in this example is e. There are methods for determining the genotype from the phenotype with some degree of probability, but these will not be discussed here.

Usually a person does not have antibodies that correspond to antigens in the Rh system, unless he or she has previously been sensitized. Sensitization occurs through exposure to red cells containing antigens that a person lacks. For example, a patient who does not have D antigen on his or her red cells can, if exposed to red cells with this antigen, produce anti-D antibody. This antibody will attach to red cells containing the D antigen. The coated cells are destroyed more rapidly than normal, and an antigen-antibody reaction leading to hypotension and renal failure may result. Thus, in this system, the antibodies are produced by prior sensitization and are not naturally occurring. They are 7S bivalent antibodies of smaller size than the ABO agglutinins and cannot usually be detected by direct agglutination of cells of known Rh type. Instead, maneuvers that facilitate agglutination must be performed. In most cases this means that the reaction between a red

Table 7-2 : ABO Genetics: Results of Matings between Individuals with Type AB Erythrocytes and Individuals with Other ABO Types

Phenotype	Genotype	Result of Mating with AB		
		Genotype(s)		Phenotype(s)
A	AO	AA AO	AB BO	A, B, AB
A	AA	AA	AB	A, AB
O	OO	AO	BO	A, B
B	BO	AB AO	BB BO	A, B, AB
B	BB	AB	BB	B, AB

cell carrying D antigen and an antibody such as anti-D will not be detected in vitro, unless it is carried out in high protein solution or in the presence of Coombs' reagent. These maneuvers usually result in agglutination of the type D antibody–coated red cells. Antibodies can be produced which will directly agglutinate D-positive (Rh-positive) erythrocytes suspended in saline. These are used for routine Rh(D) typing.

It turns out that the most important locus in the Rh system is the D locus. Patients who lack the D antigen are referred to as Rh-negative, while those who have this antigen are called Rh-positive. People who are Rh-negative should not be transfused with Rh-positive (D-positive) red cells, because they may become sensitized, produce anti-D antibodies, and, when subsequently exposed to Rh-positive erythrocytes, undergo an antigen-antibody reaction with acute hemolysis and renal failure. Sensitization can occur from prior transfusion or from escape of fetal Rh-positive cells into an Rh-negative mother at the time of delivery. Patients who have been sensitized and produce anti-D antibodies must be transfused with Rh-negative blood, otherwise they will probably have an acute hemolytic reaction.

It is perfectly safe to transfuse Rh-positive individuals with Rh-positive or Rh-negative blood. Although transfusion of Rh-positive blood into Rh-negative individuals should be avoided, it can be done in an emergency, if the patient has not been sensitized previously. Sensitization may or may not result from the first incompatible transfusion, but an acute transfusion reaction usually does not occur. Delayed hemolysis may begin days later and cause hemoglobinuria, bilirubinemia, or even renal failure. In any case all Rh-positive and Rh-negative individuals should be screened to detect the presence of Rh antibodies and antibodies to other blood group antigens such as Kell, Duffy, and Kidd. Most of the other clinically important blood group systems are similar to the Rh system. That is, patients who lack one of the antigens in the system are exposed and sensitized to this antigen by pregnancy or transfusion. Subsequent transfusion of blood to patients carrying such antibodies can cause a hemolytic transfusion reaction. To prevent this, the serum of all recipients must be screened to detect the presence of these *immune antibodies.*

The I–i Blood Group System

Neonatal red cells contain i antigens. With growth of the individual, maturation of an enzyme system takes place, so that I antigen is found on the red cell rather than i. Cold agglutinating antibodies against I antigen may appear following influenza or *Mycoplasma* pneumonia. Anti-i antibodies have been found following infectious mononucleosis. The anti-I cold agglutinin may also appear spontaneously or as part of an immunohemolytic disease, as described in regard to Coombs' test–positive hemolytic anemias, Chapter 5.

Low titers of anti-I, present for whatever cause, may complicate crossmatching. If this antibody is present in a recipient, all donor red cells will be agglutinated, suggesting that the patient cannot be transfused with compatible blood. Blood typing may also be confused, since it will appear that the red cells are being agglutinated by both anti-A and anti-B sera, when in fact they are spontaneously agglutinating because of the anti-I antibody in the recipient's serum. This can lead to serious errors in ABO and RH typing. For this reason part of the crossmatch procedure is observation of a control mixture of the patient's cells and serum for direct agglutination. If such an anti-I antibody is present in the recipient's serum, then all crossmatches will appear to be incompatible. It is possible to get around this problem by carefully washing the potential donor's red cells in warm saline prior to addition of Coombs' reagent in the last step of the crossmatch procedure; this usually makes proper ABO and Rh typing possible. These technical maneuvers are well known to blood bank technicians and can be used to obtain compatible blood. Cold agglutinins should be suspected when a patient's blood type is reported as AB but there has been difficulty in back-typing. They should also be aware that patients with low or moderate titers of cold agglutinins can receive transfusions as long as proper crossmatching has been done and the patient and donor blood cells are kept warm during the transfusion.

Typing and Cross-matching Blood

Mistakes made during the crossmatching procedure can result in catastrophic, acute, hemolytic reactions (discussed, with treatment, later). Therefore hematologists must understand each step of this procedure, which is as follows. After the indications for transfusion of red cells have been reviewed, a sample of the patient's (recipient) blood is sent to the blood bank. There the patient's blood type is determined by testing with commercially prepared anti-A, anti-B, and anti-D typing sera. The blood group is confirmed by back-typing, that is, reacting the recipient's serum with known A and B red cells. Several units of blood obtained from donors of the same ABO and Rh blood type as the recipient are then crossmatched with the donor's blood. A sample of the donor's red cells is reacted with the recipient's serum. This is called the *major side of the crossmatch,* for if there is any incompatibility between the donor's cells and the recipient's serum, all the donor's cells may be lysed or heavily coated with antibody (or complement), which would lead to hemolysis. The *minor side of the crossmatch* refers to the reaction between the donor's serum and the recipient's cells. An incompatibility, other than in the ABO system, detected here is usually not important, since any donor serum containing an incompatible antibody would be rapidly diluted in the patient's own plasma.

If the ABO blood grouping has been correct, there should be no direct agglutination between the donor's cells and the recipient's serum. If the recipient's serum contains 7S antibodies against erythrocyte antigens (due to prior sensitization), no agglutination will be seen, but antibody will have coated the donor's cells. This is detected in the last two steps of the crossmatch. A high concentration of protein (albumin), which promotes agglutination, is added to the mixture, and the cells are observed for agglutination. Then, after careful washing of the red cells to remove any loosely bound γ-globulin, Coombs' reagent is added to promote agglutination of antibody- (or complement-) coated red cells. Similar procedures are performed as part of the major and minor side of the crossmatch, although in many laboratories the final addition of Coombs' reagent is omitted on the minor side. If agglutination is detected during any part of the crossmatch, the donor blood is said to be incompatible and under normal circumstances should not be transfused into the donor. It should be noted that a *direct Coombs' test* (DAT) may not be performed as part of the crossmatch.

So that Rh-compatible red cells will be given to the patient, the Rh group is also determined prior to the crossmatch. Furthermore an *antibody screen,* or what is actually an indirect Coombs' test, is performed on the recipient's serum. To do this *test (or reagent) cell suspension* is made up of erythrocytes from various individuals, so that all clinically important antigens are present. These test cells are reacted with the recipient's serum, and the three steps in the major crossmatch are performed. If agglutination is detected, it is evidence that an antibody to one of the antigens on the test cells is present in the recipient's serum. If the antibody screen is negative, it is unlikely that the major side of the crossmatch will show incompatibility. Occasionally, however, the antibody screen does not pick up an incompatibility, but the major side of the crossmatch does: both procedures therefore are performed as part of all crossmatches.

In summary, then, as part of the crossmatch procedure, the donor and recipients are ABO- and Rh-typed and their sera screened for antibodies. Blood that is ABO- and Rh-compatible with the recipient is then crossmatched by observing for agglutination after direct mixing; after addition of high protein solution; and, finally, when red cells have been thoroughly washed after addition of Coombs' reagent. The washing step prior to addition of the Coombs' reagent is critical. If unbound γ-globulin remains, it will neutralize the Coombs' reagent and lead to a falsely negative Coombs' test.

Blood Transfusion Reactions

There are three common abnormal reactions to the infusion of blood or blood components. The first, hives, is not usually associated with fever nor with evidence of hemolysis. It is easily treated with antihistamines such as Benadryl (50 to 100 mg orally or parenterally).

The second type of transfusion reaction is usually manifested by fever and chills and complicated by bronchial constriction or other signs of anaphylaxis. The first matter of concern is to stop the transfusion and investigate the patient for evidence of hemolysis. Usually hemolysis is not detected, because the fever is caused by white cell or platelet antigen–antibody reactions. These can be prevented by using another donor and by removing the buffy coat from the red cells. Washed or frozen-washed red cells may be required for patients who are particularly sensitive to small quantities of platelet or leukocyte antigens.

The third and most feared type of reaction is the hemolytic transfusion reaction due to infusion of incompatible erythrocytes. It is usually caused by either an error in typing and crossmatching or by misidentification of the recipient. Acute hemolysis with hemoglobinemia and hemoglobinuria can take place immediately, along with fever, abdominal pain, and possibly shock. Another form of hemolytic reaction occurs when blood is crossmatched and infused in an entirely appropriate manner, but a low titer serum antibody in the recipient goes undetected. If the transfused blood contains the corresponding antigen to this antibody, there is an anamnestic response with increase in antibody titer. A *delayed transfusion reaction,* characterized by fever, abdominal pain, chills, and the appearance of red urine, then happens hours or days after the blood infusion. The diagnosis of a hemolytic transfusion reaction is confirmed by spinning down a microhematocrit tube filled with the patient's blood; breaking off the top part of the tube, which contains plasma; and testing the plasma for blood. The patient's urine is spun to bring down red cells, and the supernatant is also tested for blood. Positive results to these tests, particularly the plasma test, indicate a presumed hemolytic transfusion reaction. The antibody screen usually is positive at this time. Any antibody(ies), if present, can be characterized by reacting the patient's serum with a panel of cells containing different, but known, red cell antigens. After the antibody specificity has been identified, red cells lacking these antigens can be transfused safely into the patient.

Treatment of Hemolytic Transfusion Reactions

When the recipient's serum contains antibody against one of the donor's red cell antigens, a reaction between that serum and the donor red cells may result in hypotension (low blood pressure) and renal failure. The renal failure is thought to be secondary to the hypotension and not to the hemoglobin precipitates in the renal tubules. In some cases the acute lysis of donor red cells will lead to the release of thromboplastic substances, triggering disseminated intravascular coagulation. This will lead to a consumption of platelets, fibrinogen, and clotting factors and to bleeding from venipuncture sites and into skin, mucous membranes, and elsewhere. It may be necessary to treat the patient with heparin, an anticoagulant that inhibits intravascular clotting, in order to save his life from acute, diffuse hemorrhage.

After the incompatible transfusion has been stopped, blood pressure stabilized, and the diagnosis of a hemolytic reaction made, some experts advise the use of mannitol. This substance is an osmotic diuretic, and appears to prevent renal failure if renal output is adequate. Mannitol, 25 or 50 gm, mixed with saline or 5% dextrose-in-water solution are infused slowly into the patient. If the patient does not make urine, continued infusion of mannitol may lead to withdrawal of water from the patient's cells and further damage to kidneys and other organs. Therefore, if mannitol and fluids do not induce a diuresis, they should be discontinued, and measures to treat oliguric renal failure and prevent fluid overload instituted. Renal dialysis for removal of toxic substances is often required. If the patient is treated properly, fluid overload prevented, and renal dialysis begun when appropriate, these patients will usually recover without sequelae.

Hemolytic Disease of the Newborn (Erythroblastosis Fetalis)

An Rh-negative mother can be sensitized by the escape into her circulation of Rh-positive cells from her child at delivery. These cells pass through the fetal–maternal circulation and cause the production of anti-D antibody in the mother. The antibody produced is small enough to travel back into the placenta and pass into the fetus during a subsequent pregnancy to cause destruction of fetal red cells, anemia, congestive heart failure, and ultimately death of the infant (hydrops fetalis). Less severe cases result in jaundice at the time of birth with high levels of indirect, unconjugated bilirubin, which may affect brain metabolism and lead to neonatal death or retardation. The sequence of events is usually as follows: The Rh-negative mother has had several pregnancies, during which her Rh-positive children have released red cells into her circulation and sensitized her. With later pregnancies the titer of anti-D in her serum reaches a very high level, passes through the placenta, and causes an acute hemolytic anemia in the fetus. This results in fetal death or neonatal complications of indirect bilirubinemia.

To prevent this sequence of events in Rh-negative mothers, anti-D serum (Rhogam) obtained from previously sensitized individuals is injected into the *mother* immediately after delivery of an Rh-positive child. This prevents sensitization by stopping the D antigen from igniting the mother's immune system. Since anti-D serum must not be given if there is evidence of prior maternal sensitization, the mother's serum and the baby's cord blood are first tested for existence of anti-D. Since some fetal red cells escape into the mother during pregnancy, why doesn't sensitization occur then, prior to delivery? For reasons that are not entirely clear, pregnant women are relatively insensitive to some immune stimuli and therefore do not become sensitized until after delivery.

The serum used to prevent Rh-related erythroblastosis fetalis is known commercially as Rhogam and generically as anti-D or Rh-immune globulin. It must be emphasized that it is administered to the mother and not to the child. Since it is a powerful anti-D antiserum, it will rapidly hemolyze Rh-positive cells. The mother, however, being Rh-negative, will have no reaction to the intramuscular administration of this immune serum. It must be administered within 3 days of delivery to be sure of its effectiveness in preventing sensitization. Normally it is at least 99 percent effective.

A phenomenon similar to that of Rh-mediated erythroblastosis fetalis can occur with ABO incompatibility between baby and mother. For example, a type O mother with a type A child may produce high maternal titers of anti-A of small enough size to pass through the placenta and cause hemolytic anemia in the fetus. These reactions are usually milder than those seen in Rh sensitization. ABO incompatibility can prevent Rh sensitization: since ABO-incompatible fetal cells are rapidly cleared from the mother's blood by isoagglutinins, the chances of her being sensitized to the D antigen on them are decreased. There is no preventing ABO incompatibility, but luckily it is rare and, if recognized, the fetus usually survives and can be treated with phototherapy or exchange transfusion to prevent the development of dangerously high, toxic levels of indirect bilirubin.

Very rarely other blood group antigens cause hemolytic anemia of the newborn, but these will not be discussed here.

Blood Component Therapy

Modern-day blood banking is based on the use of blood components (*component therapy*) rather than whole blood for the treatment of hematologic diseases. Only that component of whole blood that is necessary to treat the patient's particular problem is used. This has many advantages. An important one is that, from a single unit of whole blood, components are available to more than one patient. One patient may receive red cells and another receive platelets or coagulation factors made from the same unit of whole blood.

Packed Red Cells

Reduced red cell mass is better replaced by packed red cells than by whole blood. All patients suffering from anemia, except those undergoing acute blood loss, require only the erythrocytes in a unit (450 ml of blood and 50 ml of anticoagulant) of whole blood and not the plasma or coagulation factors. If plasma is removed prior to transfusion, a decreased quantity of potentially toxic products such as hemoglobin, potassium, citrate anticoagulant, and food or drug allergens is administered. There is unconfirmed evidence that use of packed red cells decreases the incidence of serum hepatitis. Probably 80 to 90 percent of transfusions can be given as packed red cells. Even bleeding patients can receive their first unit of blood as this component, since most individuals can easily replace 250 ml of plasma from extracirculatory stores.

Buffy Coat-Poor Packed Red Cells

By removing not only the plasma but also the buffy coat from whole blood, the number of transfused leukocyte and platelet antigens can be greatly reduced. This is important to patients who have developed antibodies to these blood elements and who have febrile transfusion reactions. Most febrile transfusion reactions that are not hemolytic can be prevented by the use of buffy coat-poor red cells. A certain number of red cells are wasted by removal of the buffy coat, but this is not clinically important.

Washed Red Blood Cells	By washing red cells, either by continuous flow centrifuge or by adding and removing isotonic saline after centrifugation, packed red cells with an even further reduced amount of platelet and leukocyte antigens can be produced. This will decrease the number of antigens delivered to sensitized patients. However, if a continuous flow centrifuge is used, the price of the product is usually quite high. Once the red cells in a unit of blood have been washed, they must be infused within one day or discarded in order to prevent growth of contaminating bacteria. These disadvantages must be considered before ordering washed red blood cells. Often buffy coat-poor red cells, which are no more expensive, much more easily produced, and carry no risk of bacterial contamination, will prevent most febrile transfusion reactions that arise from leukocytes or platelets.

Frozen Red Cells   It is possible to freeze red blood cells by first mixing them with glycerol. The glycerol enters the red cell and prevents the formation of ice crystals, which would rupture the cell membrane. Transfusion of large amounts of glycerol into individuals may be toxic, and for this reason it is necessary to wash red cells thoroughly after they have been frozen and thawed. The washing process is time-consuming, cumbersome, and expensive. Various washing techniques have been developed that use continuous flow centrifugation. The washing procedure results in a product that has a very low quantity of granulocyte, lymphocyte, and platelet antigens and therefore a low incidence of febrile reactions. It also appears to decrease sensitization of individuals to HLA antigens on lymphocytes. In patients who are being prepared for kidney grafts, frozen red blood cells are used to try to prevent production of HLA-related antibodies, which might interfere with grafting. Since freezing and washing reduces the hepatitis risk to nil, high risk areas like kidney transplant centers and such patients as pregnant women who cannot tolerate hepatitis under any circumstances are supplied with frozen blood. The major limiting factors to the use of frozen cells are the time consumed in washing them, so that they are not readily available for emergency situations; their limited shelf life after defrosting, one day; and their cost.

Platelet Transfusions   Platelets are prepared by sedimentation or centrifugation of individual units of blood, removal of the plasma, and subsequent concentration of the platelets into a pellet. They are then resuspended in plasma and pooled prior to infusion. A continuous flow centrifuge is available that separates platelets, white cells, plasma, and red cells. There is gross contamination of one blood product with the other, but large amounts of platelets can be obtained from a single donor. Using a single donor reduces the number of antigens to which a recipient is exposed, thereby allowing him to receive effective platelet infusions for a longer period of time. HLA matching of the donor and the recipient may also allow more frequent and effective platelet transfusion, but it is difficult and expensive to obtain HLA-identical donors.

Platelets are usually administered to thrombocytopenic patients with platelet counts of less than 20×10^9 per liter, to prevent hemorrhage. Some patients who are already bleeding and have platelet counts of less than 50×10^9 per liter, require immediate platelet transfusion. Patients whose platelet function has been adversely affected by agents such as aspirin may require platelet transfusions even though their platelet counts are normal. The amount a unit of platelets (quantity in 450 ml of whole blood) raises the platelet count in a recipient depends on the losses encountered during preparation; on whether the patient is infected or febrile, since platelet life span is then reduced; and on the nature of the disease for which the patient is being treated. In diseases in which there is abnormal platelet sequestration or destruction — for example, hypersplenism or idiopathic thrombocytopenic purpura — the increment in platelets may be low. On the other hand, in patients with aplastic anemia a transfusion of 4 to 6 units will usually result in a platelet count well above 50×10^9 per liter.

Granulocyte Transfusions

Granulocytes can be obtained from normal or leukemic individuals by a continuous flow cell separator or by capture on special nylon filters and subsequent elution. They are best used to treat marked neutropenia, less than 0.5×10^9 cells per liter, or infections in leukopenic patients. They have proved most helpful for patients who have been rendered aplastic by anticancer medications and whose granulocyte counts will presumably be depressed for a limited period of time, rather than chronically, and for patients with aplastic anemia.

Bank Plasma and Albumin

Over a period of hours or days plasma stored in the refrigerator will lose most of its coagulation properties. It can still be used to replace lost blood volume, but it carries a relatively high risk of serum hepatitis. No means of reducing this risk has been demonstrated. For this reason pooling of plasma is not recommended; instead it is suggested that single donor units be used for volume replacement, if hepatitis-free serum albumin solutions are not available.

Hepatitis-free albumin is produced from plasma by Cohn alcohol fractionation. The albumin can be suspended in saline for use as a blood volume expander. Similar solutions of protein, plasminate and plasma protein fraction, have been prepared that contain not only albumin but also other amino acids and contaminants. These solutions are equally efficacious as albumin for restoring blood volume and are hepatitis-free.

Fresh Frozen Plasma (FFP)

Fresh frozen plasma is prepared from donor plasma at the time of phlebotomy. The immediate freezing results in a product that contains all the soluble coagulation factors and that can be used to treat patients with mild or moderate deficits in clotting factors. Plasma that has been stored without freezing for several days may still contain adequate amounts of Factors VII, IX, X, and XI, but *fresh* frozen plasma is absolutely necessary if labile clotting factors, V and VIII, are needed. The major problems with FFP are the volume of plasma required to deliver large quantities of coagulation factors to severely deficient patients and the risk of hepatitis. Unlike the available concentrates of the clinically important factors, fresh frozen plasma units have the advantage of being prepared from a single donor rather than from pools of plasma that may be contaminated with hepatitis virus.

Clotting Factor Concentrates

Factor VIII may be concentrated by freezing a unit of freshly obtained plasma and then allowing it to thaw slowly. A resulting cryoprecipitate is removed by centrifugation. Precipitates are pooled, further concentrated, and lyophilized, so that large concentrations of coagulation Factor VIII are available in small quantities of fluid. Each cryoprecipitate from a single donor contains approximately 75 units of Factor VIII activity, and lyophilized concentrates can contain up to 800 units per vial, which are diluted into 50 ml of fluid. Factor IX concentrates are also available but have an unusually high risk of hepatitis and of thrombosis from activated coagulation factors. They should be used only in emergency situations.

Fibrinogen

Fibrinogen can also be obtained by Cohn fractionation. It has been used in obstetric hypofibrinogenic patients, but carries such a high risk of hepatitis that it is rarely employed today. Units of fresh frozen plasma are recommended instead in the rare instances where fibrinogen replacement is indicated.

Immunoglobulins

Immunoglobulin for passive immunization can also be prepared from plasma. Except for hypogammaglobulinemia it is not used to treat hematologic conditions. It is usually not possible to give an adult enough γ-globulin to obtain clinically detectable levels. In the case of children, however, it is possible and may prevent serious infections in congenitally immunoglobulin-deficient patients.

Fresh Whole Blood

The practice of calling for fresh whole blood (drawn within 24 hours prior to administration) for patients who are bleeding on the operating table is to be condemned. In the past this was used as an expensive panacea for all bleeding problems. It is now clear that such patients must be evaluated by appropriate clotting studies and examination of the blood smear for platelets, so that they can be treated rationally with the component or components they lack.

Two anticoagulant solutions, acid-citrate-dextrose (ACD) and citrate-phosphate-dextrose (CPD), are approved for storage of blood. CPD has several advantages over ACD, including better preservation of 2,3-diphosphoglycerate levels and less acid load on infusion. ACD solution is better for preparation of platelet concentrates, since it causes less platelet clumping.

Case Development Problems: Blood Banking

1. Mrs. Landsteiner's red cells agglutinate when mixed with the plasma obtained from a patient known to have type A blood and another patient known to have type B blood. Mrs. Landsteiner's plasma agglutinates red cells known to be type A and red cells known to be type B. Are these findings expected or unusual? Why?

   The findings are unusual, because her red cells react with anti-A and anti-B, indicating she is blood type AB, but back-typing reveals the presence of anti-A and anti-B in her plasma. These antibodies should not be found in type AB blood. A cold agglutinin might explain these results.

2. Mr. Jones's red cells have been typed as A and Mrs. Jones's as B. One of their children has type O red cells. Can the child really be theirs? Why?

   Yes. Their genotypes may be AO and BO, so that one in four children can be expected to be type O.

3. Mr. Levine, who has type O blood, receives a transfusion from Mr. Weiner, who also has type O blood. A hemolytic transfusion reaction occurs. Since they are both type O, how can you explain the reaction? How would you confirm your hypothesis in the laboratory?

   The reaction is due to a blood group system other than ABO; for example, Rh, Kell, or Duffy. An antibody screen using test cells should demonstrate the presence of an immune antibody.

4. Mr. Smith has a hemolytic transfusion reaction while receiving blood from Mr. Ford, and antibody is detected in Mr. Smith's serum. Using Coombs' reagent, Mr. Smith's serum is reacted with a panel of cells. In the following table, red cell

antigens in each member of this panel are shown, along with an indication of whether agglutination (using Coombs' reagent) occurred or not. What is the likely specificity of this antibody?

Cells	Antigens					Indirect Coombs' Test
	D	c	C	Kell	Duffy	
1	+	+	0	+	+	positive
2	+	0	+	0	+	negative
3	+	+	0	+	+	positive
4	0	+	0	0	+	negative
5	+	+	0	+	0	positive
6	+	0	+	+	0	positive

Anti-Kell

5. How would you crossmatch blood if it were necessary to continue to transfuse this patient?

By using anti-Kell typing sera, ABO- and Rh-compatible cells lacking Kell antigens can be identified and crossmatched with Mr. Smith's blood.

6. Mrs. Fine has blood type A Rh(D)- and gives birth to a child who has blood type A Rh(D)+. She has had several pregnancies. Mrs. Fine's indirect Coombs' test is positive and the child's direct Coombs' test is positive. Can you explain these findings? What is the danger to a subsequent fetus? Will anti-D serum given to the mother prevent these dangers?

Mrs. Fine has been sensitized to red cell antigen D by Rh positive cells from her children, which entered her circulation during delivery. If her anti-D titer rises high enough, hydrops fetalis or jaundice may affect her subsequent fetuses. Since she is already sensitized, anti-D serum (Rhogam) will not prevent these complications.

7. Mrs. Reid has also had several pregnancies and is blood-typed O Rh(D)-. She gives birth to a child who is blood-typed A Rh(D)+. The Coombs' tests done on mother and child both give negative results. Can you explain why Mrs. Reid's Coombs' tests are negative while Mrs. Fine's (question 6) were positive?

The ABO incompatibility between Mrs. Reid's serum (which contains anti-A isohemagglutins) and her present baby's erythrocytes (type A) protects her from fetal-maternal transfusion and sensitization to the D antigen. Rh(D)+ cells will be agglutinated by the anti-A in her serum and removed from her circulation.

8. Mrs. Blank, whose blood type is A Rh(D)– and whose husband has B Rh(D)+, gives birth to a child who has AB Rh(D)–. Is Mr. Blank the father of this child? In this situation, can you predict whether a child will be Rh(D)+ or Rh(D)–?

He may be the father, since his genotype could be D/d for the D sublocus. One-half of pregnancies from mating with phenotype Rh(D)– (genotype *d/d*) will be Rh(D)–. The father's genotype (*D/D* vs. *D/d*) can be predicted from tables available that are based on Rh gene frequencies and require subtyping with anti-E, -e, -C, and -c antisera.

9. The following are commonly available blood components.

Fresh whole blood (drawn less than 24 hours prior to use)
Whole blood
Packed red cells
Buffy coat-poor red cells
Washed packed red cells
Frozen red cells
Fresh frozen plasma
Serum albumin
Bank plasma (single unit)

Which of these blood components would be appropriate for each of the following patients?

a. A 75-year-old patient with chronic aplastic anemia.
b. A 25-year-old man with severe gastrointestinal bleeding.
c. A severely anemic 45-year-old patient with severe renal disease and renal failure.
d. A 24-year-old gastrointestinal bleeder for whom no blood will be available immediately because of difficulty in crossmatching.
e. A 60-year-old woman who has febrile transfusion reactions but in whose plasma no hemolytic antibody can be found.

Answers:

a. Packed red cells
b. Whole blood (packed red cells initially)
c. Frozen red cells (avoid hepatitis and sensitization to HLA antigens)
d. Serum albumin
e. Buffy coat–poor red cells (washed or frozen red cells, if necessary)

10. A 40-year-old man develops fever, chills, and abdominal pain while receiving a transfusion. He suddenly starts bleeding from his nose, mouth, and venipuncture sites. Can you explain this complication?

Disseminated intravascular coagulation has occurred due to release of thromboplastic substances from hemolyzed red cells. It may require treatment with heparin, platelets, or fresh, frozen plasma.

SECONDARY ANEMIAS

Anemia of Liver Disease and Alcoholism

The anemia of alcoholism and liver disease — or, most often, of the two conditions together — is most severe in patients who are bleeding due to such complications as esophageal varices, gastric or duodenal ulcers, or gastritis. Occasionally a patient with chronic cirrhosis presents with a higher than normal PCV, and in such a case a hepatoma should be suspected.

Iron deficiency anemia due to blood loss often complicates and contributes to the anemia of chronic liver disease. Thrombocytopenia secondary to hypersplenism and coagulation factor deficits contributes to the bleeding tendency. Hemodilution due to greater than normal plasma volume also may complicate the anemia of patients who have portal hypertension and enlarged spleens.

In liver disease the red cells are normochromic, and *thin macrocytes* with increased mean cell diameter but normal MCV and target cells (Plate 11) with increased cell diameter and normal MCV are found in the peripheral blood. The macrocytosis is probably related to uptake of cholesterol into the erythrocytes' membranes. Spur or burr (Plate 26) cells are found in more severe forms of liver disease. These poikilocytes have a high cholesterol content in their membranes, are rigid, and undergo splenic sequestration and fragmentation, thereby contributing a hemolytic component to the anemia of chronic liver disease. Very often patients with these marked red cell abnormalities succumb to the liver disease within a year.

Practically all patients with chronic liver disease have a mild decrease in red cell life span associated with reticuloendothelial cell hyperplasia similar to that of the anemia of chronic disease. In Zieve's syndrome there may be marked degrees of hemolysis consisting of jaundice, hyperlipemia (elevated triglycerides), hypercholesterolemia, and hemolytic anemia following binge drinking of alcohol. The decrease in erythrocyte survival has been correlated with increased red cell lipids but not with plasma lipid changes. Its exact pathogenesis is unknown.

Since patients with alcoholism and cirrhosis often have poor dietary intake of folate, unless they drink beer or wine, they often develop megaloblastic anemia secondary to folate deficiency. Beer has some folate, and wine also; however, hard liquors usually have none. Increased erythropoiesis secondary to chronic hemolysis, malabsorption; and abnormal folate metabolism in the liver secondary to alcoholism may also contribute to the deficiency. *Thick macrocytosis,* with increased mean cell diameters and MCVs, along with hypersegmented neutrophils and megaloblastic bone marrows, is commonly prominent in these folate-deficient individuals.

Alcohol may directly suppress the bone marrow. Binge drinking is often associated with vacuolization of erythroid precursors and the presence of ringed sideroblasts (Plate 8). The latter disappear after cessation of alcohol ingestion or after administration of pyridoxal phosphate, suggesting an alcohol-induced defect in heme synthesis. It is possible that in certain cases alcoholism causes permanent damage to the bone marrow, but usually reticulocytosis and return of the hematocrit to normal is seen in patients recovering from a bout of alcoholism.

The response of the bone marrow to the anemia of liver disease is usually not optimal. A normal individual increases bone marrow production of red cells to a far greater degree than the patient with moderate-to-severe cirrhosis. Thus, these patients have some degree of functional bone marrow failure and often have other diseases as well, including infections that suppress the bone marrow. If the underlying liver disease and its complications are treated, the anemia will improve. Unfortunately in many cases the patients continue to drink alcohol and their liver disease, along with their anemia, progress.

The Anemia of Chronic Renal Disease

Patients with chronic renal failure and uremia usually develop anemia when their BUN goes above 40 mg per deciliter, their creatinine above 3 mg per deciliter, and their glomerular filtration rate below 25 percent of normal. The anemia is usually normocytic and normochromic and is associated with reticulocytosis despite the failure of the hematocrit to rise. Although there is a correlation between the severity of renal failure and anemia, in some cases relatively mild renal failure will cause severe anemia.

Bone marrow suppression, perhaps related to decreased production of erythropoietin or unresponsiveness of erythroid precursors to the hormone, appears to be the primary problem in uremic patients. Erythropoietin is produced in the kidney, and patients with diseased kidneys have lower than normal levels of urinary erythropoietin. As some erythropoiesis is maintained in complete renal failure, however, it has been suggested that there are extrarenal sites for its production. Patients without kidneys can have reticulocyte responses to hypoxia; their erythropoietin titers may rise in response to hemorrhage or administration of testosterone; and they manifest a relative hyporesponsiveness of marrow cells to erythropoietin, thought due to toxic metabolites building up in the plasma. Often an increased plasma volume and hemodilution complicates their anemia.

An extracorpuscular hemolytic component is found in patients with chronic renal disease. Reticuloendothelial cell hyperplasia is reportedly present, but its pathogenesis and contribution to the anemia is unknown. Inefficient phosphoglyceromutase activity with diminished activity of the pentose phosphate shunt has been suggested as a metabolic cause of hemolytic anemia in the presence of renal failure. Presumably, the red cells have an acquired metabolic defect that renders them more susceptible to oxidant stresses, including contaminants in hemodialysis fluids such as copper, nitrate, and chloramines. Perhaps related to these observations is the amelioration of anemia in uremic patients following splenectomy. Red cells from these patients have decreased deformability, so it is possible that toxic uremic products lead, via depression of the pentose phosphate pathway and subsequent production of Heinz bodies, to abnormally rigid red cells that cannot pass through splenic sinusoids and are therefore destroyed.

In a few patients hemolytic anemia is overt and severe. In children the combination of severe hemolytic anemia and renal failure is called the *hemolytic-uremic syndrome*. Reticulocytosis and schistocytes (Plate 13), small, irregularly contracted red cells characteristic of a microangiopathic hemolytic anemia, are present. The etiology of this syndrome is unknown and treatment unsatisfactory. Many uremic patients without overt hemolytic anemia also have irregularly contracted red cells in their blood.

Blood loss and iron deficiency anemia may develop from bleeding into the urine, gut, or hemodialysis apparatus. Mild thrombocytopenia and toxic metabolites, such as guanidinosuccinic acid, which reduces platelet function, probably contribute to the bleeding tendency. Dialysis and oral iron therapy are recommended for these complications.

The anemia associated with renal disease is usually ameliorated by dialysis or successful kidney transplantation. Patients who cannot improve by these means can sometimes be helped by administration of androgens. These compounds increase erythropoietin titers to high levels, perhaps by stimulating extrarenal sites of production. Three to six months of androgen therapy is usually required before the hematocrit rises. The usual oral dose is 30 mg of fluoxymesterone per day for men and 10 mg per day for women.

Patients treated by long-term dialysis may lose folate in the dialysis fluid. For this reason they should be maintained on folic acid supplements. Since it is difficult to maintain a hematocrit level by transfusions alone, and the risk of hepatitis is high, blood transfusion is recommended only for severe, symptomatic anemia.

Anemia Associated with Chronic Inflammatory Diseases, Malignancy, and Infection

Patients with the *anemia of chronic disease* usually have a mild-to-moderate, normochromic, normocytic anemia. In some patients the anemia is hypochromic or microcytic. It is often associated with low serum iron levels, low total iron-binding capacities, and transferrin saturations generally above 10 to 15 percent, unless there is concurrent iron deficiency. The hematocrit is usually about 0.30 percent, and the reticulocyte production index is low. The bone marrow is unremarkable, although there may be an increase in plasma cells, reticuloendothelial cells, and eosinophils (*irritated bone marrow syndrome*). Marrow iron stores are usually normal or increased, and most of the iron is in the retriculoendothelial system rather than in the normoblasts. The reason for the failure of transfer of iron from reticuloendothelial cells to normoblasts is unknown. This defect in the release of iron from the reticuloendothelial cells may contribute greatly to the anemia of chronic disease.

Lower than normal erythropoietin production has been reported in patients with chronic diseases, particularly in patients with active rheumatoid arthritis. This abnormality may partially account for the failure of the marrow to respond adequately to the anemia. The anemia often has an extracorpuscular hemolytic component, perhaps due to hyperplasia of the reticuloendothelial system. This hemolytic component is relatively mild and could be compensated for by a normal marrow response, which, however, is not present.

Certainly folic acid deficiency and iron deficiency may complicate anemia associated with chronic inflammatory diseases, malignancy, and infections. For example, in rheumatoid arthritis, excessive aspirin ingestion may lead to gastrointestinal bleeding; in malignancies of the colon, blood loss causes iron deficiency; and in chronic inflammatory diseases, dietary intake of folic acid is poor.

Infiltration of the marrow by malignant cells certainly depresses marrow function. It is not clear whether physical displacement of normal marrow cells or an unknown, toxic substance(s) secreted by these cells, or both, cause this marrow suppression.

Certain infections are associated with specific hemolytic syndromes. Organisms such as *Claustridium welchii* produce hemolysins and lead to lethal intravascular hemolysis. Direct infection of erythrocytes by *Bartonella bacilliformis* causes splenic trapping and acute hemolytic anemia. Cold agglutinins or hemolysins appear in association with infections such as influenza and *Mycoplasma* pneumonia and may, rarely, lead to acute or chronic hemolytic anemia. Chronic infections can stimulate the reticuloendothelial system and cause hypersplenism and hemolysis. Infectious hepatitis has been reported to cause acute hemolysis in patients with glucose-6-phosphate dehydrogenase deficiency. Rare patients with viral hepatitis alone develop fatal aplastic anemia.

The anemias associated with inflammatory diseases, malignancy, and infection respond to treatment of the underlying disease. The anemia is chronic but usually not disabling. If symptoms develop, transfusion of packed red cells, not whole blood, is indicated.

The Anemia of Systemic Lupus Erythematosus (SLE)

Systemic lupus erythematosus is a disease of unknown etiology. Fever, arthritis, pleuritis, pericarditis, skin rashes, and renal failure are characteristic of its many systemic manifestations, and it is associated with circulating anti-DNA antibodies and immune complexes. Cytopenias, qualitative abnormalities of platelet aggregation, and circulating anticoagulants are common hematologic abnormalities.

The anemia is most often normochromic and normocytic with the pathophysiologic characteristics of the anemia of chronic disease (see p. 237). Autoimmune hemolytic anemia (AIHA) affects about 10 percent of patients and is revealed by warm antibodies, complement, or both on their red cells. Occasionally drug-induced, Coombs' test-positive hemolysis due to penicillin, α-methyldopa, cephalosporin, or quinine occurs. Less common mechanisms of anemia are splenic enlargement with hypersplenism, renal disease, iron deficiency secondary to gastrointestinal blood loss (probably related to renal failure), and bone marrow depression induced by cytotoxic agents sometimes used to control the disease.

Adrenal corticosteroids are used to treat the systemic manifestations and any associated AIHA. As in idiopathic autoimmune hemolytic anemia, splenectomy and drugs such as azathioprine and cyclophosphamide are used to treat steroid-unresponsive AIHA.

Leukopenia and thrombocytopenia due to hypersplenism, autoantibodies, and marrow depression are also present in patients with SLE, and these cytopenias will respond to the same therapies as those used for AIHA. Circulating anticoagulants active against Factors XI, IV, VIII, prothrombin, and antithrombin have been described (see p. 408). Bleeding, when it occurs, is most often associated with thrombocytopenia and renal failure, not circulating anticoagulants.

The LE cell is formed in the peripheral bood of patients with this disease. This unusual cell is a granulocyte with a large, purple, homogenous, cytoplasmic inclusion body. Usually the blood from a suspected SLE patient is first traumatized by rotation with glass beads, centrifuged, and the buffy coat (the white cell layer between plasma and red cells) examined after a 20- to 40-minute incubation period (LE test) for these cells.

Cells similar to the LE cell but with a chromatin structure remaining in the inclusion body are seen in patients with drug reactions. Pronestyl, hydralazine, penicillin, tetracycline, and anticonvulsants are some of the drugs associated with a false positive LE test.

Myelophthisic Anemia

Myelophthisic anemias are those caused by replacement of the marrow by tumor, fibrosis, granulomas, or abnormal cells arising in lipid or other storage diseases such as Gaucher's and Niemann-Pick disease. Physical replacement of normal bone marrow cells is only part of the explanation for this type of anemia. Often the anemia of chronic disease or hypersplenism or both are present. Whether substances toxic to hematopoietic cells or to the microenvironment of the marrow are released by tumor or other cells infiltrating the marrow is uncertain.

In all myelophthisic anemias teardrop-shaped red cells (Plate 12) immature erythrocytes (nucleated red cells, Plate 4), and immature granulocytes are found in the peripheral blood, sometimes with difficulty. Certainly if this *leukoerythroblastic blood picture* is present without a known reason, marrow aspiration and biopsy are indicated.

Gaucher's disease is caused by lack of the enzyme β-glucocerebrosidase resulting in accumulation of cerebroside in histiocytes of affected patients (Plate 61). These cells are found in the bone marrow, in the patients' greatly enlarged spleens, and in other organs of the RES. Infiltration of the bone marrow, hypersplenism, functional marrow suppression, and ineffective erythropoiesis all contribute to the anemia. Splenectomy is the only therapy available to correct the anemia or the cytopenia that arises from the greatly enlarged spleens.

The typical Gaucher's cell is large (20–80 μm), with several eccentric nuclei and a characteristic fibrillar cytoplasm. Similar cells are found in the marrow of patients with chronic myelocytic leukemia and, infrequently, with thalassemia and multiple myeloma. As the enzyme defect is not present in CML patients, it is thought that the cerebroside accumulation is related to excessive granulocyte turnover.

When myelophthisic anemia is due to tumor cells, the cells (Plate 72) are seen in bone marrow preparations, either in smears or, more easily, in clot sections or biopsies. They are large cells, usually appearing in clumps. The nucleus-to-cytoplasm ratio is high, and the cytoplasm, when seen, is filmy. It is not possible to identify the site of origin of the tumor cells from their morphology. The only treatment is therapy directed at the primary neoplasm.

The myelophthisic anemias due to fibrosis (myeloproliferative syndrome), lymphoma, and myeloma will be discussed in Chapters 9 and 10. The anemia associated with granulomatous diseases such as tuberculosis is seldom seen today. Occasionally granulomas are found in marrow clot sections or biopsies of patients with unsuspected granulomatous diseases.

Anemias Associated with Endocrine Abnormalities

Hypothyroidism

A mild, normochromic, normocytic anemia is associated with hypothyroidism. Reduced red cell production probably explains the anemia and the low reticulocyte production index. The anemia improves after treatment with exogenous thyroid.

Iron deficiency anemia may be associated with hypothyroidism in women, because these patients have abnormal menstrual periods with increased blood loss. Achlorhydria, which is often present, prevents facilitation of iron absorption by hydrochloric acid.

Megaloblastic anemia can also be associated with hypothyroidism and is caused by either folate or vitamin B_{12} deficiency. The former may be due to decreased dietary intake of folates and the latter to pernicious anemia. It is interesting that thyroid and intrinsic factor autoantibodies are often found in the same patient.

Hypopituitarism

A mild, normochromic, normocytic anemia is often associated with hypopituitarism. It responds to replacement therapy with thyroid and adrenocorticoids. A full response in males may require testosterone therapy. The anemia is believed to arise from the absence of target organ secretion rather than from a specific lack of a pituitary hormone. As in hypothyroidism it may be an adaption to lowered tissue oxygen requirements and reduced production of erythropoietin.

TOPICS FOR DISCUSSION

Aplastic and Secondary Anemias

Stem cell physiology

Bone marrow cultures

Microcirculation of bone marrow

Therapy of aplastic anemia

Etiology of aplastic anemia

Congenital aplastic anemias

Immunologic features of pure red cell aplasia

Pancytopenia with hypercellular marrow

Relationship of thymoma to pure red cell aplasia

Differential diagnoses of aplastic, megaloblastic and myelophthisic anemia

Relationship between hypoplastic anemia, leukemia, chloramphenicol, and paroxysmal nocturnal hemoglobinuria

Factors influencing prognosis of aplastic anemia (monocytes, hemoglobin F, bone marrow cellularity, etc.)

Methodology of bone marrow transplantation for aplastic anemia

Histocompatibility testing

Use of immunosuppressives in bone marrow transplantation

Graft-versus-host problems in bone marrow transplantation

Pathogenesis of anemias of endocrine diseases

Pathogenesis of anemias of chronic diseases

Blood Banking

Anticoagulants for blood storage

Component therapy in blood transfusion

Diagnosis, prevention, and treatment of hemolytic disease of the newborn (erythroblastosis fetalis)

Genetics and structure of ABO, Rh, and other blood groups

Methods of freezing, storing, and defrosting blood components

Pathogenesis and treatment of hemolytic transfusion reactions

Production and standardization of typing and Coombs' reagents

Storage defect in red cells

SELECTED REFERENCES

Aplastic Anemia

Bach, F. H., and Van Rood, J. J. The major histocompatibility complex — genetics and biology. *N. Engl. J. Med.* 295:806; 872; 927, 1976.

Bauman, A. W. Management of Bone Marrow Failure. In R. I. Weed (ed.), *Hematology for Internists.* Boston: Little, Brown, 1971.

Boggs, D. R., and Boggs, S. S. The pathogenesis of aplastic anemia: A defective pluripotent hematopoietic stem cell with inappropriate balance of differentiation and self-replication. *Blood* 48:71, 1976.

Dameshek, W. Riddle: What do aplastic anemia, paroxysmal nocturnal hemoglobinuria (PNH) and "hypoplastic" leukemia have in common? *Blood* 30:251, 1967.

deGruchy, G. C. *Drug-Induced Blood Disorders.* Oxford, Engl.: Blackwell, 1975.

Kesse-Elias, M., Gyftake, E., Alevizou-Terzake, V., and Malamos, A. ^{59}Fe and ^{51}Cr studies in aplastic anemia and myelosclerosis. *Acta Haematol.* (Basel) 39:139, 1968.

Krantz, S. B. Pure red-cell aplasia. *N. Engl. J. Med.* 291:345, 1974.

Lajtha, L. G. Haemopoietic stem cells. *Br. J. Haematol.* 29:529, 1975.

Thomas, E. D., Fefer, A., Buchner, C. D., and Storb, R. Current status of bone marrow transplantation for aplastic anemia and acute leukemia. *Blood* 49:671, 1977.

Van Rood, J. J. (ed.) Histocompatibility, immunosuppression and bone marrow transplantation. *Semin. Hematol.* 11:229, 1974.

Vilter, R. W., Janold, T., Will, J. J., Mueller, J. F., Friedman, B. I., and Hawkins, V. R. Refractory anemia with hyperplastic bone marrow. *Blood* 15:1, 1960.

Williams, D. M., Lynch, R. E., and Cartwright, G. E. Drug-induced aplastic anemia. *Semin. Hematol.* 10:196, 1973.

Wilson, H. E. Aplastic and Refractory Anemias. In C. E. Mengel, et al (eds.), *Hematology: Principles and Practice.* Chicago: Year Book, 1972.

Wintrobe, M. M., et al Pancytopenia, Aplastic Anemia and "Pure Red Cell" Aplasia. In M. M. Wintrobe, et al (eds.), *Clinical Hematology* (7th ed.). Philadelphia: Lea & Febiger, 1974.

Wintrobe, M. M., et al Origin and Development of the Blood and Blood-Forming Tissues. In M. M. Wintrobe, et al (eds.), *Clinical Hematology* (7th ed.). Philadelphia: Lea & Febiger, 1974.

Yunis, A. A. Chloramphenicol-induced bone marrow suppression. *Semin. Hematol.* 10:225, 1973.

Blood Banking

Giblett, E. R., et al Part VI, Replacement Therapy. In W. J. Williams, E. Beutler, A. J. Erslev, and R. W. Rundles (eds.), *Hematology* (2nd ed.). New York: McGraw-Hill, 1977.

Goldfinger, D. Acute hemolytic transfusion reactions — A fresh look at pathogenesis and considerations regarding therapy. *Transfusion* 17:85, 1977.

Hoyer, L. W., and Lichtman, M. A. Recent Advances in Transfusion Therapy. In R. I. Weed (ed.), *Hematology for Internists.* Boston: Little, Brown, 1971.

Miller, W. V. (ed.) *Technical Methods and Procedures of the American*

Association of Blood Banks (6th ed.). Washington, D.C.: J. B. Lippincott, 1974.

Mollison, P. L. *Blood Transfusion in Clinical Medicine* (5th ed.). Oxford, Engl.: Blackwell, 1972.

Schmidt, P. J. Blood Transfusion and Blood Groups. In C. E. Mengel, et al (eds.), *Hematology: Principles and Practice*. Chicago: Year Book, 1972.

Secondary Anemias   Blomgren, S. E. Drug-induced lupus erythematosus. *Semin. Hematol.* 10:345, 1973.

Budman, D. R., and Steinberg, A. D. Hematologic aspects of systemic lupus erythematosus. *Ann. Intern. Med.* 86:220, 1977.

Dubois, E. L. (ed.) *Lupus Erythematosus.* Los Angeles: University of Southern California Press, 1974.

Eichner, E. R. The hematologic disorders of alcoholism. *Am J. Med.* 54: 621, 1973.

Erslev, A. J. Chapter 44, Anemia of Chronic Disorders. In W. J. Williams, E. Beutler, A. J. Erslev, and R. W. Rundles (eds.), *Hematology* (2nd ed.). New York: McGraw-Hill, 1977.

Erslev, A. J. Chapter 31, Anemia of Chronic Renal Failure; Anemia of Endocrine Disorders. In W. J. Williams, E. Beutler, A. J. Erslev, and R. W. Rundles (eds.), *Hematology* (2nd ed.). New York: McGraw-Hill, 1977.

Erslev, A. J. Chapter 29, Aplastic Anemia; Chapter 30, Pure Red Cell Aplasia. In W. J. Williams, E. Beutler, A. J. Erslev, and R. W. Rundles (eds), *Hematology* (2nd ed.). New York: McGraw-Hill, 1977.

Harris, J. W., and Kellermeyer, R. W. The Anemias of Bone Marrow Failure. In J. W. Harris (ed.), *The Red Cell-Production, Metabolism, Destruction, Normal and Abnormal.* Cambridge: Harvard University Press, 1970.

Israels, M. C. G., and Delamore, I. W., (eds.) Hematological Aspects of Systemic Disease. London: W. B. Saunders, 1976.

Laszlo, J. Chapter 45, Anemia Associated with Marrow Infiltration. In W. J. Williams, E. Beutler, A. J. Erslev, and R. W. Rundles (eds.), *Hematology* (2nd ed.). New York: McGraw-Hill, 1977.

McCredis, K. B., and Hester, J. P. White blood cell transfusions in the management of infections in neutropenic patients. *Clin. Haematol.* 5:379, 1976.

Sawitsky, A. (ed.) Reticuloendothelial disorders: The lipidoses I. *Semin. Hematol.* 9:225, 1972.

Sawitsky, A. (ed.) Reticuloendothelial disorders: The lipidoses II. *Semin. Hematol.* 9:349, 1972.

Sheehy, T. W., and Berman, A. The anemia of cirrhosis. *J. Lab. Clin. Med.* 56:72, 1960.

Straus, D. J. Hematologic aspects of alcoholism. *Semin. Hematol.* 10:183, 1973.

Wintrobe, M. M., et al The Normocytic, Normochromic Anemias. In M. M. Wintrobe, et al (eds.), *Clinical Hematology* (7th ed.). Philadelphia: Lea & Febiger, 1974.

Yawata, Y., and Jacob, H. S. Abnormal red cell metabolism in patients with chronic anemia: Nature of the defect and its persistence despite adequate hemodialysis. *Blood* 45:231, 1975.

8 : Leukocytes

Leukocytes prevent and fight infections: granulocytes (granular leukocytes) do this by their ability to phagocytize bacteria, and lymphocytes (nongranular leukocytes) by their role in immunity and antibody production. Qualitative and quantitative disorders of granulocytes and lymphocytes are discussed in this chapter; proliferative and malignant diseases of leukocytes are discussed in Chapters 9 and 10. For each of the cells classified as leukocytes — neutrophilic granulocytes, basophils, eosinophils, lymphocytes, and monocytes — a description of known origin, morphology, function, and cell kinetics, and the differential diagnosis of quantitative abnormalities, such as leukopenia or leukocytosis is given. Only a small number of laboratory procedures useful for diagnosing abnormalities of leukocytes are available: total white blood cell count, white blood cell differential, and peripheral blood and marrow morphology.

Many of the diseases that cause anemia also affect leukocytes. Often a quantitative abnormality of leukocytes is directly related to a concurrent and clinically more important anemia. For example, in megaloblastic anemia there is frequently an associated depression of the total white blood cell count and in particular the granulocyte count. Once the diagnosis of megaloblastic anemia is made and treatment instituted, the white blood cell count returns to normal, usually without infectious complications.

Table 8-1 summarizes leukocyte abnormalities found in peripheral blood.

GRANULO-CYTES

Morphology of Granulocyte Development

It is rare for granulocyte precursors to appear in the peripheral blood of normal persons. Peripheral blood granulocytes are predominantly segmented neutrophils (polymorphonuclear leukocytes), although occasionally nonsegmented, less mature neutrophils are also found in normal blood.

In the bone marrow the earliest recognizable white cell precursor, the *myeloblast* (Plate 32) has scant blue-gray cytoplasm, a large nucleus-to-cytoplasm ratio, and a nucleus with one or more nucleoli. There are no visible black or purple promyelocytic

Table 8-1 : Abnormalities of Leukocytes and Diseases Associated with These Abnormalities

Abnormality	Description	Associated Diseases
Leukocytosis	White blood cell count $> 11.0 \times 10^9$/L	Any physiologic or pathologic stress, corticosteroids
Neutrophilic leukocytosis (granulocytosis)	Neutrophilic leukocyte count $> 7.5 \times 10^9$/L	Infection, intoxication, tissue necrosis, myeloproliferative syndromes, leukemia (e.g., chronic, myelocytic), leukemoid reaction, hemorrhage, hemolysis
Neutropenia or granulocytopenia	Neutrophilic count $< 1.5 \times 10^9$/L	Drugs, infection, congenital megaloblastic anemia, aplastic anemia, leukemia, lupus erythematosus, postirradiation hypersplenism, myelophthisic anemia
Toxic granulation (Plate 43)	Coarse black or purple cytoplasmic granules	Infections or inflammatory diseases
Döhle bodies (Plate 40)	Small (1–2 μm) blue cytoplasmic inclusions in neutrophils	Infections or inflammatory diseases, burns, myelocytic leukemia, myeloproliferative syndromes, cyclophosphamide therapy
Pelger-Huët anomalies (Plates 41 and 42)	Neutrophil with bilobed nucleus or no segmentation of nucleus. Chromatin is coarse and cytoplasm is pink with normal granulation.	Hereditary, myelocytic leukemias, myeloproliferative syndromes
May-Hegglin anomaly	Basophilic, cytoplasmic inclusions of leukocytes. Similar to Döhle bodies.	May-Hegglin syndrome (hereditary), includes thrombocytopenia and giant platelets.
Alder's anomaly	Prominent azurophilic granulation in leukocytes. Similar to toxic granulation. Granulation is seen better with Giemsa stain.	Hereditary, gargoylism
Chédiak-Higashi anomaly	Gray-green, large cytoplasmic inclusions resembling Döhle bodies.	Chédiak-Higashi syndrome (see p. 252
LE (lupus erythematosus) cells	Neutrophilic leukocyte with a *homogenous* red-purple inclusion that distends the cell's cytoplasm	Lupus erythematosus and other collagen diseases, chronic hepatitis, drug reactions, serum sickness
Tart cell	Neutrophilic leukocyte with a phagocytized nucleus of a granulocyte that retains some nuclear structure.	Drug reactions (e.g., penicillin, procainamide)
LE "rosette"	Homogenous nuclear material surrounded by neutrophilic leukocytes	Lupus erythematosus, collagen disease, drug reactions, serum sickness
Eosinophilia	Eosinophil count $> 0.6 \times 10^9$/L	Allergic disorders, collagen diseases, parasitic infections, Hodgkin's disease, chronic myelocytic leukemia, pernicious anemia, tissue necrosis (e.g., postirradiation), sarcoid, malignancies, tuberculosis, chronic skin diseases, eosinophilic leukemia

Table 8-1 (Continued)

Abnormality	Description	Associated Diseases
Basophilic leukocytosis	Basophil count $> 0.05 \times 10^9$/L	Chronic myelocytic leukemia, myeloproliferative syndrome
Myeloid "shift to left"	Presence of bands, myelocytes, metamyelocytes, or promyelocytes	Infections, intoxications, tissue necrosis, myeloproliferative syndrome, leukemia (chronic myelocytic), leukemoid reaction, pernicious anemia, hyposplenism
Hypersegmented neutrophil (Plate 18)	Mature neutrophil with more than 5 distinct lobes	Megaloblastic anemia, hereditary constitutional hypersegmentation of neutrophils; rarely, iron deficiency anemia, malignancy, or infection
Lymphocytosis	Lymphocytes $> 9.0 \times 10^9$/L in young children, 7.0×10^9/L in older children, and 4.0×10^9/L in adults	Infectious mononucleosis, infectious lymphocytosis, pertussis, viral infections, chronic lymphocytic leukemia, syphilis
Atypical lymphocytes (Plates 49-51)	Lymphocytes, some with vacuolated cytoplasm and others containing lobulated (monocytoid) nucleus and sometimes nucleoli	Infectious mononucleosis, viral hepatitis and other viral infections, tuberculosis, drug (e.g., penicillin) sensitivity, posttransfusion syndrome.
Monocytosis	Monocyte count $> 0.75 \times 10^9$/L in children, 0.50×10^9/L in adults	Infectious and inflammatory diseases, tuberculosis, bacterial endocarditis, recovery from bone marrow suppression, drug reaction, infectious mononucleosis, leukemia, lymphomas, solid tumors, myeloma
Plasmacytosis (Türk cells) (Plate 65)	Plasma cells present (none are normally seen) in peripheral blood	Multiple myeloma, plasma cell leukemia, malignancy, chronic renal disease, aplastic anemia, tuberculosis, any severe infectious or inflammatory condition
Leukemic cells (lymphoblasts, myeloblasts, etc.)	Presence of lymphoblasts, myeloblasts, monoblasts, myelomonoblasts, promyelocytes (none normally present in peripheral blood)	Leukemia (acute or chronic), leukemoid reaction, severe infectious or inflammatory diseases, myeloproliferative syndrome, intoxications, malignancies, recovery from bone marrow suppression, infectious mononucleosis, myelophthisis
Auer bodies (Plate 53)	Round or rodlike, 1-6 μm long, red-purple, refractile inclusions in neutrophils	Acute myelocytic leukemia
Histiocytosis (Plate 45)	Presence of reticuloendothelial or phagocytic cells (none normally seen in peripheral blood)	Severe infectious (e.g., subacute bacterial endocarditis) or inflammatory diseases, leukemias, lymphomas, malignant histiocytosis, malignancy, hemolytic anemia, agranulocytosis
Smudge cell	Disintegrated lymphocyte	Chronic lymphocytic leukemia

granules; cell diameter is 15 to 20 micrometers (μm); and the nucleus is large, round, or oval. It is often impossible to distinguish myeloblasts from lymphoblasts.

Promyelocytes (Plate 33) develop from myeloblasts and have the same nuclear and cytoplasmic characteristics. The promyelocyte, however, has large oval or spheroidal, azurophilic granules scattered throughout the cytoplasm.

The next developmental stage is the *myelocyte* (Plate 34). Myelocytes vary in size from 16 to 24 μm. Maturation occurs in both cytoplasm and nucleus. The azurophilic or primary granules can no longer be seen in the cytoplasm by light microscopy, although they can be detected by electron microscopy. The blue-gray color of the cytoplasm is modified by the appearance of small pink granules, usually in the perinuclear region. These granules are called *neutrophilic* or *secondary granules*. In the nucleus, nucleoli are absent or much less distinct, and the nucleus-to-cytoplasm ratio has decreased.

During the next stage of development the *metamyelocyte* or *juvenile* (Plate 35) is formed. Its cytoplasm is pink, neutrophilic granules are prominent in it, and nucleoli are absent. The nucleus in indented or kidney-shaped, and there is often a yellow "sunburst" appearance to the cytoplasm at the point of nuclear indentation. The metamyelocyte, unlike earlier granulocyte precursors, does not divide.

The process of metamyelocyte maturation into a *band* or *stab* (Plate 36) and then into a mature granulocyte or polymorphonuclear leukocyte (*poly*) (Plate 37) consists of nuclear elongation and segmentation. The stab or band is very similar to the metamyelocyte, except that the nucleus has become horseshoe-shaped. It may sometimes be seen in the peripheral blood of normal persons. The mature, segmented neutrophil or poly, approximately 12 to 14 μm in diameter, is formed and released from the bone marrow. Its cytoplasm is pink, with small neutrophilic granules, and the nucleus is segmented into two to five (usually three) lobes connected by thin chromatin strands.

Eosinophils

The *eosinophil* (Plate 38) is similar to the mature neutrophil except that its cytoplasm is filled with large, bright red, refractile granules that cover a two-lobed nucleus. These granules appear first during the promyelocytic stage of development. The eosinophils go through essentially the same stages of development as neutrophilic granulocytes. Thus the difference between the neutrophil and the eosinophil is in the nature of the granules in their cytoplasm. The poly has neutrophilic, or pink, small granules, whereas the eosinophil has large, red, refractile granules.

Causes of eosinophilia

Allergic disorders
Hodgkin's disease
Idiopathic
Inherited
Leukemia, eosinophilic
Löffler's syndrome and pulmonary infiltration with eosinophilia (PIE)
Malignancy
Myelocytic leukemic (chronic) and polycythemia vera
Necrosis of tissue
Parasitic infections
Pernicious anemia
Skin diseases
Tropical eosinophilia
Vasculitis
X-irradiation therapy

Normally there are 0.05 to 0.45 $\times$ 10^9 eosinophils per liter in the peripheral blood of adults.

Eosinophilia (greater than 0.60 $\times$ 10^9 cells per liter) is a common abnormality most often due to allergic or dermatologic disorders (see p. 249). Occasionally parasites, Hodgkin's disease, chronic myelocytic leukemia, vasculitis, or infiltrative eosinophilic syndromes are present. Eosinophilia can follow necrosis of tissue, particularly after radiotherapy. Eosinophilia in association with scattered lung infiltrates (Löffler's syndrome) is probably caused by parasites. Unless an obvious cause of eosinophilia is present, the workup of a minimally or moderately elevated eosinophil count is usually unrewarding.

The diagnosis of eosinophilic leukemia is quite difficult to make. These patients have marked eosinophilia and hepatosplenomegaly with infiltration by immature eosinophils. There is argument over whether this syndrome is due to an allergic vasculitis or is a true leukemia.

The function of the specific granules in eosinophils is unclear. However, several substances associated with anaphylaxis are selectively chemotactic for eosinophils. Low eosinophil counts, less than 0.05 $\times$ 10^9 cells per liter, are seen following stress and after secretion or administration of adrenocorticosteroids.

Basophils

A third type of leukocyte with specific granules is the *basophil* (Plate 39). The cytoplasm of this cell is filled with large, coarse, blue or black granules that often cover the nucleus. The granules are morphologically similar to those of *mast cells, (tissue basophils)*. Mast cells are generally seen only in the bone marrow, however, basophils are seen in the peripheral blood; and the mast cell's granules usually do not cover the nucleus and are tightly packed into the cytoplasm.

Basophils have a high content of heparin and histamine and play an important role in acute, systemic, allergic reactions. Degranulation, release of histamine, and wheal formation occur when IgE or *reaginic antibody* attaches to basophils. The release of histamine-containing granules requires energy and probably does not result in the loss of viability of these cells.

Normally 0.02 to 0.05 $\times$ 10^9 basophils per liter are found in adult peripheral blood. Patients with low basophil counts (less than 0.02 $\times$ 10^9 cells per liter) usually have had acute hypersensitivity reactions such as anaphylaxis. Thyroid hormones, epinephrine, radiation, chemotherapy, infections, pregnancy, and aging can all depress the basophil count. Elevation of the basophil count, or *basophilia,* (greater than 0.05 $\times$ 10^9 cells per liter), may be due to asthma. Often basophils are seen in greater numbers in myeloproliferative disorders, including myelocytic leukemia, particularly the chronic type. Tuberculosis, estrogens, postsplenectomy state, carcinoma, Hodgkin's disease, inflammatory bowel disease, and hypothyroidism all may be associated with basophilia. Except for hypersensitivity reactions and chronic myelocytic leukemia, basophilia is of little diagnostic importance.

Systemic mast cell disease is characterized by pancytopenia, hepatosplenomegaly, and dermatographism. Skeletal lesions consisting of infiltrates of mast cells are a common finding. The diagnosis is usually made from skin manifestations (urticaria pigmentosa) or from mast cell hyperplasia found on marrow examination.

Abnormal Granulocyte Morphology

Döhle bodies (Plate 40) are blue, single or multiple, cytoplasmic inclusions about 0.5 μm in diameter. They are often seen in patients with bacterial infections, burns, trauma, pregnancy, cancer, and following the administration of anticancer agents such as cyclophosphamide. Döhle bodies are believed to consist of ribonuclear proteins. Similar blue cytoplasmic inclusion bodies in neutrophils are seen in an inherited disorder called *May-Hegglin anomaly,* in which the patients have low white blood cell and platelet counts and giant platelets. The acquired Döhle bodies seen in infections are different ultrastructurally from the inclusion bodies in the May-Hegglin anomaly.

The Pelger-Hüet anomaly takes two forms, acquired and inherited. In the heterozygous inherited condition (Plate 41) the mature neutrophil is characterized by two nuclear lobes, both of which are round and connected by a thin strand of chromatin, giving a dumbbell or *pince-nez* appearance. In the homozygous inherited form (Plate 42), the nuclear chromatin is mature, but the nucleus is round rather than segmented. Both these anomalies, the dumbbell-shaped and the round, nonsegmented nucleus, may be seen in acquired conditions such as myelocytic leukemias, either acute or chronic. Occasionally *Pelgeroid anomalies* are found in patients with severe infections, metastatic cancer to bone, and drug reactions to colchicine and sulfa drugs. In these cases the acquired changes may be reversible.

Toxic granulations (Plate 43) — dark, black or purple, cytoplasmic granules — are often seen in polys from patients with infections. They are found in association with Döhle bodies and vacuolization of granulocyte and monocyte cytoplasm. Döhle bodies, cytoplasmic vacuolization, and toxic granulation are often evidence for viral infection or bacterial sepsis; but these characteristics can also be seen in metabolic disorders and conditions unrelated to infections.

In *Alder's anomaly,* a rare abnormality, cytoplasmic inclusions resembling toxic granules are found in the granulocytes. Similar inclusions are seen in lymphocytes of children with familial disorders called *mucopolysaccharidoses.* Abnormally large, mature neutrophils called *macropolycytes* may be seen in patients with megaloblastic anemia, chronic infection, granulocytic leukemias, following administration of anticancer agents, or as an inherited abnormality. *Hypersegmentation of the neutrophil nucleus* may also be inherited. Sepsis can cause vacuolization of granulocytes, nuclear pyknosis, and loss of normal neutrophilic granules. The very rare *Chédiak-Higashi anomaly* is a familial disorder characterized by abnormally large primary granules in the cytoplasm of mature granulocytes. Affected patients have partial albinism, susceptibility to bacterial infections, and photophobia, and usually die with a lymphoma-like illness. The function of their unusual leukocytes is abnormal and probably contributes to their susceptibility to pyogenic infections.

Quantitation of Leukocytes

The total *white blood cell* (WBC) or *leukocyte count* in the peripheral blood is usually determined by manually counting the number of white cells in a known volume of solution or by using an electronic, automatic counter. In the manual method, peripheral blood from a patient is diluted with Türk's solution (2% acetic acid) using standard white cell pipettes. This is thoroughly mixed, and in the process hemoglobin is leached from the erythrocyte because of membrane swelling secondary to the low ionic strength of Türk's solution. After mixing, an aliquot is placed in a counting chamber of known volume. The chamber is 0.1 mm high and consists of nine squares, each 1.00 sq mm in area. Four squares, or a volume of 0.4 cu mm, are usually counted. The white cells are distinguished from the red cells by their dark-appearing nuclei. Since hemoglobin has been leached from the red cell, the erythrocyte ghosts are very difficult to see. The number of white cells in this volume, when multiplied by 50×10^6 [50 is derived from 2.5×20 (dilution factor)], yields the number of white cells per liter of whole blood. In the electronic method, the Coulter counter enumerates white cells as they pass between electrodes and create a pulse due to displacement of electrolytic solution. A lysing agent, rather than acetic acid alone, is required to rupture the red cell membranes, so that red cells will not be counted. The total leukocyte or white blood cell count is normally 4.0 to 11.0×10^9 per liter.

White cell differential counts are performed by placing a drop of blood on a slide or coverslip and smearing it into a thin film. This film is stained with Wright or Giemsa stain. At least 100 cells are identified and classified as neutrophils, lymphocytes, monocytes,

**Table 8-2 : Normal Human Peripheral
Blood White Cell Differential Count**

Cells	Ranges (%)	Cells ($\times 10^9$/L)
Total WBC	....	4-11
Neutrophils	40-75	1.50-7.50
Lymphocytes	15-45	0.60-5.00
Monocytes	1-10	0.00-0.80
Eosinophils	1-7	0.05-0.60
Basophils	0-2	0.02-0.05

eosinophils, or basophils. Any cells that are not usually seen in the peripheral blood and that are therefore abnormal, such as nucleated reds or "blast" cells, are also counted and classified. The results are expressed as a percentage. Table 8-2 shows easily remembered adult, upper and lower limits of normal for each cell type.

Nucleated red cells are counted as white cells by both manual and electronic methods. The WBC can be corrected for the presence of nucleated reds by using the nucleated red cell differential count, e.g.,

Total WBC = 6.0×10^9 per liter

nucleated reds = 10 per 100 WBC

then $(6.0 \times 10^9) - (0.1 \times 6.0 \times 10^9)$ = corrected WBC
$$= 5.4 \times 10^9 \text{ per liter}$$

Granulocytopenia

Leukopenia means a total white blood cell count of less than 4.0×10^9 per liter. *Granulocytopenia,* or *neutropenia,* is present when the "absolute" granulocyte count (WBC $\times$ neutrophil fraction) is less than 1.5×10^9 granulocytes per liter, counting only neutrophilic granulocytes at the stab or mature cell (poly) maturation level. Severe and frequent infections do not appear until the "absolute" granulocyte count falls to 0.5×10^9 per liter or less. Some increase in infections may be seen in the range of 0.5 to 1.0 $\times 10^9$ granulocytes per liter. As will be seen, granulocytopenia and leukopenia may be caused by a large variety of disorders.

The term *agranulocytosis* refers to a syndrome consisting of the abrupt disappearance of circulating granulocytes, fever, sore throat, necrosis of oral mucous membranes, and a severely depressed granulocyte count. If the granulocytopenia is not corrected, bacteremia and sepsis may occur. Although agranulocytosis may be caused by a variety of disorders, it is usually associated with drugs or cancer chemotherapy.

Although there is a good direct correlation between the peripheral blood "absolute" granulocyte count and bone marrow reserves of neutrophils, in certain situations — for example, prior to cancer chemotherapy with cytotoxic drugs — estimation of actual reserves may be required. Examination of a bone marrow specimen may suggest normal reserves, if cellularity and the myeloid-to-erythroid ratio are normal and no abnormal cells are found. Occasionally bone marrow morphology does not correspond to functional ability to produce and release granulocytes. Functional tests are available although seldom performed. They involve agents that promote release of marrow granulocytes, such as endotoxin, etiocholanolone, and adrenocorticosteroids. These agents are administered and the increment in peripheral blood granulocyte count measured. Etiocholanolone is preferable but difficult to obtain. It can be given intramuscularly, whereas endotoxin must be given intravenously. Endotoxin administration is associated with sudden lowering of blood pressure (hypotension). Corticosteroids are the easiest to use, because all that is necessary is ingestion of 40 mg of prednisolone and measurement 5 hours later of the increment in granulocyte count. The only problem with corticosteroids is that they not only promote release of granulocytes but also interfere with normal egress of granulocytes from blood vessels into tissues, thereby complicating the interpretation of any increment in circulating granulocytes.

Pathophysiology of *Granulocytopenia*
Granulocytopenia is caused primarily by either decreased production of normal granulocytes or increased destruction of circulating neutrophils (see p. 255).

Decreased Production of Granulocytes. Drugs and ionizing radiation are common causes of decreased marrow production of granulocytes. Examination of a marrow specimen shows aplasia or hypoplasia with absent or decreased myeloid precursor cells. Any remaining granulocytes are usually immature, because mature neutrophils are released immediately into the circulation. The absence of mature cells gives the marrow the morphologic appearance of a *maturation arrest,* although functionally the maturation process remains normal. Dose and duration of therapy often have a correlation with severity of marrow injury.

Damage to stem cells, interference with normal DNA metabolism, and destruction of marrow stroma and microcirculation have been suggested as possible causes of drug-induced marrow aplasia. Study of the phenothiazine drugs indicates that they cause myeloid hypoplasia or aplasia by interfering with DNA synthesis.

Causes of granulocytopenia

I. Decreased Production of Normal Granulocytes
   A. Marrow hypoplasia or aplasia
   B. Drugs, including anticancer agents
   C. X-irradiation
   D. Inherited and cyclic neutropenias
   E. Myelophthisis or marrow replacement (e.g., by leukemia or lymphoma)
   F. Megaloblastic anemia
II. Increased Destruction of Circulating Granulocytes
   A. Familial causes
   B. Hypersplenism
   C. Phagocytosis in RES
   D. Viral and bacterial infections
   E. Leukocyte antigen-antibody reactions
   F. Drug-induced, antibody-mediated destruction

Even small doses can cause neutropenia. Unexplained host factors may affect susceptibility to the marrow-damaging effects of the phenothiazines. Although less carefully studied, the drugs listed here (p. 257), except those incriminated in antibody-mediated granulocytopenia, have been shown to cause myeloid hypoplasia and decreased production of neutrophils. Cessation of drug therapy usually results in recovery after two or more weeks. Sometimes the marrow is irreversibly damaged, perhaps because of stem cell injury. In other cases, for example, when a patient is taking antithyroid drugs, the leukopenia may be benign and not progress or lead to infections. However, when possible, suspect drugs should be discontinued.

Ionizing radiation probably owes its effect on granulocyte production to its DNA-damaging ability. Very high doses may inflict irreversible damage on marrow stroma or microcirculation, preventing regeneration. Fortunately the damage done by carefully planned radiotherapy is reversible, with leukocyte counts returning to normal in a few weeks following cessation of therapy.

Inherited and cyclic neutropenias are also associated with myeloid hypoplasia. Rare familial diseases, such as infantile genetic agranulocytosis, familial benign neutropenia, and cyclic neutropenia, may be caused by hypoplasia or aplasia of granulocyte precursors. Cyclic neutropenic patients usually oscillate at intervals of 15 to 35 days. At the nadir of the leukocyte count their marrows are devoid of myeloid precursors, and infections develop. Between attacks the bone marrow appears normal. It has been suggested that cyclic neutropenia is due to damage to marrow stem cells, the cycling being an expression of deranged granulocyte control mechanisms. Acquired diseases resembling these three familial disorders are known and may also result from marrow damage.

Myelophthisic anemia with replacement of the bone marrow by lymphoma, myeloma, carcinoma, granuloma, or fibrosis is another not uncommon cause of granulocytopenia, particularly in older patients.

Ineffective myelopoiesis (production of abnormal granulocytes, which die prior to their release from the marrow) occurs in patients with megaloblastic anemia and is characterized by hypercellularity of marrow spicules and elevation of white cell breakdown products, such as uric acid and lysozyme, in the sera.

Increased Destruction of Granulocytes. Six types of granulocytopenia due to increased leukocyte destruction are discussed here. The first is rare inherited or acquired neutropenias that have been found associated with hypercellular bone marrow but not

Common drugs causing granulocytopenia

Alcohol
Alkylating agents: nitrogen mustard, chlorambucil, etc.
Allopurinol
Aminopyrine*
Antibiotics: chloramphenicol, nitrofuradantin, sulfa drugs,* ampicillin,
    and other penicillins, cephalosporins, gentamycin, metronidazole,
    griseofulvin, pyrimethamine
Anticonvulsants: diphenylhydantoin, phenobarbital
Antithyroid compounds: thiouracils, methimazole, carbimazole
Benzene
Cancer chemotherapy agents: methotrexate, vincristine, vinblastine,
    procarbazine, hydroxyurea, cytosine, arabinoside, daunomycin, 5-
    fluorouracil, 6-mercaptopurine, 6-thioguanine, azathioprine, etc.
Cinchona alkaloids: quinine, quinidine
Diazepam
Gold salts*
Imipramine
Indomethacin
Phenothiazines
Phenylbutazone*
Tolbutamide

*Antibody-mediated in at least some patients

with splenomegaly. Granulocyte survival studies indicate a decreased life span of circulating neutrophils.

A second type is caused by hypersplenism and is usually corrected by splenectomy. Almost any disease that enlarges the spleen can lead to hypersplenism and early sequestration or destruction of mature neutrophils. This is often seen in association with cirrhosis of the liver, congestive or infiltrative splenomegaly, and *Felty's syndrome* (rheumatoid arthritis with high latex fixation titers and splenomegaly). Felty's syndrome may also include a marrow production defect, and the clinical course characterized by infections is sometimes not ameliorated by splenectomy.

A third type of granulocytopenia due to peripheral blood destruction is seen with leukemias and related disorders, in which excessive ingestion of white cells by the reticuloendothelial cells may cause neutropenia. Marrow infiltration, hypersplenism, and chemotherapy also contribute to this neutropenia associated with leukemia.

Although the mechanism is unclear, viral and bacterial infections have been associated with neutropenia. In many cases not only is increased peripheral destruction or utilization of leukocytes present, but other unknown factors act to depress the granulocyte count in this fourth type of granulocytopenia.

A fifth type is due to leukocyte antigen–antibody reactions. In a few neonates maternal isoimmunization and transplacental passage of leukoagglutinins from the mother to the fetus result in destruction of fetal neutrophils. In such cases the mother has been sensitized during previous pregnancies by fetal leukocytes carrying the father's antigenic determinants or by prior transfusion therapy. The antibodies may be directly cytotoxic or cause leukocyte agglutination and subsequent destruction or removal from the circulation. In adults similar white cell antibodies are a common cause of febrile transfusion reactions but seldom are associated with sustained neutropenia.

Autoantibodies directed against a patient's own leukocyte antigens may produce neutropenia in patients with diseases such as systemic lupus erythematosus.

A sixth type is caused by drugs like aminopyrine that act as haptens against which antibodies are developed. When these antibodies and the drug are present together, an immediate reaction takes place, characterized by fever, chills, and destruction of peripheral blood neutrophils. All the complications of agranulocytosis can then occur. The bone marrow appears hyperplastic, and the peripheral blood contains immature neutrophils. The reaction ceases after discontinuation of the drug. Presumably the reaction between drug and antibody causes granulocyte destruction either by agglutination of granulocytes; by coating neutrophils with antibody, which causes their subsequent destruction in the RES; or by a direct cytotoxic effect of the antigen–antibody reaction on or near the cell membrane. Actually there have been very few documented case reports of this type of reaction as a cause for granulocytopenia. This drug-antibody mechanism must be distinguished from granulocytopenia due to drug-induced leukocyte antibodies that do not require presence of the drug for their action and that are directed against leukocyte antigens and not against the drug itself. Possibly the drug combines with or alters the granulocyte membrane, so that the host reacts against a non-self antigen by forming a leukocyte autoantibody. (Drugs suspected of causing neutropenia by an antibody-mediated mechanism are marked with an asterisk in the list on p. 257.)

Approach to the Patient with Granulocytopenia

The patient's history, with particular emphasis on ingestion of drugs, exposure to radiation, and previous cytotoxic cancer chemotherapy, is very important in evaluating possible marrow damage. The physical examination, with attention to signs of cancer, leukemia, lymphoma (for example, lymphadenopathy or splenomegaly), bleeding, or infection, is helpful in determining whether the marrow is possibly infiltrated, as in leukemias, or whether granulocytes are being excessively used or destroyed, as with hypersplenism or infection.

The hematocrit, platelet count, and reticulocyte count give some indication of the overall functional capacity of the marrow. Examination of the peripheral blood smear may suggest acute or chronic leukemia, megaloblastic anemia, aplastic anemia, or other primary diseases as the underlying cause for granulocytopenia. Occasionally study of the cyclic pattern of the white cell count or investigation of family members may be helpful.

The bone marrow examination is often most helpful. If there is complete or partial absence of myeloid precursors, acute or chronic injury to the bone marrow is likely. Maturation arrest, a "shift-to-the-left" with mainly immature granulocytic precursors present, suggests peripheral neutrophil utilization with exhaustion of the marrow granulocytic reserve. A more severe shift-to-the-left with presence of only blast cells, promyelocytes, and occasional mature forms is usually diagnostic of acute leukemia or recovery from marrow aplasia. Splenomegaly accompanied by a hypercellular bone marrow with normal proportions of granulocyte precursors is usually all that is needed to suggest hypersplenism as the cause of the granulocytopenia. Special bone marrow studies such as microbial cultures or genetic karyotyping for leukemia chromosomes are only occasionally useful.

Approach to patient with granulocytopenia

I. History
    A. Drugs
    B. Anticancer therapy
    C. Radiation exposure
    D. Family history

II. Physical Examination
    A. Cancer signs
    B. Lymphadenopathy
    C. Splenomegaly
    D. Signs of megaloblastic anemia
    E. Signs of bleeding or infection

III. Laboratory Tests
    A. Blood counts (serial granulocyte counts)
    B. White cell differential
    C. Peripheral blood smear for red and white cell morphology
    D. Bone marrow examination

IV. Other Procedures to Consider When Relevant and Available
    A. Leukocyte survival study (^{51}Cr, ^{32}DFP)
    B. Leukocyte kinetics (^{51}Cr, ^{32}DFP)
    C. Test for marrow reserves following etiocholanolone, endotoxin, or corticosteroids
    D. Marrow cultures for tuberculosis
    E. Marrow cytogenetics

Therapy for Granulocytopenia

Rapidly progressive and overwhelming infection remains the most serious complication of granulocytopenia. Patients with neutropenia and febrile illnesses must be treated with antibiotics immediately after appropriate cultures are obtained. If the diagnosis of infection is not bacteriologically confirmed, and if the febrile episode continues despite antibiotic therapy, it may be necessary to stop therapy, obtain new cultures, and look for localization of the infection.

Isolation of the patient is usually not helpful, unless specialized equipment and techniques that permit almost complete protection from microbes are available. "Life islands" — plastic tents with specially designed ports to prevent environmental contamination — or isolation rooms with laminar air flows that remove airborne infectious agents should be used, if available, when the granulocyte count is 0.5×10^9 cells per liter or less. Sterilization of food, limited human contact, and suppression of bowel flora with antibiotics are imposed in conjunction with life islands and laminar flow rooms.

Since many infections originate in the gut, antibiotic treatment of bowel flora to reduce their numbers is logical, but seldom effective alone. Prophylactic systemic antibiotics are not indicated in afebrile, granulocytopenic patients, because superinfection with resistant organisms becomes a distinct possibility.

Androgen therapy, as used for aplastic anemia, i.e., oxymethalone 100 to 300 mg per day orally, has been successful in a few patients with myeloid aplasia. Adrenocorticosteroids are of no value and may actually inhibit important phagocytic functions of the neutrophil. Certainly any suspected drugs or toxic agents should be stopped or removed.

Patients acutely ill with granulocytopenia and sepsis may benefit from granulocyte transfusion. The granulocytes are usually obtained, by use of a cell separator (centrifuge) or special nylon filter to which they stick, from normal individuals or patients with leukocytosis due to chronic myelocytic leukemia. Infusions of 10^{10} to 10^{11} white cells should be given for a period of 3 to 5 days. Occasionally noninfected, severely granulocytopenic patients are treated with white cell transfusions to prevent sepsis. This therapy is expensive, often ineffective, and can lead to sensitization to leukocyte antigens. If antibodies do arise, fever, chills, and even anaphylactoid reactions may result from subsequent infusions of leukocytes.

Granulocyte Function-Phagocytosis

The prime function of granulocytes is ingestion of bacteria, or *phagocytosis,* through which they play a major role in combating pyogenic infection. The monocyte and the macrophage of the reticuloendothelial system, which also phagocytize bacteria but about which less is known, are discussed later (p. 269).

The first stage of phagocytosis is the production of leukocytes in the bone marrow, their release from the marrow, and their mobilization in large numbers. The morphologic maturation of leukocytes in relation to their marrow and blood kinetics will be discussed later. The release of leukocytes may be related to their ability to transverse the small-diameter pores of the marrow sinuses located between hematopoietic cords. Nucleated cells, which are relatively rigid, have difficulty passing through these narrow channels, and only with maturation and gain of sufficient plasticity can they escape and enter the circulation. In granulocytopenic patients, these channels may also change in ways that favor granulocyte release. The mature neutrophil in the peripheral blood is most efficient at phagocytosis. Polys held in reserve in the bone marrow and immature granulocytes in the peripheral blood are less efficient as phagocytes.

During the second stage of phagocytosis *chemotaxis,* or the attraction of leukocytes toward sites of infection, injury, or inflammation, is mediated by substances in serum called *chemotaxins,* which are released by bacteria or tissues. Antibody–antigen reactions with activation of complement components also play a role in the release of chemotaxic substances that attract leukocytes. The complement system, as well as the blood coagulation system and agents such as kallikrein and plasminogen activator, may react and interact to cause chemotaxis. Neutrophils themselves may release chemotaxic substances, and lymphocytes have been found to elaborate lymphokines that have chemotactic activity.

As a result of chemotaxis phagocytes crawl toward inflamed sites. This leukocyte migration is characterized by the throwing out of pseudopods. The pseudopods may be quite filmy and thin, and, as they stream forward, the granules in the main body of the leukocyte move with them, followed last by the cell's nucleus. Neutrophils contain in their plasma membrane actin filaments and microtubules. The reaction of actin with myosin and adenosine triphosphate (ATP), as in muscles, or the interaction of microtubules with subunits of their constituent protein, *tubulin,* may play a role in the ability of granulocytes to move.

The third stage involves a process called *opsonization* (preparation for eating). Opsonization is important for allowing granulocytes to recognize which particles should be ingested and which should not; for example, leukocytes should ingest bacteria, but not normal erythrocytes. Immunoglobulin G antibodies and complement participate in a process by which particles to be ingested are coated and perhaps thereby recognized by the leukocyte as particles to be ingested. Opsonization also leads the phagocyte to prepare its metabolic machinery for engulfment and digestion.

During the fourth stage of phagocytosis, *ingestion,* the leukocyte pseudopods engulf microorganisms and encase them within phagocytic vesicles or *phagosomes.* The vesicles move from the cell periphery into the more central part of the leukocyte, where they will fuse with first neutrophilic and then azurophilic granules as part of the fifth stage of phagocytosis. Just as leukocyte motility is energy-dependent, so too is ingestion, and as a result glycolysis and glycogenolysis are increased in phagocytizing leukocytes.

During the fifth stage of phagocytosis, *degranulation,* the fusion of phagosomes and granules results in the disappearance from the cytoplasm of the azurophilic, or primary (these are not seen under the light microscope), and neutrophilic, or secondary, granules. As a result of this process digestive enzymes are delivered to the phagosome without affecting the cytoplasm of the phagocyte itself. The cytoplasmic granules release enzymes, including acid and alkaline phosphatase, ribonuclease, deoxyribonuclease, and lysozyme. These and other enzymes break down the various constituents of organisms and other ingested particles. A most important enzyme, myeloperoxidase, is also released into the phagosome.

In the sixth and seventh stages of phagocytosis, the phagocytes generate hydrogen peroxide and other oxygen metabolites that kill and digest microorganisms. Superoxide (O_2^-) and free hydroxyl radicals ($OH\cdot$) participate in these killing operations. It appears likely that the enzyme glucose-6-phosphate dehydrogenase (G-6-PD) and the hexose monophosphate shunt are necessary to produce NADPH in order to make hydrogen peroxide, superoxide, and free hydroxyl radicals. The microbicidal activity of hydrogen peroxide is potentiated by myeloperoxidase, which reacts with halide (iodide) to produce the oxygen metabolites that are even more toxic to microorganisms than hydrogen peroxide itself. Catalase and other enzyme systems are required by the phagocyte to detoxify peroxides and prevent autoperoxidation. The hydrogen peroxide–myeloperoxidase–halide antimicrobial system is very important, since patients who have an abnormal system have difficulty destroying microorganisms such as staphylococci, gram-negative bacteria, and *Candida* pathogens.

Disorders of Granulocyte Function

Defective granulocytic function occurs in many inherited and acquired diseases. If the patient suffers from infections, usually more than one function of the phagocytic cell is impaired. Abnormal serum opsonization due to decreased complement activity or hypogammaglobulinemia and disorders related to defective hydrogen peroxide formation are most commonly found.

Some patients with diabetes mellitus, Chédiak-Higashi anomaly, or myeloproliferative disorders have an impaired cellular response to chemotaxis. The basis for this abnormality is unknown. Abnormal chemotactic activity is seen in patients deficient in certain complement components, in patients with sepsis, and in *Job's syndrome,* a disease associated with high serum IgE levels, recurrent abscesses, and eczema.

Leukocyte mobility may be impaired in diseases such as rheumatoid arthritis, hepatic cirrhosis, and chronic granulomatous disease. Leukocyte immobility has also been found in patients receiving corticosteroids, in patients with defective neutrophil actin function; and in the *lazy leukocyte syndrome.* This last is characterized by infections, poor granulocyte locomotion, poor chemotactic responses, and neutropenia that is presumably due to an inability to mobilize marrow granulocytes.

Defective opsonization has been documented in patients with abnormal complement components, immunoglobulin deficiency, systemic lupus erythematosus, hepatic cirrhosis, and glomerulonephritis. A humoral factor that promotes phagocytosis, *tuftsin,* a tetrapeptide, has been found to be deficient in patients and in several families of patients with absent or impaired splenic function.

Patients with diabetic acidosis, acute infections, and chronic granulomatous disease may have impaired ingestion of properly opsonized particles. Usually this dysfunction is seen in conjunction with abnormal migration and chemotaxis.

Abnormal degranulation can result from acquired or inherited deficiency of neutrophilic granules or granule enzymes or from failure of granules to secrete their contents into phagosomes. There appears to be an unusual abnormality in degranulation of neutrophils in the Chédiak-Higashi syndrome: giant primary granules fail to fuse with phagosomes and this leads to functional myeloperoxidase deficiency.

Chronic granulomatous disease, an often fatal disease seen mainly in young males, is characterized by dermatitis, granulomas, pulmonary infiltrates, hepatosplenomegaly, hypergammaglobulinemia, and death from overwhelming sepsis with staphylococci. The etiology is unknown, but there appears to be a defect in ability to produce hydrogen peroxide. This defect is paralleled by inability of the phagocytes to reduce a yellow dye, nitroblue tetrazolium, to a blue formazan (NBT test). Why the failure of reduction is related to hydrogen peroxide formation is unknown.

Because of their inability to form enough hydrogen peroxide to kill staphylococci and other organisms containing catalase (which breaks down hydrogen peroxide), these patients have chronic and often fatal infections. Since the hexose monophosphate shunt is required for production of hydrogen peroxide, patients who have a complete absence of G-6-PD in their white cells may suffer from a syndrome similar to chronic granulomatous disease.

Granulocyte Pools and Kinetics

Granulopoiesis has been investigated by labeling leukocytes with radioactive tritiated thymidine, chromium 51, or diisopropyl-fluorophosphate 32 (^{32} DFP). From these and other studies the functioning of the committed granulocytic stem cell and the organization of granulocytes into functional pools has been deduced. Pluripotential stem cells with ability to replicate themselves and to differentiate into committed stem cells are described in Chapter 7. A percentage of pluripotential stem cells are directed into a differentiating pathway and serve as committed stem cells for the granulocytic series. The first recognizable member of the granulocyte series to develop from the granulocytic stem cell is the myeloblast. The myeloblast, promyelocytes, and myelocytes retain the ability to divide. More greatly differentiated cells, the metamyelocytes, bands and polys, mature but do not undergo mitosis.

Once the mature granulocyte (poly) is in the bloodstream, it may exist in one of two pools, the circulating granulocyte pool (CGP) or the marginal granulocyte pool (MGP). Cells in these pools are constantly interchanging, and equilibration between pools occurs rapidly. The CGP is quantified by the routine white blood cell count. Granulocytes in the marginal pool are not counted, since they are located in the intravascular space close to the endothelium but outside the mainstream of the blood vessels. Equal numbers of granulocytes are present in each of these pools, so shifting between pools can approximately double blood neutrophil counts. Such shifting has been seen after stress or corticosteroid administration. In inflammatory diseases it is possible for the MGP to increase while the CGP remains stable. This is sometimes referred to as *masked granulocytosis*. A shift of cells from the MGP to the CGP is sometimes referred to as *pseudoneutrophilia*.

In the marrow there are also two granulocyte pools: the mitotic pool, consisting of dividing cells, myeloblasts through myelocytes; and, overlapping this pool, the maturation-storage pool, consisting of myelocytes, metamyelocytes, bands, and segmented neutrophils. Marrow neutrophil differential counts are obtained by counting at least 200, and preferably 500, cells in Wright-stained smears of bone marrow specimens. Normal percentages of each cell type are given in Table 8-3.

Table 8-3 : Normal Marrow Granulocyte Differential Count

Cell Type	Range (%)*
Myeloblast	1-2
Promyelocyte	3-5
Myelocyte	8-16
Metamyelocyte	10-20
Band forms	10-15
Mature granulocytes	6-12
Eosinophils	1-5

*Erythroid and other cell lines make up the difference from 100%.

The cells in the mitotic pool divide by going through a cell cycle consisting of the following phases: G_1 (postmitotic rest period), S (DNA-synthetic phase in which chromosomes replicate from diploid to tetraploid number), G_2 (premitotic rest period), and M (period of mitosis). The so-called generation time for cells capable of successive divisions is the time from one mitosis to the next. As we will see, knowledge about cell cycles both for normal granulocytes and in pathologic states such as leukemia is important in planning rational chemotherapy.

The normal human marrow contains 18.0×10^9 nucleated marrow cells per kilogram of body weight. Of this number, 11.4×10^9 are in the granulocytic series. The marrow granulocyte reserve (MGR), consisting of myelocytes, metamyelocytes, bands, and mature granulocytes, is put at 8.8×10^9 cells per kilogram, but there is disagreement about this number, and it may be considerably larger. The bone marrow releases into the bloodstream 1.6×10^9 cells per kilogram per day of mature granulocytes. There are 0.39 cells $\times 10^9$ per kilogram in the marginal granulocytic pool and 0.31×10^9 cells per kilogram in the circulating granulocyte pool. The total blood granulocyte pool is 0.7 cells $\times 10^9$ per kilogram of body weight.

The average age of a circulating granulocyte from time of birth to appearance as a poly in the circulation is 10 days. The half-life of the granulocyte in the peripheral blood is 6 to 7 hours according to some investigators and 16 hours according to others. It survives in tissues for 4 to 5 days. Thus its total life span is 10 to 15 days; it spends most of its time in the bone marrow, a relatively short time in the peripheral blood, and once it has entered tissues, it does not return, but dies performing its phagocytic function.

Mobilization of granulocytes into the tissues can be studied by abrading one section of the skin and, at different intervals, placing a glass slide over the injured area (*Rebuck skin window*). By allowing the leukocytes to stick to the glass and then staining them with Wright stain, an estimate of the number of cells available for mobilization to inflamed sites and their differential counts can be obtained. Normally cells appear in 2 to 4 hours. Initially the responding cells are mainly granulocytes, but at 24 hours monocytes predominate. The neutrophil response is impaired in patients who receive steroids or ethanol and in individuals with acute leukemia, diabetes mellitus, and neutropenia. Some leukopenic patients have normal skin windows despite a low CGP, their MGP and MGR being normal or near-normal.

Patients who are chronically receiving adrenocorticosteroids often develop neutrophilia due to increased egress of granulocytes from the blood. This is different from the shift of granulocytes from the MGP into the CGP that results from short-term corticosteroid administration.

Patients with sustained and chronic neutropenia due to accelerated peripheral blood loss of granulocytes show "maturation arrest" of their marrow granulocyte precursor cells. Most of the granulocyte precursors present are immature. There is, however, no functional block or "arrest" in the maturation of the myelocytes, rather, there is depletion of the MGR by greatly increased peripheral demand. This should be taken into consideration when interpreting marrows in patients with hypersplenism or overwhelming sepsis. The marrow may actually be producing normal or increased amounts of granulocytes, yet only immature cells will be seen in it. In such a case a misdiagnosis of acute or chronic leukemia should be avoided. Similarly, during recovery from drug-induced agranulocytosis, there may be marrow hyperplasia and an increased number of immature forms, a so-called shift to the left of the granulocytic series. This shift can be severe enough to be mistaken for myelocytic leukemia. The reason for the shift is not peripheral demand, but rather the starting up of granulocyte production from the stem cell level.

Granulocyte Production Control Mechanisms

The control mechanisms by which a normal blood granulocyte level is maintained are not completely known. It is believed that when the peripheral blood granulocyte count falls, stimulatory factors come into play that lead to increased production of blood granulocytes and release of granulocytes from the marrow granulocyte reserve. If the marrow granulocyte reserve is reduced, as occurs in cyclic neutropenia and following subtotal marrow suppression by cyclophosphamide, the normal, stable blood leukocyte count will be altered, and oscillations will occur in the leukocyte count. Such oscillations have been seen in some patients with marrow damage, chronic granulocytic leukemia, and cyclic neutropenia.

The rate at which cells flow from the marrow reserve pool into the blood appears to be accelerated by a neutrophil-releasing factor (leukocytosis-inducing factor) present in the plasma of animals and man. The releasing factor may affect marrow sinusoids and allow egress of less mature, more rigid cells from the marrow.

The marrow granulocyte mitotic pool also seems to be under humoral control. A *colony stimulating factor* (CSF), so called because it is required for the growth of granulocytic colonies in soft agar, is found in the plasma and urine of patients with leukopenia and leukocytosis. This material, sometimes called granulopoietin, stimulates committed granulocyte precursors (CFU_c) to increase neutrophil production. The material is probably produced by monocytes or macrophages in response to an undefined stimulus delivered by mature neutrophils. Endotoxin from gram-negative bacteria can release CSF from monocytes and macrophages, and may play a role in recovery from myeloid hypoplasia.

Opposed to the positive feedback control loop mediated by granulopoietin is a negative feedback mechanism that is dependent on the accumulation of mature granulocytes in the bone marrow. As neutrophils are released in response to infection, inhibition by this control mechanism would cease, thereby allowing production of new granulocytes.

The factors regulating the flow of pluripotential stem cells (CFU_s) into the granulocyte, committed stem cell, pools are unknown.

It is likely that increased stem cell input, stimulation of mitoses in the mitotic pool, shortening of generation time, rapid marrow transit, and increased release of granulocytes all contribute to granulocyte production during stress.

Approach to the Patient with Granulocytosis

Granulocytosis ($> 11.0 \times 10^9$ granulocytes per liter) is far more common than neutropenia. Infections and inflammatory diseases cause neutrophilia more commonly than do neoplastic conditions such as leukemia. Almost any stress to the human body can result in leukocytosis with increased granulocyte counts. Because the causes of neutrophilia are so numerous, a rational approach to diagnosis is difficult. Luckily the patient's history usually suggests a primary cause, often a nonhematologic disease. Examination of the peripheral blood and bone marrow will reveal any existing primary blood disorder. Therapy for granulocytosis is essentially treatment of the underlying disease.

MONOCYTES The monocyte (Plate 44) in the peripheral blood is a medium-sized cell with granular, blue-pink cytoplasm and a nucleus with lobulation, or folding over, of the nuclear material. This lobulation of the nucleus is most helpful in identifying the cell. The cell is produced from the committed granulocyte stem cell (CFU_c), and its maturation parallels that of the granulocyte. Mature monocytes are released into the circulation and are carried to their sites of function. They enter tissues and there transform into the macrophages of the reticuloendothelial system. These macrophages, or *histiocytes,* appear in the bone marrow as large cells with filmy cytoplasm containing inclusions and an eccentric, usually pink, nucleus with two or more small, robin's-egg-blue nucleoli (see Plate 45). Because RES macrophages are derived from monocytes, the term *mononuclear-phagocyte system* has been proposed as an alternative to *reticuloendothelial system.*

Monocytes and especially macrophages play a large role in removing foreign substances from blood and tissues. They function in a manner very similar to that of granulocytes, but there are important differences. Monocytes and macrophages are more efficient than neutrophils at phagocytizing mycobacteria, fungi, macromolecules, and sensitized erythrocytes and less effective in ingesting pyogenic bacteria. They are long-lived cells and can synthesize digestive enzymes. Complement components, transferrin, interferon, endogenous pyrogen, lysozyme, and colony-stimulating factor can be synthesized and secreted by the monocyte-macrophage system. The cells in this system assist in removal of aged or damaged cells, such as erythrocytes, and also play an important role in cellular immunity and humoral antibody production.

Monocytosis is usually defined as an "absolute" monocyte count greater than 0.50×10^9 cells per liter. In the neonate, monocyte counts may be higher, up to 1.20×10^9 monocytes per liter. On a relative basis monocytes normally account for 1 to 10 percent of blood leukocytes. Monocytosis is often found in patients with infections, such as tuberculosis and subacute bacterial endocarditis, and in inflammatory diseases, including collagen-vascular conditions and inflammatory bowel disorders. Preleukemia, myelocytic leukemias, lymphomas, and the myeloproliferative diseases are also causes of monocytosis. Patients with aplasia or hypoplasia of granulocytic marrow elements often have monocytosis. Although less efficient than polys at phagocytosis, monocytes may protect against overwhelming sepsis. In some cases of agranulocytosis with recovery, monocytosis in the blood and marrow may be so severe as to suggest leukemia. Only in a rare individual with a tremendous outpouring of monocytes, including nucleolated monoblasts, should the diagnosis of monocytic leukemia be seriously considered.

LYMPHOCYTES The precursor of the lymphocyte is generally believed to be the pluripotential, primitive stem cell that also gives rise to the common progenitor cell of the myeloid, erythroid, and megakaryocytic cell lines. Lymphoid precursor cells travel to specific sites, where they differentiate into cells capable of either expressing cell-mediated immune responses or secreting immunoglobulins. The influence for the former type of differentiation in man is the thymus gland; the resulting cells are defined as thymus-dependent lymphocytes, or *T cells*. The site of the formation of lymphocytes with the potential to differentiate into antibody-producing cells (plasma cells) has not been identified in man. In chickens it is the bursa of Fabricius, and for this reason these bursa-dependent lymphocytes are called *B cells*.

By light microscopy lymphocytes cannot be distinguished as B or T cells. They vary from the size of a red cell to two or three times as large. They have a ground-glass blue cytoplasm and clumped nuclear chromatin. If they have a small amount of cytoplasm, they are called *small or mature lymphocytes* (Plate 46); if a large amount, they are called *large lymphocytes* (Plate 47). In normal persons both small and large lymphocytes are found in the peripheral blood. The earliest recognizable lymphoid precursors, *lymphoblasts* (Plate 48), in the bone marrow are similar to the circulating forms, except that they have nucleoli in their nuclei. The nucleoli are usually single or double and have well-defined nucleolar membranes. The nucleolated lymphoblast is difficult to distinguish from a myeloblast. Atypical forms of lymphocytes have vacuolated cytoplasm (Plate 49), folded-over or monocytoid nuclei (Plate 50), and nucleoli (Plate 51). It is difficult to distinguish morphologically a nucleolated atypical lymph from a malignant lymphoblast characteristic of patients with leukemia or malignant lymphoma.

Certain surface markers have been useful in differentiating human T and B lymphocytes. B cells have membrane-bound immunoglobulins, particularly IgM and lesser amounts of IgG, detectable with fluorescent anti-immunoglobulin sera. They also have receptors for the third factor of complement (C3 receptor) and for the Fc portion of immunoglobulins. Finally, a specific B cell antigen has been described. Not all B cells have all these specific markers. Approximately 25 percent of the lymphocytes in human blood are B cells. B cells seem to have a short life span, probably of days to weeks. They are located in the germinal centers of lymph nodes and spleen and in the subcapsular medullary areas of lymph nodes. They do not transform into blast-like cells when stimulated with the mitogenic plant substance phytohemagglutinin. Poke-weed mitogen transforms both B and T cells.

Human T cells have receptors for normal sheep red blood cells. When human lymphocytes are mixed in vitro with sheep red cells, many of the lymphocytes become surrounded by erythrocytes arranged in rosette formation. A specific T cell antigen, recognized by specific anti-T serum, has also been described. This serum is prepared in animals by injection of human thymus cells and adsorption of this antiserum with B cell lymphocytes. T cells are found in blood, thoracic duct lymph, perifollicular and paracor-tical areas of the lymph node, periarteriolar areas of the spleen, and virtually all tissues to which lymphocytes have access. Be-cause of their long life and recirculation these small lymphocytes are logical candidates for antigen recognition and immunologic memory retention. In vitro, phytohemagglutinin-induced blasto-genesis (transformation) occurs. Finally, some lymphocytes have no surface markers and are called *null cells.*

Inherited B cell deficiency with congenital agammaglobulinemia and inherited T cell deficiency with abnormal cell-mediated im-munity and thymic aplasia (DiGeorge's syndrome) have been described. Patients with lymphoproliferative diseases such as leukemia and lymphoma may develop deficiency or excess of T or B cells or both.

Stimulation of B cells to produce antibody is a complex process often requiring interactions between macrophages, T cells, and B cells. Some antigens, including pneumococcal and *E. coli* polysaccharides, are capable of directly stimulating B cells to pro-duce antibody, usually of the IgM type. Many other antigens re-quire initial processing by macrophages and interaction of the processed antigen with T cells. The resulting sensitized T (helper) cells cause B cell differentiation into plasma cells capable of anti-body production. T cells and perhaps a population of long-lived B cells mediate the ability to produce a secondary, or *anamnestic,* response. This rapid and intense secondary response to antigenic stimuli occurs some time after the primary immune response to the initial antigen encounter and is the result of the immunologic memory function of long-lived lymphocytes.

The T cell plays the predominant role in cellular immunity. Cellu-lar immune phenomena result from sensitization of lymphocytes following interaction with antigen. Immunity in this case is medi-ated by these sensitized T lymphocytes rather than by humoral antibodies. Delayed hypersensitivity, allograft rejection, graft-versus-host disease, immunity to tumors and intracellular para-sites, and contact allergy are all clinical examples of cellular immune reactions.

Table 8-4 : Humoral Mediators Produced By T Lymphocytes

Mediator	Biologic Activity
Migration inhibitory factor	Inhibits migration of normal macrophages out of capillary tube
Macrophage activating factor	Increases metabolic function of macrophage, increasing ability to phagocytize
Chemotactic factors for granulocytes eosinophils lymphocytes macrophages	Attracts specified cell to areas of inflammation
Lymphotoxin	Is cytotoxic to lymphocytes and other cells
Mitogenic factors	Stimulates or transforms other lymphocytes
Skin-reactive factors (lymph node permeability factor)	Produces skin reactions resembling delayed hypersensitivity responses. Increases permeability of vascular endothelium in lymph nodes.
Interferon	Renders cells resistant to virus infection
Transfer factor	Sensitizes lymphocytes to specific antigens (transfers delayed hypersensitivity reactions).

The sensitization of T lymphocytes occurs in response to antigens initially processed by macrophages. The sensitized T lymphocyte produces humoral mediators of cellular immunity and also has the capacity to kill antigen-bearing cells on contact. The better known humoral mediators and their biologic activity are described in Table 8-4. It is clear that these humoral mediators are useful at inflammatory sites. Some will attract and activate macrophages, others will recruit and sensitize other lymphocytes, and lymphocytoxin will destroy foreign cells.

Although humoral mediators of cytotoxicity exist, it is also likely that direct contact between "killer," or sensitized, lymphocytes and target cells results in cell death. Under certain circumstances prior sensitization of the killer lymphocytes is not required. Antibodies or complement on the target cell may or may not be required for lymphocyte cytotoxicity.

Lymphocytosis   Lymphocytosis in the peripheral blood is defined as an "absolute" lymphocyte count (lymphocyte fraction $\times$ total WBC) greater than 5.0×10^9 cells per liter, including atypical lymphocytes. A finding of more than 20 percent atypical lymphocytes in the white cell differential count suggests the diagnosis of infectious

Causes of lymphocytosis

Carcinoma
Hypopituitarism
Infection (influenza, brucellosis, typhoid fever, tuberculosis, syphilis,
  pertussis)
Infectious hepatitis
Infectious lymphocytosis
Infectious mononucleosis
Lymphocytic leukemias
Malignant lymphomas
Multiple myeloma
Myasthenia gravis
Thyrotoxicosis
Toxoplasmosis

mononucleosis, infectious hepatitis, cytomegalic virus infection, or drug hypersensitivity, e.g., PAS or Dilantin. A depression of the granulocyte count may cause a relative lymphocytosis.

A low "absolute" lymphocyte count, 1.5×10^9 cells per liter or less, may be caused by cytotoxic anticancer agents, x-irradiation, or adrenocorticosteroids. Malignant diseases, including carcinomas of the lung or breasts and Hodgkin's disease, can also be responsible for lymphocytopenia (see p. 273).

CASE DEVELOPMENT PROBLEM: LEUKOCYTES

A 45-year-old woman is admitted with high fever and signs and symptoms of a kidney and bladder infection. She has been treated for psychiatric problems with a phenothiazine, Thorazine, which she has been taking up until the time of admission. Five years ago she had a gastrectomy for severe gastritis. On examination, besides signs of acute urinary tract infection, splenomegaly was the only other finding.

Laboratory Data
Hematocrit: 0.29 (29%)
White blood cell count: 1.2×10^9/L
White cell differential count:
  polys, 5%
  bands, 10%
  metamyelocytes, 5%
  myelocytes, 2%
  promyelocytes, 0
  blasts, 0
  lymphs, 20%
  monocytes, 58%
Platelets: 75×10^9/L
Reticulocyte count: 3%

1. Describe at least four pathogenetic mechanisms to explain this clinical picture.
   a. Phenothiazine-induced agranulocytosis leading to acute urinary tract infection.
   b. Leukopenia due to severe infection and excessive utilization of white cells at the site of inflammation.
   c. Leukopenia secondary to gastrectomy, malabsorption of vitamin B_{12}, and megaloblastic anemia.
   d. Splenomegaly (of unknown cause) causing hypersplenism and depression of the white count, thereby predisposing to kidney infection.

2. How would you distinguish between these pathophysiologic mechanisms?

A bone marrow examination could confirm the diagnosis of phenothiazine-induced myeloid hypoplasia or aplasia. If megaloblastic anemia secondary to vitamin B_{12} deficiency is causing agranulocytosis, then red cell precursors should be frankly megaloblastic. Hypersplenism should be manifested in the bone marrow by increased cellularity, particularly of the white cell series. Peripheral utilization of white cells at the site of infection should also lead to a hypercellular marrow. The myeloid series may be severely shifted to the left due to premature release of young white cells.

The results of a urinalysis would show whether white cells are reaching the urinary tract. Presumably if the patient can produce white cells, they would appear in the urine.

Bone marrow examination shows the erythroid series to be normal in number and morphology. Granulocytic elements are markedly depressed, and only a few blasts and promyelocytes can be found. Megakaryocytes are present. The peripheral blood smear shows only toxic granulations and Döhle bodies. Urinalysis shows five to ten white blood cells per high power field.

3. On the basis of these findings, what is the most likely diagnosis?

Phenothiazine-induced myeloid hypoplasia leading to severe leukopenia and infection.

4. If the granulocytic elements of the bone marrow are hyperplastic, how can you distinguish between hypersplenism and excessive peripheral white cell destruction due to infection?

In many cases it is necessary to treat the patient's infection and observe the white count. When infection is controlled, the white count should rise toward normal. On the other hand, if hypersplenism is present, even after control of infection the white count will remain low.

In this patient the infection is controlled with antibiotics, but the white count remains at 1.2×10^9 per liter.

5. How would you treat this patient?

All drugs potentially toxic to bone marrow should be stopped. Infections should be appropriately treated. If the first infection is difficult to control, or if recurrent infections develop, white cell transfusions should be considered for treatment of infection. Androgens and marrow transplantation should be considered if the leukopenia is severe and chronic.

TOPICS FOR DISCUSSION: LEUKOCYTES

Ultrastructural studies of granulocytes

Composition of leukocyte granules

Control mechanisms of granulocytopoiesis

Leukocyte kinetics

Metabolism of leukocytes

Ultrastructural studies of granulocytes

Mechanisms of phagocytosis

Granulocyte enzymes

Myeloperovidase-halide-hydrogen peroxide system

Granulocyte antigens and antibodies

Mechanisms of neutrophilia

Mechanisms of neutropenia

Etiology of myeloid hypoplasia

Drug-induced neutropenia

Granulocyte transfusions

Function of eosinophils

Function of basophils

Mononuclear-phagocyte system

Lymphocyte metabolism

Lymphocyte function

Lymphocyte antigens

Immunologic memory

SELECTED REFERENCES

General Considerations

Boggs, D. R. Leukocyte Physiology. In C. E. Mengel, et al (eds.), *Hematology: Principles and Practice.* Chicago: Year Book, 1972.

England, J. M., and Bain, B. J. Total and differential leucocyte count. *Br. J. Haematol.* 33:1, 1976.

Laszlo, J., and Kremer, W. B. Leukocyte Metabolism. In C. E. Mengel, et al (eds.), *Hematology: Principles and Practice.* Chicago: Year Book, 1972.

Laszlo, J., Rundles, R. W., and Bertino, J., et al Part IV, The Leukocytes. In W. J. Williams, E. Beutler, A. J. Erslev, and R. W. Rundles (eds.), *Hematology* (2nd ed.). New York: McGraw-Hill, 1977.

Lessin, L., Bessis, M., and Cline, M., et al Chapter 95, Morphology of Monocytes and Macrophages; Chapter 96, Biochemistry and Function of Monocytes and Macrophages; Chapter 97, Cellular Kinetics of Monocytes and Macrophages. In. W. J. Williams, E. Beutler, A. J. Erslev, and R. W. Rundles (eds.), *Hematology* (2nd ed.). New York: McGraw-Hill, 1977.

Lichtman, M. A. (ed.) Granulocyte and monocyte abnormalities. *Clin. Haematol.* 4:1, 1975.

Wintrobe, M. M., et al Leukocytes, Spleen, and the Reticuloendothelial System. In M. M. Wintrobe, et al (eds.), *Clinical Hematology* (7th ed.). Philadelphia: Lea & Febiger, 1974.

Granulocytes   Bainton, D. F. Neutrophil granules. *Br. J. Haematol.* 29:17, 1975.

Boggs, D. R. Transfusion of neutrophils as prevention or treatment of infection in patients with neutropenia. *N. Engl. J. Med.* 290:1055, 1974.

Cline, M. J. Granulocytes in human disease. *Ann. Intern. Med.* 81:801, 1974.

Cohn, Z. A. Monocytes and macrophages. *Semin. Hematol.* 7:107, 1970.

Crosby, W. H. What to treat in Felty's syndrome. *J.A.M.A.* 225:1114, 1973.

Dresch, C., Najean, Y., and Banchet, J. Kinetic studies of ^{51}Cr and DF^{32}P labelled granulocytes. *Br. J. Haematol.* 29:67, 1975.

Golde, D. W., and Cline, M. J. Regulation of granulopoiesis. *N. Engl. J. Med.* 291:1388, 1974.

Hohn, D. C., and Lehrer, R. I. NADPH oxidase deficiency in X-linked chronic granulomatous disease. *J. Clin. Invest.* 55:707, 1975.

Kay, A. B. Functions of the eosinophil leucocyte. *Br. J. Haematol.* 33:313, 1976.

Keller, H. U., Hess, M. W., and Cottier, H. Physiology of chemotaxis and random motility. *Semin. Hematol.* 12:47, 1975.

Klebanoff, S. J. Antimicrobial mechanisms in neutrophilic polymorphonuclear leukocytes. *Semin. Hematol.* 12:117, 1975.

Miller, M. E. Pathology of chemotaxis and random mobility. *Semin. Hematol.* 12:159, 1975.

Pisciotta, A. V. Immune and toxic mechanisms in drug-induced agranulocytosis. *Semin. Hematol.* 10:279, 1973.

Quie, P. G. Pathology of bacteriocidal power of neutrophils. *Semin. Hematol.* 12:143, 1975.

Robinson, W. A., and Mangalik, A. The kinetics and regulation of granulopoiesis. *Semin. Hematol.* 12:7, 1975.

Senn, H. J., and Jungi, W. F. Neutrophil migration in health and disease. *Semin. Hematol.* 12:27, 1975.

Stohlman, F., Queensberry, P. J., and Tyler, W. S. The regulation of myelopoiesis as approached with in vivo and in vitro techniques. *Prog. Hematol.* 8:259, 1973.

Stossel, T. P. Phagocytosis. *N. Engl. J. Med.* 290:717, 774, 833, 1974.

Stossel, T. P. Phagocytosis: Recognition and ingestion. *Semin. Hematol.* 12:83, 1975.

Wintrobe, M. M., et al Variations of Leukocytes in Disease; Quantitative, Morphologic and Functional Disorders of the Granulocyte and Monocyte — Macrophage Systems. In M. M. Wintrobe, et al (eds.), *Clinical Hematology* (7th ed.). Philadelphia: Lea & Febiger, 1974.

Lymphocytes

Chessin, L. N. Lymphocytes and Plasma Cells: Newer Views of Their Relationships, Life Cycles, and Functions. In R. I. Weed (ed.), *Hematology for Internists*. Boston: Little, Brown, 1971.

Craddock, C. G., Longmire, R., and McMillan, R. Lymphocytes and the immune response. *N. Engl. J. Med.* 285:324; 378, 1971.

Kay, H. E. M. Lymphocyte function. *Br. J. Haematol.* 20:139, 1971.

Parker, C. W. Control of lymphocyte function. *N. Engl. J. Med.* 295:1180, 1976.

Podleski, W. K. Cytodestructive mechanisms provoked by lymphocytes. *Am. J. Med.* 61:1, 1976.

Wybran, J., and Fudenberg, H. How clinically useful is T and B cell quantitation? *Ann. Intern. Med.* 80:765, 1974.

Zacharski, L. R., and Linman, J. W. Lymphocytopenia: Its causes and significance. *Mayo Clin. Proc.* 46:168, 1971.

9 : Leukemias and Other Myeloproliferative Disorders

LEUKEMIAS

Leukemias are malignancies characterized by the presence of large numbers of leukocytes in the peripheral blood. Equally important is the pathologic infiltration of many tissues and organs by mature and immature leukocytes. There are two types of leukemia, acute and chronic. In the acute type the bone marrow and peripheral blood are filled with immature granulocytes or lymphocytes, whereas in the chronic type large numbers of mainly mature granulocytes or lymphocytes are present. The acute leukemias run a short course (months) in comparison to chronic leukemias (years). The leukemias are also usually divided into lymphocytic and myelocytic types. The lymphocytic is characterized by the presence of large numbers of mature or immature lymphocytes and the myelocytic by large numbers of mature or immature granulocytes or related cells such as monocytes.

Various terms are used to describe different forms of the leukemic condition. *Aleukemic leukemia* refers to acute leukemias, both lymphocytic and myelocytic, in which the peripheral blood is free of immature forms and the total white blood count is normal. The diagnosis of aleukemic leukemia is made from the bone marrow specimen, which shows infiltration by immature myeloid or lymphoid cells. In *subleukemic leukemia* immature lymphoid and myeloid cells are present in the peripheral blood, but the total white count is still within normal limits. *Hyperleukocytosis* and a *leukemoid reaction* often must be differentiated from leukemia. In hyperleukocytosis the leukocyte count in the peripheral blood is very high and mature granulocytes and band forms are present. Generally the same diseases that produce granulocytosis cause hyperleukocytosis. The heavy influx of white cells into the peripheral blood leads to total white cell counts greater than 100×10^9 per liter. In leukemoid reactions the total white count may be as high as in hyperleukocytosis, but there are more immature granulocytic or lymphocytic forms in the peripheral blood. The differentiation from true leukemia is difficult and will be discussed in a later section. *Preleukemia* is a clinical syndrome that in a number of cases evolves into true lymphocytic or granulocytic leukemia (see p. 282).

Etiology of Leukemias

The etiology of the acute and chronic leukemias is unknown. Viruses, genetic predisposition, chromosomal abnormalities, drugs, x-irradiation, and immunologic deficiencies have all been implicated in the development of leukemia.

At present there is much interest in viruses as the cause of leukemia. It has been suggested that drugs, irradiation, or other predisposing agents activate latent human leukemia viruses. However, it cannot be stressed too much that no human leukemia virus has yet been identified. The virus theory of leukemia gains its greatest support from studies of animals. In animals leukemia can be reliably produced by the inoculation of many different viruses. Even the higher mammals, exclusive of man, have been found to be susceptible to readily identified animal leukemia viruses. In man the problem is complicated by the fact that latent nonleukemogenic viruses can be activated in leukemic tissues. The question remains as to whether a virus that is found in a human leukemic is an etiologic agent or rather a latent virus activated by the leukemic process.

At present, the RNA oncornaviruses are the prime candidates for human leukemia-inducing agents, although none have actually been demonstrated in human leukemic cells. Investigators are looking for their characteristic enzymes, complementary DNA, and specific tumor antigens and are using culture methods designed to recover virus from tumors. A virus originally not recoverable may be detected through activating agents, such as x-rays or ultraviolet light, or by the use of helper viruses, which supply a coat protein enabling the RNA to emerge from a doubly infected cell. This process is called *genome rescue.* It is not clear in man whether the postulated viral agent is transmitted vertically, that is, by a zygote containing a viral genome integrated into the DNA or by maternal milk, or horizontally, for example, by aerosol between contacts.

Marrow transplantation for treatment of acute leukemia has yielded some evidence to support the virus theory of human leukemogenesis. A female leukemic patient treated with whole body irradiation and infusion of marrow from her histocompatible brother later developed recurrent leukemia. Most importantly, cytogenetic studies indicated that the leukemia recurred in the donor's rather than in the recipient's cells. This suggested the transmission of a leukemic virus from the woman to the transplanted donor's cells. An alternative possibility is that a leukemic virus in the donor's cells was activated in some unknown way to cause the leukemia.

Even if human leukemia is caused by viruses, it is likely that certain agents or conditions predispose to the development of the disease. Inherited factors or a genetic predisposition is suggested from studies of identical twins that describe an increased incidence of leukemia in the initially unaffected identical twin. Leukemia is even more common in identical twins than it is in dizygotic twins. More than genetic factors must play a role, since in the vast majority of cases only one of the identical twins is affected. Incidentally, nontwin siblings of leukemic patients stand a greater chance of developing leukemia than do individuals with no family history.

Certain diseases (Down's syndrome, or trisomy 21, and Fanconi's anemia), drugs (benzene), and irradiation (following atomic bombing or treatment of ankylosing spondylitis) cause chromosomal breaks and predispose to the development of acute and chronic leukemias. Drugs, including amidopyrine, chloramphenicol, phenylbutazone, and alkylating agents, may cause a similar predisposition. Only a small percentage of patients receiving these drugs develop acute leukemia.

It is interesting, and of some clinical importance, that chromosomal abnormalities are associated with acute leukemia. In patients with preleukemia, the finding of chromosomal abnormalities can predate the appearance of malignant cells. Patients in remission from acute leukemia may lose their chromosomal abnormalities, but these recur with relapse. Some investigators use these chromosomal changes to determine when to reinstitute or continue leukemic chemotherapy.

Finally it should be stressed that in most patients with leukemia no cause or predisposition is found.

Cell Kinetics in Acute and Chronic Leukemias

Knowledge of the cell kinetics of the immature blast (lymphoblast or myeloblast) cells in acute leukemia is, to say the least, in a state of flux. From the study of animal acute leukemias one would suspect that the high peripheral blood counts and the infiltration of tissues by leukemic cells are secondary to rapid proliferation of stem cells and precursor cells. Study of the cell kinetics of humans with fully developed acute leukemias indicates, however, that a large number of the blast cells are not proliferating at all and that those that are dividing have cell cycle times that are normal or longer than normal but certainly not shorter. Some authors have suggested that this finding is characteristic of the advanced state rather than the early leukemic state. They suggest that in early leukemia there is a great deal of hyperproliferation, but that with the development of a large leukemic cell load, a large number of cells become inactive and nonproliferating.

There appears to be general agreement that the leukemic blast cells do not differentiate into normally functioning cells. They have less motility, metabolic activity, and responsiveness to chemotactic agents. Their phagocytic ability is also defective.

Not only do they not mature nor mobilize into sites of tissue injury, but they appear to recirculate into blood, marrow, spleen, and other tissues. This latter characteristic is atypical of the normal granulocyte, which, once it leaves the bone marrow, seldom if ever returns and usually meets its death intravascularly or at the site of tissue injury. Not only are the blast cells in acute leukemia immature, they also remain in the bloodstream for a longer period of time than normal. Because of this greater circulation time the cell number in the peripheral blood is enormously elevated.

It is probable that normal stem cells are present along with the abnormal leukemic blast cells. This is likely because, although after therapy a leukemic blast cell line may be suppressed or even eliminated, a new normal cell line may then appear that is able to differentiate and repopulate the marrow and blood with normal, mature, functioning granulocytes or lymphocytes. Either the normal precursor cells are "crowded out" by the leukemic cells, or humoral agents associated with the leukemic cells inhibit normal cell proliferation.

The concept that most leukemic cells are in a so-called G_0, or nonproliferating, state is important to chemotherapy. It is clear that drugs that act on rapidly dividing cells will be of limited use against resting leukemic cells. Drugs that destroy leukemic cells in the G_0 phase or agents that bring nonproliferating cells into the cell cycle and make them therefore susceptible to cycle-active drugs are required for successful leukemic chemotherapy.

In chronic lymphocytic leukemia there appears to be an accumulation of long-lived, slowly dividing lymphocytes that are functionally abnormal. In contrast chronic myelocytic leukemia is characterized by hyperproliferation of myeloid precursor cells. Although cell cycle times are normal, the mass of cells undergoing proliferation is much greater than normal. The leukemic cells appear to proliferate not only in bone marrow but also in peripheral blood, spleen, and other organs. The blood circulation time and perhaps the life span of the granulocytes produced are greater than normal. As in acute leukemia there may be recirculation of the leukemic cells back into the marrow and into other organs such as the spleen. The myelocytic precursors mature into nearly normal functioning granulocytes. Thus in chronic myelocytic leukemia the high leukemic cell counts are due to hyperproliferation and prolonged circulation time.

Preleukemia

The diagnosis of preleukemia can be made for certain only in retrospect. When the diagnosis is correct, the clinical and morphologic features of acute leukemia develop. Many patients who appear to have this syndrome do not develop clinically apparent acute leukemia, however, and in some cases the preleukemic changes actually disappear. Many patients are elderly and die before it is possible to reach a conclusion as to whether the diagnosis of preleukemia was correct.

Patients with the preleukemia syndrome have anemia, leukopenia, or thrombocytopenia. Anemia unresponsive to the usual hematemics, so-called *refractory anemia,* is most commonly found. The peripheral blood and bone marrow findings are often suggestive of megaloblastic anemia. There is macrocytosis in the peripheral blood and megaloblastic changes in the erythroid precursors of the bone marrow. Giant myeloid forms may also be present, and in some cases ringed sideroblasts are found in the marrow. These patients do not respond to folic acid or vitamin B_{12} therapy.

Leukopenic patients with this syndrome often have other abnormalities, such as mild anemia with megaloblastic changes, increased numbers of immature bone marrow granulocytes, and monocytosis in the peripheral blood. Sometimes their neutrophils are hypersegmented or show Pelger-Hüet features. Their leukocyte alkaline phosphatase scores may be low. Auer rods are not present.

The patients who present with thrombocytopenia, with or without associated anemia or neutropenia, often have morphologically abnormal platelets with great variation in size or shape.

Experience has taught us that the patients most likely to go on to develop clinically apparent acute leukemia are those with more than one abnormality. They usually do not have anemia or leukopenia alone but have two or more cytopenias as well as other abnormalities of the erythroid, granulocytic, or megakaryocytic cell line. Some have evidence of ineffective erythropoiesis and decreased red cell survival. They usually react negatively to the Coombs' test.

Chromosome studies have been used to try to determine which patients will develop acute leukemia. The abnormalities most frequently observed are aberrations in the group C chromosomes, but they are not diagnostic.

There appear to be interrelationships between paroxysmal nocturnal hemoglobinuria (PNH), drug-induced aplastic anemia, preleukemia, acute leukemia, and other myeloproliferative diseases. Some patients with aplastic anemia secondary to drug-induced marrow injury develop cells unusually sensitive to complement-mediated lysis and later go on to develop acute leukemia. Patients with paroxysmal nocturnal hemoglobinuria sometimes develop acute leukemia. Some patients with preleukemia develop a population of cells with PNH-like biochemical characteristics.

In the search for biochemical tests that might confirm the diagnosis of preleukemia some investigators have grown blood cells in soft agar cultures. In the case of acute leukemia it appears that the leukemic blast cell is unable to grow normally in soft agar under the conditions selected by the investigators. There has been some attempt to show that patients with preleukemia have a population of cells that behave in a similar manner. These studies, however, have not been confirmed.

The Acute and Chronic Leukemias and Their Variants

Acute Myelocytic Leukemia (AML)

Clinical Description. Patients with acute myelocytic leukemia usually present with anemia, infection, or bleeding. They may give a history of unexplained fevers, infections, and bone tenderness, particularly in the ribs or sternum. A common early finding on routine examination is unexplained cytopenia.

Pallor, spontaneous hemorrhages, particularly into the skin (*petechiae,* or splinter hemorrhages, and *purpura,* or black-and-blue marks), and minimally enlarged lymph nodes or spleen are found on physical examination. In contrast to chronic myelocytic leukemia, the lymph nodes and spleen, although enlarged, do not reach massive proportions.

The patients are anemic due to infiltration of their bone marrow, bleeding, and sometimes secondary iron deficiency. The peripheral white blood cell count is almost always greater than 10×10^9 cells per liter. In a few patients the white blood cell count is normal or even low. Even in these patients circulating blast cells are found. In the occasional patient the peripheral blood is completely free of immature white cells (aleukemic leukemia).

Rarely, a patient has a normal platelet count at the time of diagnosis. More often, because of thrombocytopenia, there is bleeding and even fatal intracranial hemorrhage. Contributing to the risk of intracranial hemorrhage are large numbers of promyelocytes and blast cells. It appears that when the total white cell count in a leukemic patient reaches 100×10^9 cells per liter, there is an increased risk of intracranial bleeding, even if the platelet count is normal. Leukostasis and infarction of small cranial blood vessels are found in these patients.

Fever and infection are often present; therefore prior to initiation of leukemic chemotherapy, cultures of blood, urine, and stool are collected. These cultures may help in selecting antibiotics. If the patient has a high fever and appears toxic, broad spectrum antibiotic coverage is initiated before the results of cultures are available. If, after several days, cultures are negative, the antibiotics can be stopped. New cultures must be obtained if fever persists or becomes more severe. If an organism is isolated, then appropriate, specific antibiotic therapy based on microbial sensitivity assays should replace the broad spectrum antibiotics. No systemic antibiotics are administered prophylactically.

Because of the use of immunosuppressive agents — such as corticosteroids — and cytotoxic drugs, infections with gram-negative bacteria, fungi, tuberculosis, and other esoteric agents will commonly occur. Candidiasis, aspergillosis, mucormycosis, cryptococcosis, histoplasmosis, and *Pneumocystis carinii* respiratory tract infections commonly complicate the treatment of patients with leukemia.

Bone Marrow and Peripheral Blood. The diagnosis of AML is made on the basis of the characteristic changes in the peripheral blood and bone marrow (Plate 52). Blasts are numerous, and some show differentiation toward the promyelocytic stage. The presence of cells with typical blue-black promyelocytic granules helps distinguish myelocytic from lymphocytic leukemia. (Also, lymphocytic leukemia tends to occur in the younger age groups, while patients teenaged and older generally have myelocytic rather than lymphocytic leukemia.)

In the peripheral blood the blasts may be accompanied by some mature granulocytes. Often these mature forms are abnormal and have acquired pelgeroid anomalies (Plates 41 and 42) consisting of dumbbell-shaped nuclei or rounded nuclei in otherwise typical mature granulocytes. Auer rods or bodies (Plate 53) are needlelike or round cytoplasmic inclusions that have a refractile, pink appearance and are characteristically found in AML blast cells.

In the bone marrow, besides infiltration by myeloblasts, there may be prominent pronormoblasts, and the late stage normoblasts may have megaloblastic changes including abnormal nuclear chromatin patterns. Iron staining often reveals ringed sideroblasts. When erythroid precursors with megaloblastic change are prominent, along with huge, bizarre, multinucleated, erythroid cells (*gigantoblasts,* Plate 22) and myeloblasts, the diagnosis of *erythroleukemia* is made.

Some patients with typical blood and bone marrow features of AML may have only mild anemia and little in the way of infection or bleeding tendency. These patients are usually elderly, and the leukemia often smolders along for many years, even without treatment. Patients with *smoldering leukemia* have mildly elevated white counts with relatively few myeloblasts in the peripheral blood. They definitely have leukemia and can easily be distinguished from patients with preleukemia, who do not have increased numbers of myeloblasts in their bloodstream.

The blasts seen in acute myelocytic leukemia can usually be distinguished from lymphoblasts by the presence of Auer rods and by their differentiation toward promyelocytes. Certain stains such as peroxidase have also been used to distinguish the more mature myeloid precursors from lymphoid. Peroxidase is present in myeloid cells and to a lesser extent in monocytic cells but will not stain lymphocytes. Unfortunately, when morphologic identification is equivocal, cytochemistry is also.

Another feature of acute myelocytic leukemia is overproduction of uric acid secondary to nucleic acid turnover. Occasionally, in response to therapy, urates will precipitate in the ureters and renal pelvis or tubules and cause obstructive uropathy. Bone pain and arthritis may be a presenting symptom of leukemia. The arthritic joints are red and tender. Areas of fibrosis and infarction often are found in AML patients' bones at the time of autopsy.

In some patients with AML, tumors consisting of myeloblasts arise in bones and soft tissues. These tumors appear green because of the presence of myeloperoxidase in the leukocytes and are therefore called *chloromas.* Hematoxylin- and eosin-stained sections of these tumors can be mistaken for reticulum cell sarcoma. The clinical features and treatment of this tumorous form of acute myelocytic leukemia are not different from typical AML. X-irradiation of the chloromas is sometimes used to control their growth.

Hyperplasia of the gums can occur in acute myelocytic leukemia but is more common in the myelomonocytic and monocytic forms of acute myelocytic leukemia.

Acute Promyelocytic Leukemia (APL)

Acute promyelocytic leukemia is a variant of AML and is characterized by infiltration of the bone marrow by promyelocytes rather than myeloblasts (Plate 54). There are also large numbers of promyelocytes in the peripheral blood. APL may be complicated by hypofibrinoginemia, thrombocytopenia, and a severe bleeding tendency, manifested by purpura and intracranial or gastrointestinal hemorrhage. It appears that promyelocytic cells contain thromboplastic substances that can be released into the bloodstream and activate the soluble coagulation factors. This results in consumption of fibrinogen and platelets, and in increased levels of fibrin split products in the blood. The whole process is called *disseminated intravascular coagulation* (DIC). There is some debate as to whether DIC accounts for the hypofibrinogenemia, and it is possible that, in at least some cases, primary fibrinolysis is initiated rather than DIC. In any case APL must be treated carefully, since hypofibrinogenemia and bleeding have followed the initiation of chemotherapy.

Unusual clinical manifestations of acute myelocytic leukemia

Dental abscesses
Gastrointestinal ulceration
Hearing loss or dysequilibrium due to hemorrhage into middle or inner
 ear
Hypercalcemia
Hypothalmic or pituitary leukemic infiltrates causing endocrine
 deficiencies
Infiltration of genitourinary organs
Kidney enlargement secondary to infiltration
Leukemic infiltrates into liver leading to hepatomegaly
Leukemic infiltrates of skin
Leukemic infiltration or hemorrhage into pericardium or myocardium
Leukemoids or nonspecific rashes
Meningeal leukemia
Mouth ulcerations
Perirectal abscesses
Retinal hemorrhages and infiltrates
Splenic infarction or rupture associated with leukemic infiltration
Tonsillar, salivary, and lacrimal gland infiltrates (Mikulicz's syndrome—
 bilateral painless enlargement of the salivary glands leading to dryness
 of mouth and reduced tearing)
Tonsillitis and pharyngitis

Prior to the availability of daunomycin this variant of AML was thought to have a worse prognosis than typical acute myelocytic leukemia.

Acute Myelomono-cytic Leukemia (Naegeli Type of Monocytic Leukemia)

Cells in the peripheral blood and bone marrow of patients with acute myelomonocytic leukemia have characteristics of both myeloblasts and monoblasts (Plate 55). These blast cells have nuclei that are folded over and lobulated like those in monocytes. They may arise from a precursor cell common to granulocytes and monocytes. (See the discussion of the interrelationships among granulocytes, monocytes, reticuloendothelial cells, and phagocytic cells in Chapter 8.) The clinical characteristics of this leukemia variant are similar to those seen in typical acute myelocytic leukemia.

The enzyme *lysozyme* is found in large amounts in serum and urine from patients with this form of AML. Lysozyme can most easily be detected by electrophoresing a concentrated urine specimen: the protein appears as a cationic, monoclonal "spike." It may be excreted in amounts up to 2 to 3 gm per day. Lysozyme is normally found in mature neutrophils and monocytes but not in lymphocytes, eosinophils, or basophils. It is quantitated by its ability to lyse the cell walls of certain bacteria. It is present in the serum and concentrated in the urine of patients with diseases characterized by rapid granulocyte turnover. The highest amounts are found in the myelomonocytic and pure monocytic leukemias; lesser quantities are present in urine from patients with AML. Sometimes associated with heavy lysozymuria is renal tubular dysfunction characterized by hypocalcemia, hyperkaluria, and azotemia.

Although acute myelomonocytic leukemia is treated similarly to AML, some therapists believe the response rate is poorer than in typical AML.

Acute and Chronic Monocytic Leukemia (Schilling Type of Monocytic Leukemia)

Monocytic leukemias are characterized by large numbers of monocytes in the peripheral blood and bone marrow (Plate 56). Many of the cells have prominent nucleoli and should therefore be called monoblasts. In contrast to acute myelomonocytic leukemia, cellular features suggestive of granulocytes are missing.

Pure monocytic leukemia is rare. Gum hyperplasia, skin infiltration, hepatosplenomegaly, and perirectal infections are common clinical manifestations. In the chronic form of monocytic leukemia fatigue, pallor, and weight loss are prominent, and many of the clinical features of preleukemia are found. Patients may live for months or years but are usually quite resistant to treatment. A few have responded to the same drugs that have been successful in treating acute myelocytic leukemia.

Erythroleukemia

In all variants of acute myelocytic leukemia one can usually find abnormalities in the erythroid precursors. Macroovalocytosis, marrow megaloblastosis, and hypersegmented polys are found, although the folic acid and vitamin B_{12} levels are normal. Some nucleated reds with megaloblastic features may even escape into the peripheral blood. Erythroleukemia, or Di Guglielmo syndrome, is characterized by severe megaloblastic changes along with the appearance of large, bizarre, multinucleated erythroid precursors (gigantoblasts) in the bone marrow (Plate 22). Anemia and ineffective erythropoiesis, thrombocytopenia, and leukopenia are present at some time during the course of the disease. It terminates in a picture not different from that of acute myelocytic leukemia. Hemoglobin H and fetal hemoglobin levels are sometimes elevated. There is usually iron overload in the bone marrow, with prominent ringed sideroblasts. The periodic acid–Schiff (PAS) reaction may reveal cytoplasmic inclusions in marrow erythroblasts.

Eosinophilic Leukemia

Eosinophilic leukemia, a rare form of AML, is characterized by immature eosinophils in the bone marrow and peripheral blood. The condition is often hard to distinguish from early chronic myelocytic leukemia, in which large numbers of eosinophils may be present, and from collagen vascular diseases, in which there is a diffuse infiltration of organs by eosinophils. Eosinophilic leukemia patients with lung infiltrates suffer from shortness of breath, cyanosis, and pleural effusions. Eosinophils also infiltrate the heart, liver, and central nervous system, causing a wide variety of symptoms.

Basophilic or Mast Cell Leukemia

Patients with chronic myelocytic leukemia may have large numbers of circulating basophils, and mast cells are not uncommonly found in elderly people with osteoporosis and in response to inflammatory diseases. But there is also an extremely rare type of leukemia, *basophilic* or *mast cell leukemia* that is characterized by a great number of basophils in the blood and by mast cells in marrow and other tissues. These cells release heparin, histamine, and serotonin. In one syndrome, *urticaria pigmentosa,* brown skin nodules infiltrated with mast cells are prominent. Trauma to the skin produces urticaria or dermatographism due to liberation of histamine. In another form of the disease, *systemic mastocytosis,* the mast cells infiltrate all tissues and organs, producing destructive changes. Besides dermatographism there are osteolytic and osteosclerotic changes in the bones, and flushing, edema, itching, hypotension, and tachycardia may also be present. These vascular reactions have been attributed to the release of histamine. Peptic ulcer and malabsorption, and hemorrhagic manifestations thought to be secondary to the release of heparin, have also been described. The diagnosis of mast cell leukemia is made on the basis of huge numbers of basophils in the peripheral blood and mast cells in the bone marrow.

Known treatment of the mast cell diseases is completely unsatisfactory. It should be stressed again that eosinophilic and basophilic leukemias must be distinguished from the intense eosinophilia or basophilia sometimes seen in chronic myelocytic leukemia.

Undifferentiated or Stem Cell Leukemia

Some patients lack morphologic features characteristic of the variants of myelocytic leukemia described here. The predominant cell in the bone marrow and blood is a blast form without Auer rods or maturation. If the patient is young, acute lymphocytic leukemia may be suspected. Special stains, such as peroxidase, and the aid of an experienced morphologist can sometimes help in classifying the leukemia, but despite this a group of acute leukemias exist that cannot be diagnosed as myelocytic or lymphocytic and are therefore called *undifferentiated* or *stem cell leukemia*. If the patient is an adult, he or she will often respond to therapy used for AML.

Chronic Myelocytic Leukemia (CML)

Etiology. Exposure to radiation appears to be the only known predisposing agent to the development of chronic myelocytic leukemia. Studies of radiologists, Japanese atomic bomb victims, and patients with ankylosing spondylitis treated by radiotherapy to the spine indicate that after a latent period of approximately 3 to 6 years an increased incidence of chronic granulocytic leukemia is found. It should be emphasized, however, that only about 5 to 10 percent of patients who have chronic granulocytic leukemia give a history of excessive radiation exposure. When radiologists were first tested for exposure, they had an incidence of leukemia nine times that of doctors with little radiation exposure. This incidence has fallen with the use of modern x-ray shielding methods. In atomic bomb victims the incidence depends on the closeness of the survivor to the center of the explosion. Although there is an increased incidence of leukemia in atomic bomb victims, their offspring do not appear to carry any increased risk of developing the disease. Patients treated for ankylosing spondylitis run a risk approximately ten times that of the general population. The chances of developing leukemia from x-irradiation given for other medical conditions is probably higher than normal also, but ankylosing spondylitis seems to have the highest incidence and to have been investigated most thoroughly.

In approximately 90 percent of patients with chronic myelocytic leukemia an acquired chromosomal abnormality — the Philadelphia chromosome, with missing genetic material — has been found. It was thought formerly that the Philadelphia chromosome was chromosome G21, but it is now becoming clear that the defect is in chromosome G22 and that it involves translocation of genetic material, usually to chromosome 9. A study of pairs of identical twins, one of whom had CML, indicated that only the twin having the disease carried the Philadelphia chromosome, whereas the other did not. This provides evidence that the disorder is acquired. It is entirely unclear how the Philadelphia chromosome abnormality comes about and how it produces or influences the course of chronic myelocytic leukemia.

The Philadelphia chromosome is found in the erythroid, myeloid (including monocytic, eosinophilic, and basophilic), and megakaryocytic cell lines but not in lymphocytes or fibroblasts.* This has been used as evidence for a single stem cell precursor for the erythroid, myeloid, and megakaryocytic cell lines. Other explanations, however, are possible but will not be discussed here.

Clinical Features. The typical patient with chronic myelocytic leukemia is relatively asymptomatic. Usually the leukemia strikes in middle age, but it also is found in infants, children, and young adults. On physical examination splenomegaly is found to be prominent, but lymph nodes are rarely enlarged. Examination of the patient's peripheral blood reveals leukocytosis and a whole spectrum of mature and immature granulocyte precursors (Plate 57). The bone marrow is hypercellular, with an increased number of myeloid and megakaryocytic elements and an increased number of immature granulocytic cells. Although teardrop and nucleated red cells in the peripheral blood (Plate 58) and fibrosis in the bone marrow (Plates 59 and 60) may be seen at the time of diagnosis, they are more often present in the late stages of the disease or not at all. Anemia often develops. The platelet count is initially high, but, with time, thrombocytopenia often ensues. As the disease progresses, massive splenomegaly and cytopenias complicate its course. Finally, about 60 to 70 percent of patients develop a *blastic crisis* indistinguishable from acute myelocytic leukemia.

Infarction of spleen or bone should be suspected if a patient has an enlarging spleen and unexplained left upper quadrant pain or has a sudden onset of unexplained pain in the pelvic or long bones. No specific treatment for these painful infarctions is available. An enlarged spleen may give upper gastrointestinal discomfort and bloating and decreased appetite. Splenectomy is advocated as treatment for enlarged or painful spleens, but the perioperative mortality and morbidity are high, and in some cases the white cell and platelet counts rise precipitously.

*Recent evidence suggests that a precursor cell common to the myeloid and lymphoid cell lines exists and may carry the Philadelphia chromosome.

Chronic myelocytic leukemia can also be associated with hypercalcemia, a concurrent lymphoproliferative disease, breast masses consisting of accumulation of mature and immature granulocytes, or a clinical picture almost identical to that of acute myelocytic leukemia. In this last case the patients have the abnormal Philadelphia chromosome but have morphologic findings and a clinical course more consistent with acute myelocytic leukemia.

A minority of patients in the blast crisis phase of Philadelphia chromosome-positive CML have morphologic features of ALL, respond to ALL-type therapy, and have an enzyme marker (terminal transferase) characteristic of lymphoblasts. It is considered possible that a very primitive stem cell exists that can give rise to lymphocytes as well as to erythroid, myeloid, and megakaryocytic cell lines and that accounts for the transformation of CML to ALL.

Some patients with chronic myelocytic leukemia go through cyclic changes in the total white blood cell count. Their counts rise as high as 100×10^9 per liter and then in several weeks are normal, with few or no immature forms. With time the white count less often returns to normal, and finally the patient develops a noncycling blood picture typical of chronic myelocytic leukemia. The reasons for this cycling are unclear. Some authors have suggested that it is an exaggeration of the cycling present in normal individuals. Cycling toward normal should not be mistaken for a response to therapy.

Histiocytes similar to those in Gaucher's disease (Plate 61) are occasionally found in the bone marrow of patients with chronic myelocytic leukemia. They are believed to be related to increased white cell turnover and ingestion of leukocyte membrane lipids into histiocytes. The enzyme defect seen in typical Gaucher's disease is absent. Pelgeroid cells may also be present in the peripheral blood and marrow.

Besides the Philadelphia chromosome, several other laboratory abnormalities are common in CML. For example, serum uric acid may be so high, secondary to breakdown of granulocytes, as to require treatment. A neutrophil enzyme, alkaline phosphatase, is often absent or low. Its histochemical assay involves the use of an organic substrate that precipitates and turns blue or brown in the presence of alkaline phosphatase. Mature white cells (polys or bands) in the peripheral blood are scored from 0 to 4+ depending upon the amount of precipitate present. One hundred cells are evaluated. A value from 0 to 400 is computed by multiplying the score by the number of cells with this score and summing the five results. A value of 20 to 100 is considered normal. Many patients with chronic myelocytic leukemia have no leukocyte alkaline phosphatase. A biochemical method of measuring leukocyte alkaline phosphatase is also available. Unfortunately some nonleukemic conditions such as liver disease, diabetes, gout, and paroxysmal nocturnal hemoglobinuria may be associated with low or absent leukocyte alkaline phosphatase scores. Leukemoid reactions, polycythemia vera, Hodgkin's disease, infections, pregnancy, and myeloproliferative diseases may increase leukocyte alkaline phosphatase levels. Usually with treatment of CML the leukocyte alkaline phosphatase score returns toward normal. There is no relationship between the Philadelphia chromosome and the activity of this enzyme. In fact, in CML patients in remission, the Philadelphia chromosome remains while the leukocyte alkaline phosphatase score often returns to normal, presumably because a normal clone of granulocytes replaces the leukocytes that have absent or low alkaline phosphatase content.

As discussed in Chapter 3 it is thought that vitamin B_{12} binder is produced in white cells. There is an increased production of transcobalamin I in chronic myelocytic leukemia, so that the unsaturated vitamin B_{12} binding capacity and serum B_{12} levels are high. Serum lactic dehydrogenase levels may also be elevated. Pseudohyperkalemia due to release of potassium from platelets during clotting has been reported.

The onset of the blast or terminal phase of chronic myelocytic leukemia may be heralded in several ways. Aneuploidy, or the presence of an abnormal number of chromosomes, multiple Philadelphia chromosomes, marrow fibrosis, unexplained fever, basophilia, an increased leukocyte alkaline phosphatase score not due to therapy, sudden enlargement of the liver or spleen, or cytopenias may all be present just prior to the onset of a blast crisis. Then the white blood cell count rises rapidly to hundreds of billions per liter with 30 percent or more myeloblasts and promyelocytes. A few patients may develop some of the poor prognostic signs without developing the high peripheral white blood count typical of blast crisis. The diagnosis is *accelerated phase of CML* when patients develop signs of a blast crisis but not the peripheral blood immature granulocytosis.

The immediate prognosis of chronic myelocytic leukemia is good, but the moderate- to long-term prognosis is poor. Generally patients die within 1 to 4 years. Patients who lack the Philadelphia chromosome often have leukopenia and thrombocytopenia, respond less well to therapy, and have early blast crises. Their median survival is approximately one year as compared to three to four years for patients with the Philadelphia chromosome.

Chronic myelocytic leukemia must often be differentiated from a leukemoid reaction. Leukemoid reactions are due to infections such as active tuberculosis and inflammatory or malignant diseases. The white cell count is high, but usually there are only relatively few immature forms. In a leukemoid reaction the alkaline phosphatase level should be increased and the Philadelphia chromosome absent. In a few cases the "shift to the left" in the peripheral blood granulocytes is severe enough to make the differential diagnosis from CML difficult, but usually the underlying cause for the leukemoid reaction — for example, sepsis — is obvious.

Acute Lymphocytic Leukemia (ALL)

Acute lymphocytic leukemia is a rare disease characterized by the presence of large numbers of lymphoblasts and immature lymphocytes in the bone marrow, peripheral blood (Plate 48), lymph nodes, and spleen. Its etiology is unknown; ideas under investigation have been discussed under Acute Myelocytic Leukemia. The disease usually affects children from age 1 to 4 years and is the most common type of acute leukemia through age 15. Perinatal or congenital leukemias in children under age 1 are more frequently of the acute myelocytic type. The lymphocytes in ALL usually lack both B and T cell markers. A minority of ALL patients have T-lymphoblastic leukemia, which runs a more aggressive course and is relatively resistant to treatment.

As in acute myelocytic leukemia the evidence suggests that the leukemic cells do not proliferate more rapidly than normal. The number of cells dividing is actually less than normal, and the cell cycle time is normal or longer. Morphologically, the acute leukemia cells appear to outgrow and replace normal elements, but the cell kinetic data that would explain this finding are not available.

Also as in acute myelocytic leukemia, the patient usually presents with fever, infections, anemia, or bleeding. Unlike the case with adult, acute myelocytic leukemia, the lymph nodes and spleen are often enlarged. Examination of the peripheral blood shows close to 100 percent lymphoblasts, lymphocytes, and smudge (basket) cells, which last are probably the remains of damaged, fragile, leukemic lymphocytes. The patient often has severe thrombocytopenia, which is responsible for skin and mucous membrane petechiae and purpura. A number of immature granulocytes are often seen in the peripheral blood as a response to leukemic replacement of bone marrow.

A bone marrow specimen is difficult to obtain, and dry taps are not infrequent. Bone marrow biopsies must sometimes be done in order to demonstrate infiltration by lymphocytes and lymphoblasts. Normal bone marrow elements are generally scanty and appear to be replaced by the leukemic lymphocytes. Megaloblastic changes are not prominent, nor is there evidence of involvement of the erythroid, granulocytic, or megakaryocytic cell lines.

The complications of acute lymphocytic leukemia are similar to those of acute myelocytic leukemia, except that central nervous system involvement is considerably more common. This becomes important, as we will see, in planning therapy for these children. Headaches, vomiting, excessive weight gain suggestive of hypothalamic involvement, stiff neck, papilledema, or seizures may be the first signs or symptoms of meningeal leukemia.

There is little difficulty in establishing the diagnosis, since the peripheral blood and bone marrow morphology are easy to interpret. In a few patients, particularly teenagers, it may be difficult to decide whether the leukemia is lymphocytic or myelocytic. Occasionally chronic lymphocytic leukemia and lymphosarcomas, very rarely seen in children, are confused with ALL.

Chronic Lymphocytic Leukemia (CLL)

Chronic lymphocytic leukemia generally occurs in the elderly. It is characterized by the accumulation of abnormal, mature appearing B lymphocytes. These lymphocytes appear to have a very long life span but are functionally incompetent. They do not respond normally to antigens or to phytohemagglutin, a plant substance that transforms normal lymphocytes into lymphoblastlike, or *lymphoblastoid,* forms. Often associated with chronic lymphocytic leukemia is a defect in ability to produce normal immunoglobulins. Most of the clinical manifestations of the disease are a result of the accumulation of abnormal, functionally incompetent lymphocytes.

The etiology and predisposing conditions for the development of chronic lymphocytic leukemia are unknown. There does appear to be a greater than normal incidence of CLL and related forms of lymphoproliferative diseases in families of affected patients. In some studies CLL has been associated with an increased incidence of second malignancies such as carcinoma of the breast.

Most CLL patients are discovered on routine examination of peripheral blood smears. In their blood are large numbers of mature-appearing lymphocytes that are quite fragile (Plate 62). Damage to these fragile lymphocytes results in the formation of smudge, or basket, cells. Their bone marrows are infiltrated with cells of similar appearance. In one unusual variant of CLL, *chronic lymphosarcoma cell leukemia,* or *leukosarcoma* (Plate 63), the lymphocytes are large and have distinct nucleoli in their nuclei. Clefts in the nuclei are not uncommon in patients with the usual form of chronic lymphocytic leukemia, but "cloverleafing" and very prominent clefting is characteristic of chronic lymphosarcoma cell leukemia. Another even rarer variant is *hairy cell leukemia,* or *malignant reticuloendotheliosis,* which is clinically similar to chronic lymphocytic leukemia but in which the abnormal cell resembles a reticuloendothelial cell and has hair-like

Treatment ⟩
CLL

projections of the membrane. Treatment is different from that of chronic lymphocytic leukemia, since the condition often responds poorly to cytotoxic agents. When treatment is needed, adrenocorticosteroids, splenectomy, or multiple drug chemotherapy is often recommended.

In the typical patient CLL is diagnosed from the routine peripheral blood smear; then over a period of months or years the lymph nodes, liver, and spleen become enlarged and infiltrated. In many cases it is difficult to distinguish between CLL and malignant lymphoma (see Chapter 10), because lymph node enlargement and splenomegaly are present early in the course of the disease. A great deal of discussion has gone on concerning the relationship of CLL to malignant lymphoma. It is clear that the histologic appearance of the lymph nodes in chronic lymphocytic leukemia patients is often identical to that seen in patients with a leukemic form of lymphocytic lymphoma. In fact the diagnosis is sometimes given as *CLL-lymphoma,* because it was not possible to distinguish between the two diseases.

A method of clinically staging CLL patients has been proposed that is based on the concept that CLL is a disease of progressive accumulation of nonfunctioning lymphocytes; stage 0, bone marrow and blood lymphocytosis only; stage I, lymphocytosis with enlarged nodes; stage II, lymphocytosis with enlarged spleen or liver or both; stage III, lymphocytosis with anemia; and stage IV, lymphocytosis with thrombocytopenia. Median survival time (in months) goes down with each clinical stage: stage 0, greater than 150; stage I, 101; stage II, 71; stage III, 19; stage IV, 19.

Hypogammaglobulinemia (0.2 to 0.7 gm per deciliter) is regularly present, and in some cases abnormal monoclonal immunoglobulin spikes resembling those seen in multiple myelomas (see Chapter 10) appear on serum electrophoresis. In a few cases these monoclonal spikes represent macroglobulins identical to those found in patients with Waldenström's macroglobulinemia (see Chapter 10). Hyperviscosity syndromes secondary to the production of macroglobulins or aggregated 7S immunoglobulins occur only rarely in chronic lymphocytic leukemia.

In the later stages of CLL susceptibility to infection and cytopenias develops. The susceptibility to infection apparently is related to hypogammaglobulinemia, defects in cellular immune responses, and neutropenia. The number of granulocytes, normal early in the course of the disease, may become severely diminished with the use of cytotoxic chemotherapeutic agents, increased leukemic infiltration of the bone marrow and spleen, and onset of hypersplenism.

Thrombocytopenia usually does not become a problem unless a patient is treated with cytotoxic agents, has bone marrow replaced, or develops hypersplenism. Occasionally autoimmune thrombocytopenia is prominent. In this case the thrombocytopenia is severe and is associated with increased platelet destruction that is not accounted for by hypersplenism alone and is presumably caused by an antibody.

Anemia is a common problem and is due to decreased production secondary to marrow infiltration and chemotherapy and to hypersplenism. In about 20 percent of CLL patients an autoimmune, Coombs' test–positive, hemolytic anemia does develop. In some this occurs following an infection or institution of chemotherapy. The γ-globulin or the complement, or both, Coombs' tests may be positive. Patients with autoimmune hemolytic anemia or thrombocytopenia often respond to treatment with adrenal corticosteroids.

Most of the elderly patients with this disease survive 3 to 5 years with or without treatment. A few patients with the more malignant varieties die within 1 to 2 years. A goodly number of patients survive 10, 15, or even more years. The clinical course is often complicated by infections; hemorrhage; infiltration of organs and consequent symptoms; and obstruction of ureters, bile ducts, or other body conduits. It is extremely rare for chronic lymphatic leukemia to progress to acute leukemia, but there have been occasional cases in which the terminal phase has been characterized by a clinical course and abnormal cellular morphology similar to that found in acute lymphocytic leukemia.

Principles of Therapy for Acute and Chronic Leukemias

The details of the treatment of the acute leukemias are changing constantly; however, there appears to be an overall philosophy that is held by most investigators and clinicians in this field. The methods used to obtain remission are based on the theory that if malignant cells can be eradicated or nearly eradicated, normal bone marrow elements will proliferate and resume normal function. This will, of course, reverse the complications of the acute leukemia. It appears to be relatively easy to do this in acute lymphocytic leukemia, since drugs are available that will destroy the leukemic lymphocyte and maintain intact the proliferative capacity of the erythroid, granulocytic, and megakaryocytic cell lines. On the other hand, in acute myelocytic leukemia the available drugs destroy or suppress all cell lines. In both forms of acute leukemia, drugs active against the blast cells are administered until the leukemic cells can no longer be found in the peripheral blood or bone marrow. In the case of acute myelocytic leukemia, chemotherapy often results in complete aplasia of the bone marrow. Despite this administration of drugs that are known to destroy large numbers of leukemic cells, it is likely that some remain, particularly those cells that are not proliferating. It is hoped that the body's own immune system can destroy these remaining leukemic cells. Immunologic techniques that enhance the reticulo-endothelial system are sometimes used to promote this process.

Criteria for Remission. In evaluating the end results of leukemia chemotherapy a complete remission is usually defined by the bone marrow, hemogram, physical examination, and symptoms. For remission to be considered complete, the bone marrow must be normally cellular and contain less than 5 percent blast cells. Erythropoiesis, granulopoiesis, megakaryopoiesis, and the myeloid-to-erythroid ratio must all be normal. The hemoglobin must be normal or near-normal, the granulocyte count greater than 2.0×10^9 cells per liter, and the platelet count greater than 100×10^9 cells per liter. No blast cells should be seen in the peripheral blood. On physical examination the liver, spleen, and lymph nodes must be normal. There can be no leukemic infiltrations, evidence of hemorrhage, nor infection. The patient must be asymptomatic with full normal activity. Patients with partial remissions may show changes toward normal but not the return to normal seen in complete remissions. Patients who reach only partial remission or obtain no remission often quickly succumb to the leukemia.

Phases of Treatment. The first phase in the treatment of acute leukemia is referred to as the *induction phase.* Drugs are chosen that will quickly destroy large numbers of leukemic cells. There is a tendency to use combinations of drugs and to vary both the numbers of drugs given at one time and the doses. Attempts are made to include drugs that are effective in various parts of the cell cycle. The hope is to destroy both proliferating and nondividing cells by the choice of appropriate therapeutic agents. Some attempts have also been made to use drugs (e.g., cytosine arabinoside) that will take nonproliferating cells and "push" them into a proliferative phase, where they can be destroyed by agents active against dividing cells.

In most protocols combinations of drugs are given as a series of cycles. Each cycle period consists of one or more drugs taken on certain days during a set period of time, often 14 or 28 days. This cycle may be repeated any number of times. The patient's clinical status, peripheral blood, and bone marrow are examined frequently. Once the patient's status meets the criteria for a complete remission, the induction phase has been completed. In many protocols a *consolidation phase* is then entered. The patient is cycled with the same or different drugs in an attempt to destroy as many hidden leukemic cells as possible and — perhaps along with the body defenses — eliminate them entirely. Before the consolidation phase or even during it, attempts are often made with radiotherapy or intrathecal (spinal fluid) injection of an antileukemia drug to destroy cells in such "hiding places" as the meninges of the brain and spinal cord, where they tend to accumulate. Finally, after a complete remission is secure, *maintenance therapy* is usually instituted. This may take the form of a single drug or, following a recent trend, cycles of various antileukemic drugs, singly or in combination, to maintain the remission. Patients who fail to obtain complete remission, those who obtain partial remission, and those who subsequently relapse after complete remission are often subjected to second or even third drug combinations in an attempt to obtain complete remission. This phase is called *reinduction.*

In acute myelocytic leukemia induction is usually attempted with cytosine arabinoside, daunomycin, or both. (These drugs will be discussed in detail later.) Other agents are sometimes used in combination with one or both of these. There is no agreement about which drugs to use for consolidation or maintenance. In fact, although patients who have a complete remission survive longer than those who don't, there is at present no good evidence that either consolidation or maintenance therapy prolongs survival.

In acute lymphocytic leukemia vincristine and prednisone are usually given first, to obtain a complete remission. In 80 to 90 percent of cases these drugs are all that is required; remission is almost 100 percent if daunomycin is added. In acute myelocytic leukemia the initial complete remission rate is approximately 60 percent. With each relapse the remission rate following reinduction falls, and the duration of remission is relatively shorter. It is unusual for patients with AML to be maintained in remission for more than a year and a half. Remissions in ALL usually last 2 to 3 years, and in approximately 25 percent of patients, 5 years or more.

The treatment philosophy for chronic leukemia is different from that for acute, because we do not have drugs or combinations of drugs that can eliminate all or even most of the chronic leukemic cells. At present, cure for chronic leukemia is not possible, only palliation. Treatment is aimed at relieving symptoms or preventing the onset of symptoms. Fortunately patients with chronic leukemias usually survive, even without treatment, for 3 years or more from the time of diagnosis.

Remission from chronic leukemia is symptomatic, that is, there is a relief of symptoms usually in association with a measurable decrease in organomegaly and improvement in peripheral blood counts. Despite symptomatic improvement, morphologic evidence of disease persists in blood, bone marrow, or both. When good remissions are obtained, morphologically normal marrow cell lines sometimes appear, so it is theoretically possible to eliminate chronic leukemic cell lines and yet preserve normal ones. Less hopeful, however, is the finding that in chronic myelocytic leukemia the Philadelphia chromosome persists in marrow cells even when a complete remission has been induced.

Drug Resistance. An important problem in drug therapy of the leukemias is the development of drug resistance. This may result from one or more changes in cell metabolism. Alterations in membrane transport, deletion of activating enzymes, quantitative or qualitative changes in target enzymes, development of alternate pathways, and alterations in binding of the agents to macromolecules may cause drug resistance and clinical relapse. One drug, methotrexate, inhibits the enzyme dihydrofolate reductase. Resistance develops when the levels of this enzyme markedly increase, thereby allowing folic acid metabolism to proceed without inhibition. Methotrexate may inadequately inhibit enzyme activity at these higher levels. Some attempts are being made to increase the level of methotrexate to compensate for the change in dihydrofolate reductase levels. Resistance to 6-mercaptopurine, a drug that inhibits purine biosynthesis, results from the appearance of tumor cells with low levels of the enzyme necessary to ccnvert 6-mercaptopurine to its active metabolites. Work is being done to develop ways of getting around drug resistance, but success in this area depends on first understanding the biochemical changes underlying the resistance. Attempts are also being made to predict drug resistance to antileukemic drugs by in vitro methods prior to initiating chemotherapy. Unfortunately clinically useful assays are currently unavailable.

Drug Therapy for Acute Myelocytic Leukemia

Cytosine Arabinoside. Cytosine arabinoside (CA, Cytosar, ara-C, arabinosyl cytosine) is a pyrimidine nucleoside analogue that interferes with DNA synthesis. It has been suggested that its cytotoxicity is caused by competitive inhibition of DNA polymerase by arabinoside cytidine triphosphate, which functions as an antagonist of the physiologic substrate deoxycytidine triphosphate, or by incorporation of arabinoside cytidine triphosphate into the DNA helix with production of conformational changes. CA is active during the S (DNA-synthetic) phase of the cell cycle, and there is some evidence that it can recruit nonproliferating cells into the S phase. Its absorption orally is incomplete, so it is given as a continuous infusion, intravenous injection, or, on occasion, intramuscularly.

The effects of cytosine arabinoside on normal and leukemic cells depend a great deal on the schedule of administration; the longer it is infused, the more dramatic its effects. Its major toxic effect is suppression of the marrow and often production of severe megaloblastosis. The latter may be a result of the inhibition of DNA synthesis. Nausea, vomiting, and hepatic dysfunction are other side effects. Cytosine arabinoside has been used alone in the treatment of acute myelocytic leukemia but appears to be more effective in combination with other agents such as thioguanine or daunomycin. Its many successful combinations include COAP (Cytoxan, Oncovin, ara-C and prednisone), CAT (cytosine arabinoside and thioguanine), and COD (CA, Oncovin and daunomycin) programs.

Daunomycin (daunorubicin, rubidomycin). Daunomycin is an anthracylene antibiotic derived from a fungus. It complexes with DNA, thereby inhibiting DNA synthesis (S phase) and DNA-dependent RNA synthesis. It must be given intravenously as a bolus ("IV push") or as an infusion over several hours. Extravascular injection can cause skin ulceration. In solution daunomycin has a distinctive red color. The major toxic side effects include severe bone marrow depression, ulcerations of the mouth and pharynx, hair loss, and irreversible cardiac toxicity leading to congestive heart failure. Cardiac toxicity is most often seen in adults who have had a total cumulative dose greater than 900 mg per square meter of body surface area, but this condition can also occur at lower dosages, especially in elderly patients or individuals with preexisting organic heart disease. Since daunomycin is excreted at least in part by the liver, doses should be reduced for patients with liver disease.

At present there is a trend toward using cytosine arabinoside and daunomycin together as initial treatment for acute myelocytic leukemia. As there is a great and growing number of protocols using these two agents either in combination or sequentially, we cannot discuss specific schedules of administration here. Daunomycin is reported as especially effective in the treatment of the promyelocytic and erythroleukemic variants of acute myelocytic leukemia. It is severely bone marrow–toxic but rapidly reduces the marrow leukemic cell population, so that the time required for remission induction is shorter than with other drugs. Adriamycin (Adria) is a closely related compound with similar, but perhaps less dramatic, toxicities that is now being tried for treatment of AML.

6-Mercaptopurine (6-MP, Purinethol). 6-Mercaptopurine is a purine nucleoside analogue of hypoxanthine. By way of a series of complex reactions 6-MP interferes with purine biosynthesis and thus with DNA synthesis. It is active during the S phase of the cell cycle. Because it is well absorbed by the intestine, it can be given orally. It is available only in 50-mg tablets. Since its metabolism is affected by xanthine oxidase and this enzyme is inhibited by allopurinol, a drug used to reduce serum uric acid, the dose of 6-mercaptopurine must be reduced by 50 to 75 percent for patients receiving both drugs. There is some debate about this reduction, however, and some physicians have used 6-mercaptopurine in full doses despite the concomitant use of allopurinol. In any case peripheral blood counts, buffy coat smears, and bone marrow must be followed as the prime indicators of any need for change in dosage with this and other agents used for leukemic chemotherapy. The side effects of 6-mercaptopurine include severe bone marrow depression (occasionally megaloblastosis), gastrointestinal toxicity, and cholestatic jaundice. There may also be nausea, vomiting, and oral ulceration. Except as part of the VAMP (vincristine, amethopterin, mercaptopurine, prednisone) program, 6-mercaptopurine is now seldom used for remission induction of acute myelocytic leukemia. Resistance to 6-MP results from the appearance of leukemic cells with low levels of the enzyme system necessary to convert 6-MP to its active metabolites.

6-Thioguanine. The pharmacology and toxicity of this drug, and the dosage schedule for it, are similar to what we have described for 6-MP. 6-Thioguanine is not metabolized by xanthine oxidase, and therefore allopurinol does not influence its activity. This purine nucleoside analogue is often used in combination with cytosine arabinoside (CAT program) to treat patients with AML.

Drug Therapy for Acute Lymphocytic Leukemia

Vincristine (Oncovin). Vincristine is an alkaloid of the periwinkle plant. A stathmokinetic agent that affects cellular microtubules, it thus arrests cell division in metaphase by an unknown mechanism. It is active in the M, or mitotic, phase of the cell cycle. Necrosis and sloughing of the skin are common side effects of the extravasation of this drug during intravenous infusion. It also causes peripheral neuropathy characterized by weakness, loss of reflexes, foot drop, or cranial nerve dysfunction with eyelid drooping, ophthalmoplegia, vocal cord paralysis, or hoarseness, and can bring on paralytic ileus and abdominal pain. Neuritic pains, constipation, inappropriate antidiuretic hormone secretion, and occasionally neutropenia are other side effects.

Adrenalcorticosteroids. Prednisone and dexamethasone are the common, synthetic, adrenal corticosteroids used in the treatment of leukemia. Their primary mechanism of action is unknown, but they are capable of lysing normal lymphocytes and are associated with a reduction in both normal and abnormal lymphoid tissue mass. Significantly they are active against nonproliferating cells and thus do not require cell division to be effective. They may also cause demargination of granulocytes, thereby increasing the total white blood count. This effect is offset by depression of granulocyte migration into inflammatory sites. An elevated or normal white blood cell count may be misleading in patients on corticosteroids. The chronic use of corticosteroids increases susceptibility to infection and is associated with low serum potassium levels, cushingoid features (round face and buffalo hump over upper back), obesity, acne, diabetes mellitis, peptic ulceration, hypertension, and osteoporosis with painful bone fractures.

One tablet of dexamethasone (0.75 mg) is equivalent to one tablet of prednisone (5 mg) as measured by their ability to suppress inflammation. Dexamethasone is less likely to produce electrolyte imbalance but can cause a disabling proximal muscle myopathy.

Methotrexate (Amethopterin). Methotrexate is an analogue of folic acid. It binds strongly to the enzyme dihydrofolate reductase, which is required for the metabolism of folic acid to its biologically active forms (see Chapter 3). It prevents the production of tetrahydrofolic acid, which is used to form an active coenzyme, *folinic acid* or *citrovorum factor* (leucovorin), which in turn participates in reactions leading to the production of the DNA precursor, thymidine. Therefore methotrexate by its action on dihydrofolate reductase interferes with DNA synthesis (S phase). This action can be reversed, however, by giving the end product citrovorum factor. Methotrexate is cytotoxic only to proliferating cells, including normal cells in the gastrointestinal tract and mucous membranes. Its side effects include megaloblastosis, pancytopenia, ulcerations of mucous membranes including the mouth and pharynx, nausea, vomiting, abdominal pain associated with gastrointestinal tract ulcerations, liver or renal damage, and hair loss.

The effects of methotrexate are proportional to the amount of time it remains in the body. Fortunately it is rapidly excreted in the urine. If given as a continuous intravenous infusion, however, or by mouth with slow absorption from the gastrointestinal tract, maximal effects on normal and abnormal tissues occur. Because of the severe toxicity associated with oral administration, large doses of methotrexate are usually given by a parenteral, usually intravenous, route. Smaller doses may be administered orally.

Resistance to methotrexate develops when the intracellular level of dihydrofolate reductase markedly increases and methotrexate inadequately inhibits enzyme activity. Large doses of this drug may compensate for the elevation in enzyme activity, but they increase toxicity. Citrovorum factor will reverse the effects and toxicity of methotrexate if given before the methotrexate is cleared from the blood. Other possible mechanisms of resistance have been suggested, including decreased cell membrane ability to transport the drug and appearance of dihydrofolate reductase molecules with altered affinity for methotrexate.

L-Asparaginase. L-Asparaginase converts L-asparagine to aspartic acid, thus decreasing the amount of asparagine available to cells. It has been found that leukemic cells require exogenous asparagine and that the antineoplastic effect may be related to this requirement. Leukemic cell resistance to L-asparaginase may be related to increases in asparagine synthetase activity, whereby asparagine is possibly produced by the leukemic cell and the requirement for exogenous asparagine eliminated.

L-Asparaginase is usually used in combination with other drugs for the treatment of acute lymphocytic leukemia. It may produce liver disease, pancreatitis, hypocalcemia, and azotemia and interfere with the production of albumin, fibrinogen, and insulin. Allergic reactions, including fever, chills, and anaphylactic shock, are reported side effects.

Therapy for Chronic Myelocytic Leukemia

Alkylating Agents. The alkylating agents used in leukemic chemotherapy undergo internal ionization to form highly reactive intermediates capable of combining with proteins, nucleic acids, and amino acids. In the reaction with nucleic acids, cross-linking between complementary strands of DNA occurs. Since this cross-linking interferes with DNA replication, the alkylating agents are S phase–active agents. Numerous alterations have been made in the original sulfur mustard compound to produce alkylating agents such as chlorambucil (Leukeran), phenylalanine mustard, (Alkeran), and cyclophosphamide (Cytoxan). Triethylenethiophosphoramide (Thio-TEPA), dibromomannitol, and busulfan (Myleran), have different structures, but their mechanism of action is thought to be similar. Cyclophosphamide is unusual because it must be activated by the liver before it has biologic activity against leukemic cells.

The alkylating agents busulfan and phenylalanine mustard are commonly used for the treatment of CML. The major side effect of busulfan is bone marrow depression, which may continue for days or even weeks after administration of the drug. Overtreatment with this drug may result in complete bone marrow aplasia and pancytopenia. Busulfan is also associated with fibrosis of the marrow and other organs, including the ovaries, testes, and lung. Thus menopausal symptoms, infertility, aspermia, and pulmonary insufficiency may be side effects of this drug. It also causes an unexplained darkening of the skin, which may be related to increased melanin deposition. Skin darkening, weakness, low blood pressure, and poor appetite form a *pseudohypoadrenalism syndrome* that arises after years of chronic therapy with this drug.

Dibromomannitol is similar in mode of action, response rate, and side effects to busulfan.

Phenylalanine mustard is not associated with pulmonary fibrosis, skin darkening, or the pseudohypoadrenalism syndrome. For this reason it is becoming more popular for the initial treatment of chronic myelocytic leukemia. It, too, has a prolonged effect on the bone marrow and may affect production of red cells and platelets as well as granulocytes. Gastrointestinal upset and a possible leukemogenic potential with long usage are other unusual side effects.

Chlorambucil, an alkylating agent almost devoid of side effects except for bone marrow suppression, can be used to treat chronic myelocytic leukemia. It has few of the side effects attributed to the other alkylating agents except for bone marrow suppression, which is mild to moderate and easily reversible. Although its action is persistent, chlorambucil usually does not suppress marrow function as long as phenylalanine mustard or busulfan. This drug is not frequently used to treat CML, mainly because experience with it for this disease is limited.

CML occasionally occurs during pregnancy. In such a case antileukemia therapy should be delayed as long as possible, and then alkylating agents or 6-mercaptopurine employed. Usually the mother and child survive without undue sequelae.

Splenic X-Irradiation. Before the availability of alkylating agents, chronic myelocytic leukemia was treated with x-irradiation administered to the spleen. Small doses, usually less than 100 rads and rarely up to 1,000 rads, are all that is required to cause a decrease in the size of the spleen and a return of blood counts and clinical status to normal. The distant effects of splenic irradiation are hard to explain. They may be due to the irradiation of circulating immature neutrophils or stem cells. Usually intermittent courses of splenic irradiation are required at 6- to 8-week intervals. A number of studies indicate that alkylating agents are superior to splenic irradiation, because with drugs the patient does not have to go through remissions and relapses every few months. There seems to be no significant difference in survival times between these two treatment modalities, nor does it appear that either therapy actually increases average survival time compared to no therapy. The basic reason for treating CML patients, it must be emphasized, is for palliation of symptoms.

Treatment of the blast crisis of CML is less satisfactory than even in acute myelocytic leukemia. Patients seldom live for more than several months, and remissions, if obtained, are partial and of short duration. Alkylating agents and splenic irradiation have no therapeutic usefulness.

Hydroxyurea (Hydrea). Patients refractory to treatment with alkylating agents or splenic irradiation have sometimes responded for a few months to hydroxyurea. This affects DNA synthesis by inhibiting ribonucleoside diphosphate reductase. Toxicity includes myelosuppression, nausea, vomiting, mouth ulcers, skin eruption, hair loss, and drowsiness. Dosage should be reduced in patients with renal disease.

Granulocyte Leukophoresis. Removal of excess granulocytes from peripheral blood is made possible by specially designed machines, which take blood from the vein of a patient and selectively remove granulocytes by centrifugation. The granulocyte-poor blood is reinfused into another vein. By daily leukophoresis for one or two weeks it is possible to reduce granulocyte counts and shrink spleen size in patients with CML. Remissions are best maintained by simultaneous use of an alkylating agent, such as phenylalanine mustard.

Splenectomy. Removal of the enlarged spleen early in the course of CML has been recommended, but there is no evidence that this prolongs life or ameliorates symptoms more than treatment with chemotherapy. Furthermore, a high risk is involved in removing the spleens from these patients, who, at least in the advanced stages of the disease, are prone to infections.

Therapy for Chronic Lymphocytic Leukemia

Alkylating Agents. Cyclophosphamide and chlorambucil (see p. 304) have both been used in the treatment of chronic lymphocytic leukemia. Inflammation of the bladder is a common side effect of cyclophosphamide and can be prevented or ameliorated by a large intake of fluids in order to dilute the concentration of drug reaching the bladder. Hair loss may also occur, particularly when this drug is used along with vincristine. With either cyclophosphamide or chlorambucil a return of blood counts to normal and a reduction in organomegaly is noted within a period of weeks or months.

Radiotherapy. When blockage of ureters or bile ducts means that patients require immediate treatment, x-irradiation to these sites may give quick, long-term improvement. New techniques of total body irradiation, during which several hundred rads are given to the whole body, have led to long-lasting remissions similar to those seen with successful chemotherapy. Extracorporeal irradiation has been used to lower peripheral blood lymphocyte counts in CLL and has been associated with a decrease in the size of lymph nodes and other organs. By means of cannulas blood is removed from a vessel, exposed to a source of radiation, and then returned to the body. Remissions have been short-lived, however, and there is not enough experience to recommend this therapy at the present time.

Adrenal Corticosteroids. Although patients with chronic lymphocytic leukemia are usually treated with alkylating agents alone, those who have autoimmune hemolysis or thrombocytopenia, hypersplenism, or infiltration of the bone marrow often benefit from being given prednisone along with the alkylating agent. If an alkylating agent alone is employed, marked decreases in blood counts may occur before the benefits of the alkylating agent are evident. By using prednisone or other steroids this initial depression of blood counts can be ameliorated. Because of the long-term side effects of chronic adrenal corticosteroid administration, prednisone doses are tapered as rapidly as blood counts will allow. Corticosteroids may be associated with an initial but transient rise in the circulating lymphocyte count, along with increased lymph node size. These initial effects are followed by a decrease in lymph node size and blood lymphocyte count.

Splenic Irradiation and Splenectomy. Splenic irradiation or splenectomy has been advocated for the treatment of chronic lymphocytic leukemia, but the uncertainty of the response to splenic irradiation or to perioperative morbidity has limited their use. Removal of the spleen may be necessary because of drug-resistant hypersplenism with severe cytopenia. Although some patients are definitely helped by splenectomy, particularly early in the course of the disease, there does appear to be a balancing and perhaps overriding increase in mortality and morbidity associated with this operative procedure.

Philosophic Considerations in Treatment of Acute and Chronic Leukemia

Until recently there has been great debate about whether to treat patients who have acute adult myelocytic leukemia. With the chemotherapeutic agents that were available initially, patients' life spans were shortened in some cases and good remission with longer survival was obtained in others. With the present use of the cytosine arabinoside and daunomycin approximately 60% of AML patients go into complete remission that may continue for many months. Therefore most hematologists today agree that patients under 60 years of age who do not have complicating medical problems and who are agreeable to therapy should receive antileukemic drugs. Remissions occur even in the case of older patients and those with myelocytic leukemia variants, such as promyelocytic, monocytic, and myelomonocytic and erythroleukemia. These variants were formerly thought to have a very poor prognosis even with therapy. Elderly patients often have smoldering leukemias, and in this case treatment should be delayed until symptoms begin or appear imminent.

Thus, most adult leukemics with acute myelocytic leukemia and most children with acute lymphocytic leukemia (or their parents) are informed of the nature of their disease, and with their (or their parents') permission an attempt is made to obtain an initial complete remission using antileukemic chemotherapy. It is most important that the patients be informed of the nature of their disease, for it is unfair to subject them to the complications associated with rendering the marrow aplastic without full knowledge of the nature of the disease, the risks, and the chances for complete remission. In the case of children parental consent is easy to obtain because of the good results with chemotherapy. Difficult problems arise with teenagers, since chemotherapy is usually not as successful as in the 3-to-6-year-olds, and the patients' understanding and cooperation is essential.*

Adjunctive Therapy in Acute and Chronic Leukemias

Blood Transfusion

Particularly in advanced stages of acute and chronic leukemia and after initiation of chemotherapy, erythrocyte and platelet transfusion are needed. In the absence of acute hemorrhage, packed red cells, preferably buffy coat–poor or, if there are febrile (leukocyte antibody-mediated) reactions, washed or frozen-washed red cells, should be used to treat the anemia. Usually it is not possible to maintain the hematocrits at much above 0.30 (30%) and in some cases lower hematocrits are tolerable.

Since platelets carry ABO and HLA antigens, platelet transfusions are best prepared from ABO and HLA-matched individuals, even if they are not related. These platelets appear to survive better than those from random unrelated donors but unfortunately are often unavailable. Platelets obtained from single donors by plateletphoresis are superior to platelet packs prepared from multiple donors, because they expose the patient to only one set of platelet antigens. If the patient is being considered for bone marrow transplantation, then relatives who are potential HLA-identical marrow donors should be avoided as platelet donors.

Platelet transfusions should be given to patients with platelet counts of less than 20×10^9 per liter. Patients who are actively bleeding may require platelet transfusion, even with platelet counts as high as 75×10^9 per liter. Certainly if a patient has taken drugs, such as aspirin, that interfere with platelet function, or is uremic, or if there are other reasons to suspect that his own

*For an excellent discussion of the psychological problems of the treatment of leukemia, the reader is referred to Dr. William A. Greene's chapter in *Hematology for Internists,* edited by Robert I. Weed, published by Little, Brown and Company in 1971.

platelets are not functioning properly, then platelet transfusions are indicated even if the platelet count is higher than 50×10^9 per liter.

Granulocyte transfusions have now become possible. These are used for adults with myelocytic leukemia whom treatment by chemotherapy has rendered aplastic and severely granulocytopenic. The granulocytes are obtained by special filters to which granulocytes adhere or by differential centrifugation of blood from normal donors or patients with chronic myelocytic leukemia. About 5×10^{10} granulocytes are infused each day for 4 or 5 days, usually when the granulocyte count falls below 0.2 to 0.5×10^9 per liter. HLA matching of donors to recipients will help avoid leukocyte antibody reactions, which are febrile discomforting, and, in some patients, severe or anaphylactic.

Persistent administration of platelet transfusions despite failure of platelet counts to rise can lead by an unknown mechanism to granulocytopenia. Therefore, if patients fail to respond to platelet transfusions, this treatment should be discontinued, particularly if there are febrile reactions. If the patient is toxic, infected, or has a high fever, platelet transfusions may yield a suboptimal rise in platelet count.

Antibiotic Therapy The treatment of infections acquired during the course of acute or chronic leukemias, particularly during attempts at inducing remissions, has become standardized. Since the patients often develop overwhelming sepsis quickly, it is recommended that bacteriologic workup and broad spectrum antibiotic treatment be initiated as soon as fever appears. Cultures for aerobic and anaerobic bacteria, fungus, and tuberculosis should be obtained, when appropriate, from throat, sputum, urine, and blood. A complete physical examination, including a search for rectal or prostatic abscesses is important. Chest and sinus x-rays and radiographic studies of symptomatic organs should be obtained as quickly as possible.

Once this workup has been completed, antibiotic therapy should be instituted. A penicillinase-resistant antibiotic against gram-positive organisms — for example, oxycillin or a cephalosporin — should be combined with an aminoglycoside antibiotic that is active against gram-negative bacteria including *pseudomonas*, such as gentamycin. In some circumstances treatment with clindamycin or other drugs active against anaerobes is also instituted. Although there is debate about which drugs to use, the general principle of initiating therapy quickly with a broad spectrum approach has proved important. Once culture results are available, antibiotics are continued or substituted according to bacteriologic sensitivities. If fever persists and there is no clear-cut confirmation of bacterial infection, it is quite appropriate to stop all antibiotic therapy, reculture, and observe the patient. Drug reactions or other nonbacteriologic causes of fever sometimes become evident. Appropriate therapy for tuberculosis with isoniazid and ethambutol, or for fungal infections with amphotericin B or other antifungal agents, should be instituted whenever these diagnoses are strongly suspected or confirmed.

Early in the leukemic disease febrile episodes are caused by infection or by the leukemia itself. In the later stages of the disease or after chemotherapy 70 percent or more of febrile episodes are caused by infectious agents. In general, esoteric infections with fungus, tuberculosis, *Pneumocystis carinii,* or toxoplasmosis occur in the later stages of the disease, particularly after intensive chemotherapy.

Antibiotics have also been used prophylactically. The rationale behind this approach is to use nonabsorbable antibiotics to suppress bowel flora, which frequently are the cause of sepsis. A typical regimen consists of mycostatin, paramamycin, vancomycin, polymyxin B, and amphotericin. These antibiotics are often made up in the form of a liquid elixir. The side effects include nausea, vomiting, and diarrhea. Unfortunately patients often cannot tolerate the smell nor the side effects of these antibiotics. Their efficacy is still experimental, and there is little evidence that their use increases the likelihood of remission or the survival time of the leukemic patient.

Isolation and bowel sterilization techniques, including the use of life islands or lamina flow rooms, probably have a place in reducing infectious complications during leukemic chemotherapy. However, an increased remission and survival rate has not been convincingly demonstrated. These techniques are expensive, and the psychological effects of isolation can be quite severe.

Hyperuricemia

Many of the acute and chronic leukemias are associated with hyperuricemia and uricosuria. This is thought to be due to increased turnover of white blood cells with increased breakdown of purines and pyrimidines. In a few cases leukemia may present as gouty arthropathy or nephropathy. Immediately after institution of chemotherapy, the uric acid load may greatly increase, leading to deposition of urate crystals in the renal tubules with subsequent renal failure. The nephrotoxic effects of hyperuracemia can be prevented by using allopurinol, an inhibitor of xanthine oxidase and uric acid production. Along with allopurinol it may be necessary to institute prophylactic colchicine therapy to prevent attacks of acute gout. Because of the frequency of severe, pruritic skin eruptions, we have instituted allopurinol therapy only when the uric acid level is greater than 10 mg per deciliter or during the initial induction phase of therapy. Adequate hydration of the patient is equally important for prevention of uric acid stones and nephropathy.

Radiotherapy and Chemotherapy for Central Nervous System (CNS) Complications of Leukemia

In acute myelocytic leukemia and in the advanced blastic phase of chronic myelocytic leukemia, large numbers of leukemia cells may accumulate in the small blood vessels of the brain, a condition called *leukostasis*. This may lead to necrosis of these blood vessels, intracranial hemorrhage, and often death. As this does not usually happen unless the granulocyte count is greater than 100×10^9 per liter, hydroxyurea is used to quickly lower the peripheral granulocyte count. This therapy has little effect on the bone marrow. Similar leukemic CNS nodules also arise occasionally in patients with acute lymphocytic leukemias. Whole brain irradiation has been recommended in this case.

Meningeal leukemia occurs frequently in patients with acute lymphocytic leukemia and is usually followed by recurrent bone marrow disease. Headache, raised intracranial pressure, signs of meningitis, and seizures are common presenting manifestations. Systemic chemotherapeutic agents are usually of little help in treating this complication. Meningeal leukemia is best diagnosed by cytologic examination of the spinal fluid, using a Millipore filter technique, and by the finding of low glucose and high protein levels in the spinal fluid. Treatment is not particularly effective. Intrathecal administration of methotrexate or cytosine arabinoside, or whole brain irradiation, will control meningeal leukemia, but only for a short time.

During the initial drug treatment of acute lymphocytic leukemia in children, prophylactic treatment of the central nervous system with intrathecal methotrexate and x-irradiation is employed in an attempt to sterilize leukemic cells in the brain and spinal cord. The realization of the importance of the central nervous system as a hiding place for leukemic cells has led to the development of treatment protocols that have significantly lengthened the average remission period for patients with acute lymphocytic leukemia.

Immunotherapy

The treatment of acute leukemia, as mentioned (Principles of Therapy for Acute and Chronic Leukemias), involves reducing the leukemic tumor mass to as low a level as possible and then allowing the host's immunologic defense mechanisms to destroy remaining leukemic cells. To stimulate the host's defense mechanisms, various immunologic techniques have been used. For example, BCG (bacille Calmette-Guérin) vaccine developed against tuberculosis has been given by various methods, including scarification, to boost the response of the host's reticuloendothelial system. There is debate over the best method of administration and the best strain of BCG to use. It is not yet clear whether the duration of remission is extended by the use of such techniques.

Another immunologic technique involves saving aliquots of the patient's own leukemic cells and, after remission is obtained, reinjecting the cells killed (irradiated), back into the patient. This is purported to stimulate the patient's own immunologic defense mechanisms to destroy remaining leukemic cells.

Bone Marrow Transplantation

Human bone marrow transplantation between HLA-compatible siblings remains an experimental therapy for acute leukemia. The recipient is pretreated with large doses of total body irradiation or cyclophosphamide in order to destroy the leukemia cells and provide immunosuppression. Graft-versus-host disease is treated with methotrexate and steroids. Unfortunately death from complications of transplantation and recurrence of leukemia occurs in approximately 60 percent of nontwin siblings, but better results are obtained with twins, particularly if they are identical.

MYELOPROLIF-ERATIVE DISORDERS

The *myeloproliferative disorders* are characterized by overgrowth or proliferation of erythroid, myeloid, or megakaryocytic cell lines and by proliferation of fibrocytes or reticulum cells in the bone marrow. Such proliferation may also occur in extramedullary sites, such as the spleen, liver, or lymph nodes. The proliferation in extramedullary sites can be explained if one understands that early in embryonic life hematopoiesis occurs primarily in the spleen and liver rather than in the bone marrow. Apparently the ability of these organs to give rise to bone marrow or at least to support erythroid, myeloid, and megakaryocytic cells is maintained throughout adult life.

Some of the myeloproliferative disorders have been already discussed in this chapter, for example, acute and chronic myelocytic leukemia and erythroleukemia. These three leukemias make up one of the two major subgroups of the myeloproliferative disorders. A neoplastic proliferation of a single cell type, which causes destruction and invasion of bone marrow and other organs, characterizes this subgroup. In most cases patients with these diseases die from complications of acute leukemia. The second major subgroup includes polycythemia vera, agnogenic myeloid metaplasia, and hemorrhagic thrombocythemia. Before discussing the specific features of these three diseases we shall list their common characteristics as follows.

1. Abnormality in peripheral blood counts. Although these diseases are usually proliferative, leading one to expect elevated

blood counts, anemia, leukopenia, or thrombocytopenia are often present.

2. Proliferation of reticulum cells, producing fibrotic tissue. Such fibrosis is usually most prominent in the patient's bone marrow (Plates 59 and 60). Fibrosis can also affect other potentially hemopoietic organs such as the spleen, however. Osteosclerosis with excessive calcification of the bone marrow may also occur. Perhaps as a result of the overgrowth of bone marrow elements and reticulum cells, marrow or splenic infarcts arise.

3. Liver and spleen enlargement. This may be due in part to growth of bone marrow in extramedullary sites, so-called *myeloid metaplasia;* to fibrosis; or to nonspecific reticulum cell hyperplasia. Myeloid metaplasia or islands of hematopoiesis are recognizable by the presence of megakaryocytes.

4. Blood cell morphologic abnormalities (Plate 58). Teardrop-shaped red cells, immature red and white cells, large platelets, and even megakaryocytic fragments are prominent in the peripheral blood.

5. Hyperuricemia and uricosuria. As the result of increased turnover of blood cells there is increased production of uric acid. Attacks of acute gout, gouty arthritis, tophi, and renal failure secondary to uric acid nephropathy or uric acid stones may occur.

6. Elevation of unbound vitamin B_{12}-binding protein. Perhaps because transcobolamin is produced in white cells, there are increased amounts of vitamin B_{12}-binding proteins.

Since the myeloleukemic syndromes have been discussed in a previous chapter, the following sections will be devoted to discussion of the three diseases that make up the second subgroup of the myeloproliferative disorders — polycythemia vera, agnogenic myeloid metaplasia, and hemorrhagic thrombocythemia.

Polycythemia Vera

Polycythemia vera is characterized by an increased number of mature circulating erythrocytes. The packed cell volume (normally less than 0.52 (52%) in males or 0.50 (50%) in females) and red cell mass is increased above normal. Other abnormalities associated with myeloproliferative disorders may also be present, but it is the characteristic elevation in red cell mass that sets this disease apart from the others. As a result of the increased red cell volume, hyperviscosity, vascular distention, and stasis may occur, leading to an increase in thromboembolic or hemorrhagic complications. Transition to agnogenic myeloid metaplasia or AML occurs in a small number of patients.

The clinical features of polycythemia vera including the following.

1. Occurrence in middle-aged or elderly patients, with a slight predominance in males and Jews of European extraction.

2. Symptoms ascribed to hyperviscosity, including pounding headache, dizziness, angina, visual disturbances, paresthesias, and ringing in the ears.

3. Thrombotic episodes, such as phlebitis, myocardial infarction, and cerebral vascular accidents. Thrombocythemia, as well as erythremia, predisposes to these complications.

4. Hemorrhagic phenomena, such as nose bleeds, bleeding from the gums, purpura, gastrointestinal bleeding, uterine bleeding, and bleeding from organs such as the lung or genitourinary tract. Thrombocythemia, which often affects these patients, may contribute to the bleeding and thromboembolic complications. Defective platelet function is common in these patients.

5. Itching (pruritus), especially after bathing.

6. Gastrointestinal symptoms and peptic ulcers.

7. Splenomegaly, usually due to extramedullary hematopoiesis. The spleen is often palpable at the left costal margin. If it is enlarged more than 2 or 3 cm, or if it appears to be enlarging in size, then the possibility must be considered that transition to agnogenic myeloid metaplasia or acute myelocytic leukemia is occurring.

8. Increased red blood cell count. The peripheral blood smear contains small, often hypochromic, red cells. The microcytosis and hypochromia is usually due to a concomitant iron deficiency. This iron deficiency is said to be secondary to occult gastrointestinal blood loss secondary to thrombocythemia and defective platelet function. The reticulocyte count is usually normal, and only occasional immature red cells are found in the peripheral blood. Only as the disease progresses to agnogenic myeloid metaplasia (in approximately 10 percent of patients) do significant numbers of immature red cells and teardrop forms appear in the peripheral blood.

9. Granulocytosis, thrombocythemia, and basophilia commonly present.

10. Elevated leukocyte alkaline phosphatase and transcobolamin. The leukocyte alkaline phosphatase score is usually, but not always, elevated. The vitamin B_{12} binding capacity is also increased, although not to the degree seen in chronic myelocytic leukemia.

11. Bone marrow abnormalities. The bone marrow is hypercellular, with loss of fat spaces. Megakaryocytic proliferation is often prominent. Usually there is no fibrosis, unless the patient is undergoing transition to agnogenic myeloid metaplasia.

12. Hyperuricemia. Hyperuricemia is often present, and some of the patients present with complications due to increased uric acid in blood and urine.

13. Arterial oxygen abnormalities. The arterial oxygen content is low, but arterial oxygen saturation is usually normal or near-normal. It is thought that the lower oxygen content is due to decreased diffusing capacity in the lungs secondary to multiple pulmonary artery emboli or thromboses.

Differential Diagnosis. Polycythemia vera must be distinguished from relative polycythemia due to a decreased plasma volume and from secondary polycythemia due to hypoxia and increased erythropoietin activity, or from some other known cause for an elevated red cell mass. Relative polycythemia may be seen in patients with depletion of the circulating plasma volume, in which case it is caused by loss of salt and water. The hemoconcentration that results is reflected in an elevated hematocrit, normal red cell mass, and decreased plasma volume. In many cases the cause of the decreased plasma volume is not apparent.

It is imperative to document that the red cell mass is elevated before proceeding with an extensive and expensive hematologic evaluation for polycythemia. For this reason a radiochromium red cell mass should be determined as part of the initial evaluation for all patients with elevated hematocrits. If this is not possible, then plasma volume should be determined by using radioactive albumin and an isotope dilution method. In some borderline cases there may be difficulty in deciding what is the normal red cell mass for a given patient. Tables have been published giving equations and other data helpful in determining whether measured red cell mass is truly increased.*

Once it has been established that an increased red cell mass is present, then the differential diagnosis becomes secondary polycythemia versus polycythemia vera. The causes of secondary polycythemia and their pathophysiology are discussed in the following paragraphs.

The most common causes of secondary polycythemia are cardiac or respiratory diseases, which cause reduction in arterial oxygen content and saturation. High altitude has the same effect. Another common cause of secondary polycythemia is inappropriate increased erythropoietin activity associated with a variety of renal diseases. As tissue hypoxia is probably detected in the kidney and results in increased circulating erythropoietin levels, and as erythropoietin itself may be produced by kidney cells, it should not seem strange that renal diseases are associated with erythemia. Renal cysts and renal cell carcinoma are the more common forms of kidney disease associated with high hematocrits. Hydronephrosis and practically all other renal diseases have been, in at least

*See Retzlaff, et al, Erythrocyte volume, plasma volume and lean body mass in adult men and women, *Blood* 33: 649, 1969.

one case, associated with polycythemia. Usually the systemic symptoms of polycythemia vera, such as itching and quantitative abnormalities of white cells and platelets, are not present.

Hemoglobin bound to carbon monoxide, carboxyhemoglobin, loses its ability to carry oxygen. Tissue hypoxia results, along with an increase in erythropoietin levels and red cell mass. Cigarette smoking resulting in carboxyhemoglobin, and environmental pollution with carbon monoxide, have been associated with mild erythrocytosis.

Certain cases of familial erythrocytosis appear to be due to the presence of abnormal hemoglobins. Substitutions that affect the binding of oxygen to hemoglobin's heme group occur in these hemoglobins. An increase in affinity for oxygen leads to tissue hypoxia and increased erythropoietin production. Hemoglobins with these characteristics include Chesapeake, Rainier, Yakima, Kempsey, and Ypsilanti.

Benign and malignant tumors have also been associated with inappropriate erythropoietin production. Such tumors include hypernephroma, uterine myomas, cerebellar hemangioblastoma, pheochromocytoma, adrenal adenoma, and hepatomas.

Although many of the findings compatible with polycythemia vera are not present in secondary polycythemia, some important exceptions may occur. For example, thrombocytosis and granulocytosis may also be associated with malignant tumors and may be mistakenly attributed to polycythemia vera. Splenomegaly, when present, is helpful in distinguishing true polycythemia from secondary polycythemia, since in the latter case splenomegaly is usually not present.

Therapy. A great deal has been written about the therapy of polycythemia vera, and there has been a great deal of controversy over it. Luckily the natural history of the disease usually runs a course of 10 to 15 years or more, and it appears that all the available therapies are effective in controlling symptoms and perhaps prolonging life. Controversy concerning the effect of therapy on the development of leukemia continues. It appears that there is a natural propensity for transition from polycythemia vera to malignant forms of the myeloproliferative disorders, and this propensity may be increased by the use of radioactive phosphorus or alkylating agents. It may be, however, that this increased propensity is due to the longer life of the treated compared to the untreated patient. The risk of developing acute leukemia is small and appears to be an acceptable price to pay for the chance of longer and more comfortable survival.

For patients with little or no clinical discomfort, a platelet count of less than a trillion per liter, and no history of thromboembolic or hemorrhagic complications, the treatment of choice appears to be *phlebotomy,* that is, the removal of blood at regular intervals. The idea is to correct hypervolemia and hyperviscosity and at the same time render the patient iron-deficient. An iron-deficient will produce only a limited number of erythroid cells and will require few phlebotomies or even none to keep the hematocrit at normal levels. Only in a few cases will symptoms of iron deficiency be prominent and require the cautious replacement of iron stores.

For patients with clinical symptoms, significant thrombocytosis, and thromboembolic complications, or for those who require frequent or difficult-to-obtain phlebotomies, myelosuppressive therapy with radiophosphorus (^{32}P) or alkylating agents is indicated. In most cases radiophosphorus is the simplest therapy and the easiest to administer. The patient receives 4 to 6.0 millicuries of radiophosphorus orally. By about three months his blood counts have returned to normal or near-normal, and his clinical symptoms have ameliorated. This therapy may be required once a year or, in some cases, two to three times or more annually. As previously mentioned, both radiophosphorus and the alkylating agents have been suspected of being potentially leukemogenic agents, and therefore the dose must be kept as low as possible. Once a patient gives a satisfactory response to radiophosphorus, he has no complications from the therapy and requires little follow-up by the hematologist. Blood counts and smears should be checked every 6 months. If for some reason radiophosphorus is unacceptable to the patient or the physician, alkylating agents may be used.

The initial dose of alkylating agent is given for 1 to 3 weeks, then tapered so that within 1 to 3 months the patient is on maintenance therapy. There is debate over the efficacy and speed of action of these alkylating agents and the frequency of complications with them. There is some tendency for patients receiving busulfan to be overtreated and develop aplastic bone marrows. The effects of busulfan appear to be delayed for several weeks, and if blood counts seem to be falling rapidly, it is best to taper or withhold doses until the count has stabilized. Busulfan is claimed to be more effective than other agents for patients threatened by thrombocythemia; however, the response to busulfan takes almost as long to happen as the response to radioactive phosphorus. Unless emergency measures (nitrogen mustard given intravenously or plateletphoresis) are required to control thrombocytosis immediately, radiophosphorus, busulfan, phenylalanine mustard, chlorambucil, or cyclophosphamide can be administered with more or less equal effectiveness in treating polycythemia vera.

Systemic symptoms such as pruritis may be relieved by anti-pruritic agents such as antihistamines or phenothiazines. Uric acid elevations are treated with allopurinol; however, this drug has complications such as skin rashes, gout and leukopenia, and is, therefore, recommended only for patients with complications of hyperuracemia or uricosuria.

Much of the mortality associated with polycythemia vera has been perioperative. Polycythemia must be recognized prior to any surgical procedure, and the hematocrit brought to normal, if at all possible, preoperatively.

Approach to the Patient with Erythrocytosis

The first step in the approach to the patient with erythrocytosis is to document an increase in red cell mass. Then the physical examination and a number of laboratory tests are necessary to rule out benign and malignant tumors and other diseases associated with erythrocytosis. Once the diagnosis of true erythrocytosis has been made and secondary causes have been ruled out, then polycythemia vera becomes the likely diagnosis. Leukocytosis, thrombocytosis, splenomegaly, an elevated leukocyte alkaline phosphatase score, and lack of evidence for myelofibrosis and myeloid metaplasia will all help confirm the diagnosis of polycythemia vera.

Agnogenic Myeloid Metaplasia

As in the case of polycythemia vera and the leukemic forms of the myeloproliferative disorders, the etiology of agnogenic myeloid metaplasia is not known. But, as in the other myeloproliferative disorders, it is thought that the disease results from a disorder in the stem cells of the bone marrow that give rise to peripheral blood cells and to fibrocytes. Whether the stem cell disorder is one of overproliferation or neoplastic transformation is still not clear. Some authors regard agnogenic myeloid metaplasia and polycythemia vera as nonmalignant diseases; however, since these conditions have many of the characteristics of malignant diseases, and in the case of agnogenic myeloid metaplasia often result in the demise of the patients within a relatively short period of time, they are generally considered hematologic malignancies.

Clinical Features. Most often the patient presents with abnormal peripheral blood findings, splenomegaly, or both. The peripheral blood (Plates 12 and 58) shows teardrop-shaped red cells, immature red and white cells, and large and bizarre platelets with some megakaryocytic fragments. There may be severe poikilocytosis. The patient's spleen and often the liver are enlarged. Weakness, fatigue, weight loss, and cachexia are not uncommon signs and symptoms. Abdominal distention, left upper quadrant discomfort, and decreased capacity for food, along with symptomatic splenic infarctions, are common complications in the later stages of the disease. The spleen may initially be only moderately en-

Approach to the patient with erythrocytosis

I. History
  A. Pruritis, particularly after bathing
  B. Pounding headaches
  C. Hyperviscosity syndrome
  D. Family history of polycythemia
II. Physical Examination
  A. Evidence of elevated hematocrit, including plethora, cyanosis of the nose, suffusion of the mucous membranes of the eye, conjunctivitis
  B. Evidence of uterine, renal, hepatic, or central nervous system tumors
  C. Splenomegaly (hepatomegaly or lymphadenopathy)
III. Laboratory Studies
  A. Peripheral blood counts
  B. Blood smear (teardrop, red cells, immature red and white cells, large platelets or megakaryocyte fragments)
  C. Red cell mass (radiochromium)
  D. Erythropoietin levels in serum or urine
  E. Arterial oxygen saturation
  F. Leukocyte alkaline phosphatase level
  G. Intravenous pyelogram
  H. Transcobalamin or serum vitamin B_{12} levels
  I. Uric acid
  J. Bone marrow examination (stain for fibrosis and iron)
  K. Serum iron and total iron-binding capacity
  L. Hemoglobin studies (electrophoresis, oxygen affinity, heat stability test)

larged, but it then rapidly enlarges to fill the pelvis and abdominal cavity. The serum uric acid is often elevated and complications of hyperuricemia may be encountered.

Anemia is a prominent feature of the disease. The white count may be low, normal, or high, and the platelet count may also be low, normal, or high. Leukocyte alkaline phosphatase scores are elevated or normal. The bone marrow is difficult to obtain, and usually a dry tap results. Bone marrow biopsy reveals fibrosis (Plates 59 and 60) and in some cases new bone formation or *osteosclerosis.* There is no Philadelphia chromosome. Extramedullary hematopoiesis is found in spleen, liver, lymph nodes, and other organs. Actual tumors of extramedullary hematopoiesis may be present almost anywhere. Bone x-ray reveals osteosclerosis and sometimes lytic lesions. There may be bone pain due to infarctions. The findings of anemia, characteristically abnormal blood cell morphology, myelofibrosis, and extramedullary hematopoiesis or myeloid metaplasia are the hallmarks of agnogenic myeloid metaplasia.

Complications include progressive anemia, cachexia, unexplained congestive heart failure, hypersplenism, and the development, for unexplained reasons, of portal hypertension with ascites and even varices. Sometimes spontaneously and sometimes in association with removal of the spleen, a picture resembling that of acute or chronic myelocytic leukemia may be seen.

Differential Diagnosis. Agnogenic myeloid metaplasia must be distinguished from chronic myelocytic leukemia and from myelophthisic anemia due to replacement of normal marrow elements by carcinoma or tuberculosis. Bone marrow biopsy and cultures for tuberculosis are necessary to exclude the first two possibilities. The presence of a Philadelphia chromosome is generally accepted as a distinguishing feature of chronic myelocytic leukemia. In chronic myelocytic leukemia also, the white blood cell counts are generally higher and the leukocyte alkaline phosphatase is usually zero or less. The size of the spleen and the amount of marrow fibrosis is greater in agnogenic myeloid metaplasia. In both agnogenic myeloid metaplasia and CML, however, a leukoerythroblastic blood picture, teardrop cells, marrow fibrosis, bone infarction, splenomegaly, splenic infarction, hyperuricemia, and cytopenias may be prominent.

Therapy. Patients with agnogenic myeloid metaplasia are elderly and suffer greatly from anemia. They often have evidence of heart failure or portal hypertension. Some have massive splenomegaly which interferes with nutrition. Many therapeutic modalities have been recommended for this disease, but they are all unsatisfactory. The patients usually live 1 to 3 years relatively comfortably and then enter a more progressive phase during which they develop one or more complications of their disease. Often cachexia, massive splenomegaly, heart problems, and infections and hemorrhagic complications due to cytopenias are the end result of the natural history and therapy of this disease.

Of the large number of therapies suggested, the following are most commonly used. Androgens, because of their ability to raise erythropoietin levels to supernormal heights and perhaps to influence the responsiveness of the erythroid precursors to erythropoietin, are given in the hope of correcting the severe anemia. Folic acid is also sometimes given, since megaloblastic changes and low folic acid levels have been found. A reticulocyte and hematocrit response occurs occasionally, but even when mild megaloblastic changes are present, improvement is rarely seen. Alkylating agents such as busulfan, chlorambucil, and phenylalanine mustard have been recommended. They have some ability to reduce spleen size and thereby reduce the complications of hypersplenism that interfere with the management of these patients. If a trial of these drugs is undertaken, the physician must be prepared to stop therapy as soon as it appears that the hematologic condition is worsening despite improvement in organ size. ^{32}P has been tried instead of alkylating agents, but currently the latter are preferred by most therapists. Treatment directed at congestive heart failure, poor nutrition, bleeding due to thrombocytosis or thrombocytopenia, and hyperuricemia is instituted when indicated.

A word must be said about splenectomy. Certainly if this procedure is done to correct hypersplenism and other symptoms attributed to a massively enlarged spleen, it must be undertaken early in the course of the disease, or the complications and perioperative mortality will be considerable. The advocates of splenectomy have shown amelioration of cytopenias, particularly anemia, of hypersplenism, and of symptoms referrable to the massively enlarged spleen. As already mentioned, it is not dangerous to remove a spleen containing large amounts of extramedullary hematopoiesis as long as marrow function is adequate. There is little evidence that removal of the spleen removes the chief source of blood cell production. It appears that myeloid metaplasia in the spleen does not contribute greatly to the peripheral blood count. Only when bone marrow activity is virtually absent does removal of the spleen appear to have a dangerous or even potentially fatal effect on peripheral blood counts. Bone marrow scans using radioactive indium or iron have not been very helpful in determining whether splenectomy can be undertaken safely.

Splenectomy has been advocated for patients with portal hypertension. The reason why splenectomy ameliorates this problem is entirely unclear. It has been suggested that islands of myeloid metaplasia in the liver obstruct the liver sinusoids that are necessary for portal hypertension to develop. Increased splenic vein blood flow has also been implicated. Splenectomy is sometimes associated with bleeding, infections, development of leukemia-like states, thrombosis, and thrombocytosis, and therefore it should not be undertaken lightly.

Hemorrhagic Thrombocythemia

Hemorrhagic thrombocythemia is characterized by high platelet counts associated with bleeding or thromboembolic phenomena, splenomegaly, and an increased bleeding time. It must be distinguished from polycythemia vera and secondary thrombocytosis. The causes of secondary thrombocytosis include inflammatory diseases and anoxia, inflammatory bowel diseases, polycythemia vera, Hodgkin's disease, chronic myelocytic leukemia, removal of the spleen, acute gastrointestinal bleeding and iron deficiency, and neoplasms.

Large and bizarrely shaped platelets, megakaryocytic fragments, or whole megakaryocytes circulate in the peripheral blood of patients with hemorrhagic thrombocythemia. This syndrome overlaps megakaryocytic leukemia, in which the megakaryocytes are present in peripheral blood and infiltrate such organs as the liver. The platelet count is usually a trillion per liter or more and may rise to as high as 14 trillion. Since these platelets function abnormally, iron deficiency as a result of bleeding is not uncommon. Bone marrow spicules show hyperplasia of all elements, particularly megakaryocytes.

If the secondary causes of thrombocytosis have been eliminated, and if there is not enough evidence to make the diagnosis of polycythemia vera, then a patient with thrombocytosis and splenomegaly is likely to have hemorrhagic thrombocythemia. No treatment is required if the patient is asymptomatic and the platelet count is less than a trillion per liter. If the platelet count is very high, or if the patient has developed thromboembolic complications, then treatment with ^{32}P or alkylating agents is indicated. Intravenous nitrogen mustard is given if the platelet count is dangerously high. Under no circumstances should splenectomy be undertaken, since this can result in a rapidly fatal thrombocytosis.

Approach to Patient with a Myeloproliferative Disorder

Both the clinical findings common to these disorders and the features that separate them into disease entities must be evaluated as part of the workup. Usually bone marrow scans are not available and splenic aspiration is considered too dangerous to perform.

Approach to patient with a myeloproliferative disorder

I. History
   A. Hemorrhagic or thromboembolic complications
   B. History of bone or splenic infarcts
II. Physical Findings
   A. Splenomegaly
   B. Hepatomegaly
   C. Lymphadenopathy
   D. Ascites
   E. Congestive heart failure
III. Laboratory Data
   A. Peripheral blood counts
   B. Peripheral blood smear (teardrop forms, immature white or
      red cells, large or bizarre platelet forms, poikilocytosis,
      polychromatophilia)
   C. Reticulocyte count
   D. Leukocyte alkaline phosphatase
   E. Uric acid
   F. Bone marrow aspirate biopsy
      1. Chromosome analysis (Philadelphia chromosome)
      2. Iron stores
      3. Special stains for fibrosis and increased reticulum
      4. Cellularity
IV. Other Tests to Consider
   A. Radioiron ferrokinetic studies and scan over bone marrow,
      liver, and spleen
   B. Indium III bone marrow scan
   C. Splenic aspiration (done in order to look for islands of mye-
      loid metaplasia in the spleen)
   D. Serum B_{12} and transcobalomin levels
   E. Platelet function tests
   F. X-rays of pelvis for osteosclerosis

CASE DEVEL-
OPMENT
PROBLEM:
LEUKEMIA AND
MYELOPRO-
LIFERATIVE
DISORDERS

A 65-year-old man has headaches, and his face appears flushed. His hematocrit is 0.64 (64%); hemoglobin, 16 gm per deciliter; and red blood cell count, 8×10^{12} cells per liter.

1. On the basis of these data alone, what tentative diagnoses can you make and what diagnostic procedures would you undertake to confirm them?

The symptoms, along with the elevated red blood cell count and hematocrit, suggest polycythemia. The red cell mass should be determined by a radiochromium, isotope dilution method to confirm that it is increased. Calculation of Wintrobe indices yields a mean corpuscular volume of 80 fl and a mean corpuscular hemoglobin concentration of 25 gm per deciliter. These indices indicate the presence of a hypochromic, microcytic anemia. Iron deficiency sometimes complicates polycythemia vera, so either serum iron and total iron-binding capacity should be determined or a bone marrow examination for iron stores done.

A radiochromium assay of red cell mass is performed. Twenty-five milliliters of blood are removed from the patient. Approximately 100 μCi of radioactive chromium 51 is added and the appropriate labeling procedures carried out. Ten milliliters of washed, packed, radioactively labeled red cells that have been found to contain 300,000 counts per minute of radioactivity are prepared and injected back into the patient. After 20 minutes, to allow for circulation, another sample of blood is withdrawn from the patient and 10 ml of washed, packed red cells are prepared and counted. This sample yields 1,000 counts per minute. The patient's predicted normal red cell mass, based on his height and weight, is 2,300 ml.

2. What is the patient's calculated red cell mass, and how would you interpret this finding?

The calculated red cell mass is $10 \times 300,000/1,000$, which equals 3,000 ml. As this mass is significantly above that predicted, the patient has polycythemia. A diagnosis of polycythemia *vera* cannot be made, since patients with secondary polycythemia also have an increased red cell mass. The patient does not have relative polycythemia due to a decreased plasma volume, since the red cell mass is actually abnormally high.

The patient has a red face and a slightly enlarged spleen. His white blood cell count is 30×10^9 per liter with no immature white cells or nucleated red cells seen on peripheral smear; his platelet count is 700×10^9 per liter. A leukocyte alkaline phosphatase score is 280.

3. What diagnosis is suggested by these findings, and what further tests should be done?

The high blood counts, splenomegaly, and elevated leukocyte alkaline phosphatase score strongly suggest the diagnosis of polycythemia vera. Even so, a complete physical examination, intravenous pyelogram, and determination of arterial oxygen saturation, if there is any suspicion of cyanotic lung or heart disease, should be done to rule out the common causes of secondary polycythemia. The urinary erythropoietin level, if it can be determined, is helpful, since in polycythemia vera it is normal and in secondary erythrocytosis abnormally high.

The patient gives no history of bleeding or thromboembolism (clotting of blood vessels or showers of clot thrown into the lung or another organ's blood vessels).

4. What therapy for his polycythemia would you recommend?

Since the patient is asymptomatic in spite of his high hematocrit and platelet count, there is no sense of urgency nor need to use chemotherapy or ^{32}P. Most hematologists would treat with phlebotomy alone. It can be argued that ^{32}P therapy would be just as safe and perhaps more effective in preventing complications and prolonging life. It can also be argued that use of ^{32}P increases the chance of developing acute leukemia.

The patient is treated successfully for 5 years, with his blood counts maintained at normal levels and his spleen size unchanged. He has been asymptomatic. Now, 5 years after initial diagnosis, his spleen begins to enlarge, and he becomes anemic.

5. On the basis of your knowledge of the natural history of polycythemia vera, what abnormal findings would you look for in his peripheral blood smear?

Two possibilities exist: (1) he is developing acute leukemia or (2) he is developing agnogenic myeloid metaplasia. The presence of immature white cells would be important, especially if they were mostly blasts, suggesting acute leukemia. If there were more mature forms than normally, as well as immature ones, then agnogenic myeloid metaplasia would be more likely. Changes in the red cell morphology would be of value, since teardrop forms and nucleated red cells favor the diagnosis of agnogenic myeloid metaplasia. The platelet count is usually low in acute leukemia, whereas in agnogenic myeloid metaplasia it is high or normal, falling to low levels in the later stages of the disease.

6. How would you distinguish the clinical picture of agnogenic

myeloid metaplasia from that of chronic myelocytic leukemia?

Agnogenic myeloid metaplasia sometimes develops during the course of polycythemia vera, whereas chronic myelocytic leukemia is not usually associated with polycythemia vera. Patients with agnogenic myeloid metaplasia have a high leukocyte alkaline phosphatase score and no Philadelphia chromosome. Patients with chronic myelocytic leukemia have the Philadelphia chromosome and a low or zero leukocyte alkaline phosphatase score. The most massively enlarged and firmest spleens are seen in agnogenic myeloid metaplasia, whereas in chronic myelocytic leukemia the spleen usually does not become very large until late in the course of the disease. Teardrop forms, a leukoerythroblastic blood picture, and marrow fibrosis are common in agnogenic myeloid metaplasia but may also occur in chronic myelocytic leukemia. Although in theory these two diseases should be distinguished easily, cases of Philadelphia chromosome–negative, chronic, myelocytic leukemia may be indistinguishable from agnogenic myeloid metaplasia.

Your patient now has a hematocrit of 0.25 (25%) and a white count of 30×10^9 per liter with 6 percent blasts, 10 percent promyelocytes, 30 percent myelocytes, 20 percent metamyelocytes, and the rest bands and polys. His platelet count is 600 $\times 10^9$ per liter, and his spleen is massively enlarged and fills the whole abdomen.

7. What is the likely diagnosis, and what other diseases must also be considered?

The most likely diagnosis is agnogenic myeloid metaplasia, but a leukemoid reaction, tuberculosis, and myelophthisic anemia must also be considered. The patient has none of the diseases associated with leukomoid reactions. Furthermore the platelet count is high, an unusual finding in a leukemoid reaction. Tuberculosis at one time was an important part of the differential diagnosis of agnogenic myeloid metaplasia, since the two diseases have similar peripheral blood abnormalities and enlarged spleens. Nowadays tuberculosis of the spleen is distinctly rare. If the patient is febrile, has an exposure to tuberculosis, or gives any other reason to suspect this diagnosis, appropriate cultures should be performed. Patients with metastatic cancer involving the bone marrow often have peripheral blood findings suggestive of agnogenic myeloid metaplasia. Usually they do not have splenomegaly, however, and an examination of their bone marrow shows cancer cells.

8. List the various therapies that might be used to treat your patient, and describe their advantages and disadvantages.

Androgens, alkylating agents, radioactive phosphorus, splenectomy, and folic acid. Splenectomy relieves cytopenias but is associated with a large operative risk. Androgens may improve anemia but do often affect other blood counts or shrink the spleen. Alkylating agents and ^{32}P shrink the size of the spleen but often cause more severe cytopenias.

The patient's spleen is removed in an attempt to ameliorate his anemia. This is unsuccessful however; the patient not only remains anemic but develops a white blood cell count of 100×10^9 per liter with 90 percent myeloblasts.

9. What is likely to have occurred, and how can this complication be treated?

After splenectomy some patients develop a picture not unlike that of acute myelocytic leukemia. The patient should be treated for acute myelocytic leukemia, but his response probably will be poor.

10. Besides chemotherapy for the leukemia, what adjunctive or nonspecific measures should be taken as part of general and supportive therapy in acute leukemia?

One should consider controlling the hyperuricemia with drugs such as allopurinol. Isolation in a "life island" or lamina flow room, along with bowel sterilization with nonabsorbable antibiotics, should be considered during chemotherapy. Red cell, platelets, and white cell transfusions are frequently required.

TOPICS FOR DISCUSSION: LEUKEMIA AND RELATED MYELOPRO-LIFERATIVE DISORDERS

Etiology of acute leukemia

White cell kinetics and the leukemias

Rational treatment of acute leukemia based on cell cycle

Stem cells and their relation to leukemias

Growth of leukemic cells in soft agar and liquid cultures

Transitions between myeloproliferative disorders

Patient selection for antileukemic therapy

Immunotherapy for induction and maintenance of remission in leukemia

Bone marrow transplantation for treatment of leukemia

Relationship between chronic lymphocytic leukemia and malignant lymphoma

Complications of treatment of acute and chronic leukemias with chemotherapy

Role of psychotherapy in treating leukemic patients

Use of radioactive phosphorus in treatment of acute and chronic leukemias

Splenectomy and splenic irradiation as treatment for leukemia

Bone marrow morphology during treatment for acute leukemias

Radiation as an etiological agent in leukemia

Differential diagnosis of leukemoid reactions

Differential diagnosis of leukoerythroblastic blood picture

Preleukemia and preleukemic conditions

Lysozyme, its use in diagnosis and therapy of leukemias and other myeloproliferative disorders

Cytochemical methods for identifying myeloblasts, lymphoblasts, and monoblasts

Biochemistry of leukemic cells

Regulation of erythropoiesis in erythroleukemia

Acute myeloproliferative syndromes

Platelet function in myeloproliferative disorders

Vitamin B_{12} and vitamin B_{12}-binding proteins in leukemia and other myeloproliferative diseases

Chromosomal markers in leukemia and myeloproliferative disorders

Exotic infections complicating chemotherapy of leukemias

Splenic and bone infarctions in myeloproliferative disorders

Blast crisis in chronic myelocytic leukemia

Emergency and routine treatment of thrombocytosis

Influence of splenomegaly on plasma volume

Treatment of polycythemia vera with chemotherapy, radioactive phosphorus, or phlebotomy

Ferrokinetic data, indium 111, iron 52 and technetium 99m bone marrow scans in agnogenic myeloid metaplasia

Erythropoietin assays for clinical use

Megakaryocytic proliferation and megakaryocytic leukemia

Perioperative complications of polycythemia vera

Polycythemia and malignant disease

Cigarette smoking, carboxyhemoglobin and erythrocytosis

SELECTED REFERENCES

Leukemia

Aur, R., Simone, J. V., and Hustu, H., et al Cessation of therapy in childhood acute lymphocytic leukemia. *N. Engl. J. Med.* 291:1230, 1974.

Beard, M. E. J., and Fairley, G. H. Acute leukemia in adults. *Semin. Hematol.* 11:5, 1974.

Berard, C. W., Gallo, R. C., and Jaffe, E. S., et al Current concepts of leukemia and lymphoma: Etiology, pathogenesis, and therapy. *Ann Intern. Med.* 85:351, 1976.

Bodey, G. P., and Freireich, E. J. Acute Leukemia. In C. E. Mengel, et al (eds.), *Hematology: Principles and Practices.* Chicago: Year Book, 1972.

Bodey, G., and Rodriquiez, V. Protected environment — prophylactic antibiotic programmes; microbiological studies. *Clin. Haematol.* 5:395, 1976.

Carbone, P. P., and Canellos, G. P. The Chronic Leukemias. In C. E. Mengel, et al (eds.), *Hematology: Principles and Practices.* Chicago: Year Book, 1972.

Chabner, B. A., Myers, C. E., and Oliverio, V. T. Clinical pharmacology of anticancer drugs. *Semin. Oncol.* 4:165, 1977.

Frei, E., and Zubrod, C. G. Principles of Chemotherapy for Hematologic Neoplasms. In C. E. Mengel, et al (eds.), *Hematology: Principles and Practices.* Chicago: Year Book, 1972.

Galton, D. A. G. (ed.) The chronic leukaemias. *Clin. Haematol.* 6:1, 1977.

Goh, K., and Heusinkveld, R. S. Contributions of Cytogenetics to Hematology. In R. I. Weed (ed.), *Hematology for Internists.* Boston: Little, Brown, 1971.

Greene, W. A. Psychological Problems in Leukemias and Lymphomas. In R. I. Weed (ed.), *Hematology for Internists.* Boston: Little, Brown, 1971.

Griner, P. F. Chronic Myelogenous Leukemia. In R. I. Weed (ed.), *Hematology for Internists.* Boston: Little, Brown, 1971.

Gunz, F. W. Chapter 89, Erythroleukemia. In W. J. Williams, E. Beutler, A. J. Erslev, and R. W. Rundles (eds.), *Hematology* (2nd ed.). New York: McGraw-Hill, 1977.

Gunz, F. W., and Baikie, A. G. *Leukemia* (3rd ed.). New York: Grune & Stratton, 1974.

Hall, T. C. Biochemical Therapeutics of Acute Leukemia. In R. I. Weed (ed.), *Hematology for Internists.* Boston: Little, Brown, 1971.

Henderson, E. S. Chapter 91, Acute Leukemia: General Considerations; Chapter 92, Acute Myelogenous Leukemia. In W. J. Williams, E. Beutler, A. J. Erslev, and R. W. Rundles (eds.), *Hematology* (2nd ed.). New York: McGraw-Hill, 1977.

Henderson, E. S. Chapter 113, Acute Lymphocytic Leukemia. In W. J. Williams, E. Beutler, A. J. Erslev, and R. W. Rundles (eds.), *Hematology* (2nd ed.). New York: McGraw-Hill, 1977.

Henderson, E. S. (ed.) Current status reports: Leukemia and lymphoma therapy. *Semin. Hematol.* 9:137, 1972.

Jacquillat, C. I., Weil, M., and Gemon, M. F., et al   Evaluation of 216 four-year survivors of acute leukemia. *Cancer* 32:286, 1973.

Kass, L., and Schnitzer, B.   *Refractory Anemia.* Springfield: Charles C. Thomas, 1975.

Keating, M. J., Freireich, E. J., and McCredie, K. B., et al   Acute leukemia in adults. *CA* 27:2, 1977.

Levine, A. S., Schimpff, S. C., Draw, R. G., and Young, R. C.   Hematologic malignancies and other marrow failure states: Progress in the management of complicating infections. *Semin. Hematol.* 11:141, 1974.

Lichtman, M. A.   The Kinetics of Cell Proliferation in Acute Leukemia: Future Therapeutic Implications. In R. I. Weed (ed.), *Hematology for Internists.* Boston: Little, Brown, 1971.

Linman, J. W.   Leukemia. In J. W. Linman (ed.), *Hematology: Physiologic, Pathophysiologic, and Clinical Principles.* New York: MacMillan, 1975.

Linman, J. W., and Saarni, M. I.   The preleukemic syndrome. *Semin. Hematol.* 11:93, 1974.

Meisler, A. I.   The Etiology of Leukemia. In R. I. Weed (ed.), *Hematology for Internists.* Boston: Little, Brown, 1971.

Miescher, P. A., and Farquet, J. J.   Chronic myelomonocytic leukemia in adults. *Semin. Hematol.* 11:129, 1974.

Monfardini, S., Gee, T., and Fried, J., et al   Survival in chronic myelogenous leukemia influence of treatment and extent of disease at diagnosis. *Cancer* 31:492, 1973.

Pierre, R. V.   Preleukemic states. *Semin. Hematol.* 11:73, 1974.

Rai, K. R., Sawitsky, A., and Cronkite, E. P., et al   Clinical staging of chronic lymphocytic leukemia. *Blood* 46:219, 1975.

Rowley, J.   The role of cytogenetics in hematology. *Blood* 48:1, 1976.

Rundles, R. W.   Chapter 87, Chronic Granulocytic Leukemia; Chapter 115, Monocytic Leukemia. In W. J. Williams, E. Beutler, A. J. Erslev, and R. W. Rundles (eds.), *Hematology* (2nd ed.). New York:McGraw-Hill, 1977.

Simone, J.   Acute lymphocytic leukemia in childhood. *Semin. Hematol.* 11:25, 1974.

Stryckmans, P. A.   Current concepts in chronic myelogenous leukemia. *Semin. Hematol.* 11:101, 1974.

Thomas, E. D., Buckner, C. D., and Banaji, M., et al   One hundred patients with acute leukemia treated by chemotherapy, total body irradiation, and allogenic marrow transplantation. *Blood* 49:511, 1977.

Weed, R. I.   Management of Adults with Acute Leukemia. In R. I. Weed (ed.), *Hematology for Internists.* Boston: Little, Brown, 1971.

Wintrobe, M. M., et al   Complications of Neoplastic Diseases of the Hematopoietic System and their Treatment; Principles of Therapy and Effects of Specific Drugs Used in Therapy of Neoplastic Diseases of the Hematopoietic System. In M. M. Wintrobe, et al (eds.), *Clinical Hematology* (7th ed.). Philadelphia: Lea & Febiger, 1974.

Wintrobe, M. M., et al   Classification, Pathogenesis, and Etiology of Neoplastic Diseases of the Hematopoietic System; The Acute Leukemias; Chronic Myelocytic Leukemia; Chronic Lymphocytic Leukemia. In M. M. Wintrobe, et al (eds.), *Clinical Hematology* (7th ed.). Philadelphia: Lea & Febiger, 1974.

Myeloproliferative
Syndromes

Bauman, A. W., and Schwartz, S. I. Myeloid Metaplasia: Medical Management and Role of Splenectomy. In R. I. Weed (ed.), *Hematology for Internists*. Boston: Little, Brown, 1971.

Bouroncle, B. A. Myelofibrosis and Myeloid Metaplasia. In C. E. Mengel, et al (eds.), *Hematology: Principles and Practice*. Chicago: Year Book, 1972.

Gunz, F. W. Chapter 88, Myelofibrosis; Chapter 90, Essential Thrombocythemia. In W. J. Williams, E. Beutler, A. J. Erslev, and R. W. Rundles (eds.), *Hematology* (2nd ed.). New York: McGraw-Hill, 1977.

Rundles, R. W. Chapter 86, Myeloproliferative Disorders — General Considerations; Chapter 94, Preleukemia. In W. J. Williams, E. Beutler, A. J. Erslev, and R. W. Rundles, (eds.), *Hematology* (2nd ed.). New York: McGraw-Hill, 1977.

Wintrobe, M. M., et al   Myelofibrosis. In M. M. Wintrobe, et al (eds.), *Clinical Hematology* (7th ed.). Philadelphia: Lea & Febiger, 1974.

Polycythemia

Bauman, A. W. Polycythemia Vera. In R. I. Weed (ed.), *Hematology for Internists*. Boston: Little, Brown, 1971.

Berlin, N. I. (ed.) Polycythemia I. *Semin. Hematol.* 12:335, 1975.

Berlin, N. I. (ed.) Polycythemia II. *Semin. Hematol.* 13:1, 1976.

Erslev, A. J. Chapter 73, Secondary Polycythemia. In W. J. Williams, E. Beutler, A. J. Erslev, and R. W. Rundles, (eds.), *Hematology* (2nd ed.). New York: McGraw-Hill, 1977.

Gilbert, H. S. Erythrocytosis and Polycythemia Vera. In C. E. Mengel, et al (eds.), *Hematology: Principles and Practice*. Chicago: Year Book, 1972.

Glass, J. L., and Wasserman, L. W. Chapter 72, Primary Polycythemia. In W. J. Williams, E. Beutler, A. J. Erslev, and R. W. Rundles (eds.) *Hematology* (2nd ed.). New York: McGraw-Hill, 1977.

Krauss, S., and Wasserman, L. R. Chapter 74, Spurious (Relative) Polycythemia. In W. J. Williams, E. Beutler, A. J. Erslev, and R. W. Rundles (eds.), *Hematology* (2nd ed.). New York: McGraw-Hill, 1977.

Videbaek, A. Polycythaemia and myelofibrosis. *Clin. Haematol.* 4:1, 1975.

Wintrobe, M. M., et al   Polycythemia. In M. M. Wintrobe, et al (eds.), *Clinical Hematology* (7th ed.). Philadelphia: Lea & Febiger, 1974.

10 : Lymphoma and Other Lymphoproliferative Diseases

MALIGNANT LYMPHOMA

Malignant lymphoma is a disease of the lymph nodes and is characterized by infiltration and destruction of their normal architecture by morphologically mature or immature lymphocytes or reticulum cells. This disease has a clinical course characteristic of a malignancy. It may either initially or subsequently involve any organ system, as it can arise not only in lymph nodes but also in lymphoid tissues found in all organs. In some cases it starts in the lymph nodes and spreads by various routes to involve the liver, gastrointestinal tract, and bone marrow. On the other hand *extranodal lymphomas* arise in the lymphoid tissue of the gastrointestinal tract, bones, or other organs and spread later to other areas.

There are two major types of malignant lymphoma, Hodgkin's disease and non-Hodgkin's lymphoma. Closely related to non-Hodgkin's lymphoma is multiple myeloma, a disease of the plasma cell (a B lymphocyte–derived cell), and Waldenström's macroglobulinemia, a disease that has features of the malignant lymphomas and also some of the characteristics of the plasma cell dyscrasias, including an abnormal macroimmunoglobulin. These malignant diseases and a benign infectious disease that is characterized by lymphocyte proliferation and lymph node hyperplasia, infectious mononucleosis, are discussed in this chapter.

Etiology

The etiologic agent of the malignant lymphomas is unknown. A number of possibilities are being actively investigated, however, and show promise of leading to the cause of lymphomas, particularly Hodgkin's disease. Since new data are rapidly being accumulated in this field, only current hypotheses for the pathogenesis of Hodgkin's disease and non-Hodgkin's lymphomas are discussed.

For many years investigators have been looking for an infectious agent for Hodgkin's disease. Histopathologic findings suggest an inflammatory or infectious process. Microorganisms such as the tubercle bacillus and other unusual bacterial and fungal agents have been considered as causes. However, there is no evidence that these agents are etiologic. Most likely, patients with advanced Hodgkin's disease are predisposed to infections with these unusual agents. Viruses, such as the herpes virus known as *Epstein-Barr* or *EB virus,* have been closely associated with the development of an

333

unusual condition called *Burkitt's lymphoma.* Epidemiologic and immunologic evidence suggests that this lymphoma is caused by an infectious agent present in certain parts of Africa. The same virus has been shown to be the cause of a benign disease, infectious mononucleosis. The viral etiology of malignant lymphoma receives support from animal data: inbred, genetically disposed strains of animals have developed immunologic disorders, lymph node hyperplasia, and ultimately lymphoma. Viruses are thought to mediate these changes, but similar viruses have not been found in man.

Epidemiologic studies of contact between Hodgkin's disease victims have suggested that an infectious agent with a long latent period is involved in the development of the disease, particularly in young adults. In Albany, New York, close links were described in 34 out of 42 cases of space-time–clustered lymphoma studied. In a control group of 18 patients with burns, no links could be detected. These data have been challenged, however, on the grounds that the control group and statistical analysis were inadequate. Other outbreaks of Hodgkin's disease, and familial and marital cases, have also been reported.

Further supporting evidence for the transmissibility of Hodgkin's disease comes from studies of cases in New York State schools. In five of eight secondary public schools in which cases were diagnosed during 1960–1964, further cases were diagnosed during 1965–1969. In contrast, none of the matched control schools (without cases of Hodgkin's disease in the first period) had cases in the later period. Even if transmissibility is accepted, it is clear that the risk is of low magnitude, and that no interlinking is found between most patients with Hodgkin's disease.

Another theory for the etiology of malignant lymphoma involves the host's immunologic system. This theory suggests that an agent, perhaps a virus, alters thymus-derived lymphocytes so that they undergo antigenic alteration of their surface. Normal immunocompetent T cells react against the antigenically altered cells. A chronic immune reaction (similar to graft-versus-host disease) then leads to the appearance of neoplastic (Reed-Sternberg) cells. Although it is true that there is derangement of cell-mediated immunity in the malignant lymphomas and that tumor-associated antigens have been reported in the spleen of patients with Hodgkin's disease, other assumptions made by this hypothesis have not yet proved correct. Furthermore the tumor-associated antigens may well not be specific for Hodgkin's disease. For these and other reasons the immunologic theories, although attractive, have not been universally accepted. Immunologic abnormalities do exist in Hodgkin's disease, but they may be secondary phenomena rather than etiologic. Congenital or acquired dysfunction of the immunologic systems as found in agammaglobulinemia, ataxia-telangiectasia, Chédiak-Higashi syndrome, and diseases associated with autoimmunity such as Hashimoto's syndrome, Sjögren's syndrome, and acquired hemolytic anemia have been associated with malignant lymphoma.

Histopathology of Malignant Lymphomas

The characteristic pathologic features of malignant lymphomas are (1) destruction of the normal follicular architecture of the lymph nodes by large numbers of mature and immature lymphocytes or reticulum cells, or both, (2) invasion and destruction of the lymph node capsule and the subcapsular sinuses, and (3) infiltration of the pericapsular fat by large numbers of cells similar to those that destroy the architecture of the lymph nodes. If these features are present, the diagnosis of malignant lymphoma is strongly suggested. It is sometimes difficult to distinguish these abnormalities from those seen in severe or atypical lymph node hyperplasia, in which the follicular structure, although not completely destroyed, is greatly deranged, and in which changes similar to those of lymphoma may occur in the capsule, subcapsular sinus, and pericapsular fat. In lymph node hyperplasia, however, the proliferating cells do not meet cytologic criteria for malignancy. Atypical lymph node hyperplasia is often found in lymph nodes adjacent to those involved by frank lymphoma and in lymph nodes of patients who later develop frank lymphoma. In some cases the distinction between frank lymphoma and atypical lymph node hyperplasia becomes very difficult, and there may be disagreement among pathologists. Toxoplasmosis and Dilantin-induced lymph node hyperplasia are two other diseases that can be confused with lymphoma, if one is unaware of their characteristic features.

Diffuse and nodular forms exist for each of the subtypes of malignant lymphoma. In the nodular forms there are dense clusters of lymphocytes, reticulum cells, or both, similar to lymph follicles. The lymphomas characterized by nodular aggregations carry a better prognosis, both with and without treatment, than the diffuse form of lymphoma, in which such aggregations are absent. Prognosis also depends on the histologic subtype and, most importantly, the extent of lymphomatous spread through the body. Of course these factors are interrelated and not independent.

Attempts are currently underway to further define the cell types found in lymphomatous nodes. There may be a correlation between the morphologic characteristics of a cell, particularly its nucleus, and whether it is of T cell or B cell origin. Furthermore some of the cellular characteristics may be related to whether the cell is "turned on," or *transformed*. Transformation refers to lymphoblastoid changes that occur in a cell when it is stimulated by antigens to which it has been sensitized or by plant substances such as phytohemagglutinin. These studies also cast doubt on whether the cells classified as reticulum cells are truly cells that produce reticulum fibers. It may be that only a minority are, and that the rest are actually *immunoblasts,* or lymphocytes that have been turned on to the production of immunoglobulins. We know that such cells develop nucleoli in their nuclei and other changes that make them resemble malignant cells. Further discussion of these findings will come later.

Classification of Hodgkin's Disease

The lymph nodes in Hodgkin's disease as in all malignant lymphomas, are characterized by destruction of the normal follicular architecture and invasion of the subcapsular sinus, capsule, and pericapsular space. What makes the picture different from that of the other lymphomas is the presence of Reed-Sternberg cells (Plate 64). These are very large (? reticulum) cells with two nuclei, or at least a multilobulated nucleus, and each nucleus has a dense nucleolus surrounded by a clear space. The clear space is most likely an artifact of hematoxylin-and-eosin staining. These characteristics give the Reed-Sternberg cell an "owl's eye" appearance. They are also occasionally found in other diseases, such as adenocarcinomas, rubeola, infectious mononucleosis, sarcomas, melanomas, non-Hodgkin's lymphomas, and multiple myeloma. This complicates the diagnosis but usually creates little difficulty for the experienced pathologist, since the other features of Hodgkin's lymphoma allow differentiation from nonlymphomatous diseases. These features include a pleomorphic infiltrate composed of lymphocytes and reticulum cells of various degrees of maturity, along with fibrocytes, plasma cells, monocytes, and eosinophils, as well as fibrosis and necrosis. Interestingly, the histopathologic findings of Hodgkin's disease resemble those of a chronic inflammatory reaction.

Noncaseating granulomata are seen in organs such as the spleen and liver; more importantly, the cellular infiltrate characteristic of Hodgkin's disease may not be present. Therefore, these granulomata make the findings indistinguishable from those of sarcoidosis and pose certain difficulties to the determination of the extent of disease spread. At present, when these granulomata are found in spleens and livers unassociated with the characteristic histologic findings of Hodgkin's disease, we do not presume that the organ is involved with Hodgkin's disease but rather assume that this is a granulomatous response to the tumor. Only further investigation will show whether this assumption is indeed correct.

Table 10-1 lists three classification schemes for Hodgkin's disease. The International classification derives at least in part from the

Table 10-1 : Three Classification Schemes for Subtypes of Hodgkin's Disease

Jackson and Parker	Lukes and Butler	International
Paragranuloma	Lymphocytic Lymphohistiocytic	Lymphocytic predominance
Granuloma	Mixed cellularity Nodular sclerosis	Mixed cellularity Nodular sclerosis
Sarcoma	Reticular Diffuse fibrosis	Lymphocytic depletion

classification suggested by Lukes and Butler. *Paragranuloma,* described by Jackson and Parker, or as it is called in the current international classification, *lymphocytic predominance,* is characterized by an infiltrate consisting of mainly lymphocytes with a relatively smaller number of reticulum cells. Atypical reticulum cells and Reed-Sternberg cells are rare; fibrosis is absent. Only about ten percent of cases of Hodgkin's disease are diagnosed as lymphocytic predominance. This type carries the best prognosis, when other factors are held constant.

Granuloma (Jackson and Parker) has been split in the International scheme into two classifications, *mixed cellularity* and *nodular sclerosis.* In mixed cellularity, the most common type of Hodgkin's disease, the typical pleomorphic infiltrate is found, along with necrosis and fibrosis and numerous Reed-Sternberg cells. Nodular sclerosis has the same cellular infiltrate but arranged in a unique manner. The reticulum cells are found in lacunae, giving a *starry sky* appearance to the infiltrate. Surrounding and encompassing this pleomorphic infiltrate are bands of fibrosis. It is these aggregations of cells, separated by the eosinophilic collagen, that give this Hodgkin's subtype its name, nodular sclerosis. The mixed cellularity and nodular sclerotic types make up about eighty percent of cases of Hodgkin's disease. Nodular sclerosis usually has a better prognosis than mixed cellularity.

The *sarcoma* subtype described by Jackson and Parker is characterized by a cellular infiltrate consisting mainly of reticulum cells and Reed-Sternberg cells. In some cases diffuse, dense areas of fibrosis are predominant. This *lymphocyte depletion* subtype carries the worst prognosis and is often associated with an unusual clinical syndrome consisting of fever, pancytopenia, lymphocytopenia, abnormal liver function tests, and marrow involvement with fibrosis, hypoplasia, and Reed-Sternberg cells. Abdominal lymphadenopathy predominates rather than the usual peripheral node enlargement.

**Pathology of
Non-Hodgkin's
Lymphoma**

Lymph nodes from patients with non-Hodgkin's lymphomas have the characteristic features of malignant lymphoma, but the nature of the infiltrating tissue is different from that of Hodgkin's disease. The infiltrate is usually monotypic, that is, it consists of one cell type rather than the many seen in the common forms of Hodgkin's disease. Of course Reed-Sternberg cells are not present. Many classifications have been proposed for non-Hodgkin's lymphoma. They depend upon the estimated maturity or immaturity of the infiltrating cell and also upon whether the proliferating cells are assumed to be lymphocytes or reticulum cells. The simplest classification gives three subtypes. The first is the *lymphocytic, small cell, or well-differentiated lymphosarcoma.* The tumor tissue is composed of mature lymphocytes that resemble those found in chronic lymphocytic leukemia. The lymphocytes are small with scant cytoplasm and have very dark, compact, sometimes clefted, nuclei. Nucleoli are absent in the great majority of these cells. The second type is the *lymphoblastic, large cell,* or *poorly differentiated lymphosarcoma* with predominantly large cells containing nuclei that have an open chromatin network and contain one or more nucleoli. The third morphologic subtype, *reticulum cell sarcoma* or *histiocytic lymphosarcoma,* is characterized by large cells with clear nuclei and one or more nucleoli. These cells may be surrounded by reticulum fibers that take up silver stains. Phagocytized material may be present in the cell's cytoplasm. These reticulum cells are indistinguishable by light microscopy from those seen in Hodgkin's sarcoma, but Reed-Sternberg cells are not found.

If a freshly cut surface of a lymphomatous node is touched to a slide and stained with Wright stain, lymphoblasts can more easily be distinguished from reticulum cells than after staining with hematoxylin and eosin. This procedure can help distinguish lymphoblastic lymphosarcoma from reticulum cell sarcoma.

Mixed cell lymphosarcoma is an unusual form of non-Hodgkin's lymphoma in which the infiltrate is composed of lymphocytes and histiocytes. A *lymphohistiocytic form of Hodgkin's disease* has also been described. In fact, in some patients with mixed cell lymphosarcoma, a Reed-Sternberg cell is subsequently discovered, and the patient is reclassified as having lymphocyte-predominant Hodgkin's disease. *Immature lymphocytic lymphosarcoma* is diagnosed when the cell type is a lymphocyte intermediate in maturity between a small lymphocyte and a lymphoblast. Actually this type of lymphosarcoma is found relatively frequently.

Both nodular and diffuse forms of all these types of lymphoma have been described. The nodular forms carry a better prognosis.

The Rappaport classification is one of the more extensive classifi-

Rappaport's classification of non-Hodgkin's lymphomas

NH:
Nodular, histiocytic

NM:
Nodular, mixed, histiocytic-
lymphocytic

NLPD:
Nodular, lymphocytic,
poorly differentiated

NLWD:
Nodular, lymphocytic, well
differentiated

DH:
Diffuse, histiocytic

DM:
Diffuse, mixed, histiocytic-
lymphocytic

DLPD:
Diffuse, lymphocytic,
poorly differentiated

DLWD:
Diffuse, lymphocytic, well
differentiated

DU:
Diffuse, undifferentiated

Adapted from Jones, S. E., et al, Non-Hodgkin's Lymphomas IV: Clini-
copathologic correlation in 405 cases. *Cancer* 31:809, 1973.

cation schemes for non-Hodgkin's lymphoma. It identifies nine different subtypes of non-Hodgkin's lymphoma. This scheme depends on whether the infiltrate is nodular or diffuse, lymphocytic or histiocytic (reticulum cell), and on how well or poorly differentiated the lymphocytes appear. The nodular and the mature lymphocytic types carry the best prognosis both with and without therapy. In contrast, diffuse, poorly differentiated lymphocytic and histiocytic cell types carry the worst prognosis.

Currently there is interest in defining the cellular infiltrate in terms of whether the cells carry B or T cell markers. Well-differentiated lymphocytic lymphomas and nodular lymphomas consist of B cells derived from lymph node follicular center cells. Poorly differentiated lymphocytic lymphomas may be derived from B cells and in some cases from T cells. Non-Hodgkin's lymphomas characterized by convoluted cell nuclei probably represent T cell neoplasia. Mixed cell or lymphohistiocytic lymphomas appear to originate from B cells. The characteristic cells found in lymph nodes of patients with reticulum cell sarcomas may be histiocytes, that is, phagocytes; or produce reticulum, that is, true reticulum cells; or may represent transformed lymphocytes. There is evidence that Hodgkin's disease is a T lymphocyte disorder and that Reed-Sternberg cells are in fact transformed lymphocytes.

Immunoblastic sarcomas are lymphomas of large transformed lymphocytes of either B or T cell type, often associated with immune system disorders, senescence, and a rapidly fatal course. Rheumatoid arthritis, systemic lupus erythematosus, Sjögren's syndrome, and α-chain disease are some of the immune disorders present in patients with this unique lymphoma. Plasmacytoid cellular features and monoclonal gammopathy are also commonly found.

Related to immunoblastic sarcomas is a B lymphocyte disease called *immunoblastic lymphadenopathy*. It is clinically characterized by systemic symptoms as in Hodgkin's disease, generalized lymphadenopathy, hepatosplenomegaly, and skin rash. Frequently it includes polyclonal gammopathy or a Coombs' test–positive hemolytic anemia or both. Pathologically the lymph node architecture is obliterated and the capsule invaded. Unlike malignant lymphoma it displays an entire range of cytologically benign, immunologically reactive cells, including lymphocytes, plasma cells, and immunoblasts or transformed lymphocytes. There is also marked vascular proliferation. Although it is considered a benign disease, some patients develop immunoblastic sarcoma and others die following treatment with cytotoxic drugs. Corticosteroids may be a better choice of drug for this disease.

Clinical and Pathologic Staging of Malignant Lymphomas

Clinical and pathologic staging of the malignant lymphomas are done only after an adequate history is taken to determine whether the patient has fever, weight loss (equivalent to 10 percent of his body weight), or night sweats, and after a complete physical examination has been done with particular attention to lymph node (see Figure 11 for location of clinically important lymph node groups), tonsil, liver, and spleen size. Blood counts and smear, laboratory tests for liver and kidney function, uric acid level, x-ray examination of the chest and bones (bone scan is also suggested), and bone marrow needle biopsy should also be performed and, in some cases, lymphangiography, inferior vena cavography, intravenous pyelography, and gallium 57 scanning for lymph node involvement with lymphoma. (See outline under Approach to Patient with Malignant Lymphoma, p. 353.)

A clinical stage is determined on the basis of findings from all these procedures (see p. 343). Clinically involved lymph nodes (palpation of hard or rubbery glands) at a single site on either side of the diaphragm are classified as Stage I. More than one site involvement is Stage II. In Stage III there is involvement on both sides of the diaphragm, and in Stage IV there is evidence of lymphoma outside the lymph nodes or spleen. The presence of splenomegaly should be indicated by a subscript S. If the patient has one extralymphatic site that could conceivably be cured by radiotherapy, this should be noted as a subscript E, and the disease should not be classified as Stage IV on the basis of this extranodal involvement. For example, if the patient has lung involvement adjacent to mediastinal lymph nodes, this may be cured by radical radiotherapy; therefore, the condition should be classified as Stage II$_E$. The presence of fever, weight loss, or night sweats is indicated by an A or B appearing after the Roman numeral of this stage (e.g., IIIB). Patients with advanced stages or B symptoms have a poorer prognosis than those without systemic manifestations and with localized disease.

Lymphangiography is an important x-ray technique designed to evaluate lymph nodes in the abdomen for lymphoma. Dye is injected subcutaneously into the leg and finds its way into a lymphatic. A lymph channel can then be visualized. With a tiny needle it is cannulized and radiopaque oil is injected under pressure. The oil is allowed to distribute itself for about 24 hours through the leg lymphatics into the abdominal lymph vessels and nodes. Replacement of normal lymph node structures with tumor is seen as areas of radiolucency. With this x-ray technique the lymph nodes of the groin, pelvis, and up to the lower lumbar region can usually be visualized. Side effects include allergic reactions to the oil and pulmonary insufficiency due to shunting of excessive oil into the lung lymphatics. The oil remains in lymph

Fig. 11 : Anatomic
location of clinically
important lymph
node groups. (Adap-
ted from Rubin, P.,
Comment: The re-
classification of
Hodgkin's disease.
J.A.M.A. 222:1304,
1972.)

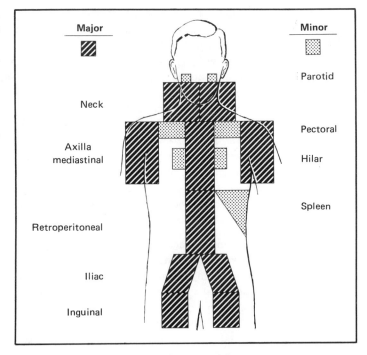

nodes for months, during which time the status of the lymph nodes and their response to therapy can be monitored by abdominal x-rays. Lymph node biopsy performed after lymphangiography is complicated by the fact that vacuoles resulting from the oil are seen throughout the lymph node, giving a Swiss cheese–like appearance. Usually it is easy for the pathologist to make a histologic diagnosis despite the presence of the lymphangiogram dye. Although there are frequent false positive results, that is, the lymph nodes appear abnormal, but biopsy shows them not to be involved with tumor, false negative lymphangiograms are rare. Clinical staging is often affected by the findings on lymphangiography. However, the pathologic stage, and therefore therapy, is usually determined by abdominal exploration and biopsy of suspicious lymph nodes.

Pathologic staging refers to the extent of disease as determined at the time of abdominal exploration. Abdominal exploration is performed by a formal laparotomy or by the use of a laparoscope and percutaneous biopsies of suspicious tissues. Removal of other tissues for histologic examination — for example, lung biopsy — is also used as part of pathologic staging. Once pathologic staging has been completed, then consideration is given to therapy.

It should be emphasized that the staging criteria described here were first developed for Hodgkin's disease. It was found that the

---

Staging of malignant lymphomas

I. Clinical Staging (CS)
  A. Stage I: Involvement of a single lymph node region (I) or of a single extralymphatic organ or site (I_E).
  B. Stage II: Involvement of two or more lymph node regions on the same side of the diaphragm (II) or localized involvement of an extralymphatic organ or site and of one or more lymph node regions on the same side of the diaphragm (II_E).
  C. Stage III: Involvement of lymph node regions on both sides of the diaphragm (III), which may also be accompanied by localized involvement of the spleen (III_S), extralymphatic site (III_E), or both (III_{SE}).
  D. Stage IV: Diffuse or disseminated involvement of one or more extralymphatic organs or tissues with or without associated lymph node enlargement.
    1. No B symptoms
    2. Weight loss, fever, night sweats.
II. Pathologic Staging (PS)
  A. Involvement found at laparotomy or by any further removal of tissue for histologic examination other than that taken for the original diagnosis. Include annotations for specific sites biopsied.
    N+ or N− For other lymph node positive or negative by biopsy
    H+ or H− For liver positive or negative by biopsy
    S+ or S− For spleen positive or negative following splenectomy
    L+ or L− For lung positive or negative by biopsy
    M+ or M− For bone marrow positive or negative by biopsy or smear
    P+ or P− For pleura or pleural fluid positive or negative by biopsy or by cytologic examination
    O+ or O− For bone positive or negative by biopsy
    D+ or D− For skin positive or negative by biopsy

Adapted from Jones, S. E., Fuks, Z., Bull, M., Non-Hodgkin's Lymphoma IV: Clincopathologic Correlation in 405 Cases. *Cancer* 31:808, 1973.

stages had a correlation with prognosis. Great weight is given to the stage of disease in deciding on therapy for Hodgkin's disease, as limited disease is potentially curable by radiotherapy. These same staging criteria were found to have a correlation with the prognosis for non-Hodgkin's lymphoma. Staging is therapeutically less useful in non-Hodgkin's lymphoma, however since the entity often presents at an incurable stage because of early bone marrow involvement.

Besides the pathologic differences between Hodgkin's and non-Hodgkin's lymphomas, there are many differences in their clinical course. Most important of all is the propensity for non-Hodgkin's lymphoma to be widespread throughout the body, particularly in the liver, gastrointestinal tract, and bone marrow, at the time of diagnosis. In many cases of Hodgkin's lymphoma, on the other hand, the disease is confined to lymph nodes, liver, and spleen at the time of diagnosis. Some authors have suggested that Hodgkin's disease begins in one lymph node group and then spreads sequentially to contiguous lymph node groups. In some cases it is necessary to postulate that the disease spreads retrograde through the thoracic duct from cervical lymph nodes to abdominal lymph nodes. Hematogenous spread by way of vascular invasion can also occur in Hodgkin's disease, so that patients with widely metastatic disease are found. In non-Hodgkin's lymphoma the disease appears to arise simultaneously in different lymph nodes and extranodal tissues. Experimental data confirming these differences and their explanations are still controversial and incomplete.

Some authors believe that in Hodgkin's disease the pattern of node involvement is not due to sequential spread but rather to a propensity for certain node groups to support the growth of Hodgkin's tumor tissue. Those investigators who believe in the sequential spread hypothesis use the pattern of lymph node involvement at time of diagnosis as evidence that sequential spread to contiguous node groups has occurred. Those who argue for a predisposition of certain node groups to tumor growth use the same data to suggest that certain lymph node areas have a predilection to Hodgkin's disease whenever the etiologic agent is present and active. Experimental data to prove or disprove these hypotheses are just not available.

Clinical Findings in Malignant Lymphoma

Various combinations of symptoms, physical findings, and disabilities may be produced by the malignant lymphomas, through pressure on, infiltration of, or replacement of organs, or by vascular or duct obstruction. The common findings in some of these organ systems are discussed in the following paragraphs.

Skeletal System

Bone involvement with lymphoma is common; and osteolytic, osteoblastic, or mixed lesions may be found in the skull, ribs, sternum, spine, and pelvis, as well as in the long bones. Other manifestations of bone disease include bone pain and high levels of serum alkaline phosphatase and serum calcium, particularly if the patient is immobilized. Severe hypercalcemia manifested by mental confusion, constipation, renal insufficiency, weakness, and lethargy may require treatment with mobilization, saline diuresis, corticosteroid administration (prednisone 30 mg daily orally), infusion of phosphates, or parenteral injection of the antibiotic mithyramycin (25 µg/kg).

Bone can be the primary site of involvement for reticulum cell sarcoma, particularly in young adults. If treated with large doses of radiotherapy, it is controllable for long periods of time and possibly curable. This prognosis contrasts with the prognosis for lymph node reticulum cell sarcoma, which is very poor. Skeletal x-rays and bone scans using radioactive polyphosphates are very helpful in determining the location of bony involvement. In advanced cases bone pain may be controlled with palliative x-ray therapy to the local lesions.

Bone pain at the site of lymphomatous involvement following the ingestion of ethanol is a symptom of Hodgkin's disease, but it is also occasionally encountered in other lymphomas and sarcoidosis.

Liver

In the advanced stages of malignant lymphoma liver involvement is quite common. The liver may be diffusely infiltrated or studded with lymphomatous nodules. The clinical picture sometimes resembles that of obstructive jaundice with elevated serum alkaline phosphatase levels. Enlarged lymph nodes obstructing the biliary tree as a cause of jaundice is unusual but has been described. The differential diagnosis between extrabiliary tract obstruction and intrahepatic infiltration is often difficult to make. Liver biopsy or percutaneous bile duct cannulation may be required. Other causes of jaundice in patients with lymphoma include viral hepatitis, hemolytic anemia, and drug sensitivity.

Determining whether the liver is involved at the time of diagnosis remains one of the most important problems in treatment of Hodgkin's disease with curative intent. Neither radiotherapy nor chemotherapy holds a promise of eradicating lymphoma when it involves the liver. For this reason it is important to exclude liver involvement by abdominal exploration or by laparoscope-directed percutaneous biopsies. Even with these procedures small foci of involvement may be missed. Pathologists sometimes have difficulty determining whether infiltrates are due to lymphoma or represent a nonspecific mononuclear cell reaction. Reed-Sternberg cells are often absent in otherwise typical infiltrates of Hodgkin's disease. Granulomas found in the liver of patients with Hodgkin's disease, if they are not associated with typical Hodgkin's disease tissue, are not considered lymphomatous infiltrates.

Spleen

Spleen involvement with lymphoma is common in the advanced stages of this disease. However, splenomegaly does not necessarily mean the spleen is involved with tumor tissue. This is particularly important in Hodgkin's disease, since palpable spleens may not contain tumor infiltrates. It appears that patients with Hodgkin's disease can develop splenomegaly as a result of nonspecific hypertrophy or congestion. Only one-half of enlarged and palpable spleens in patients with known Hodgkin's disease contain tumor when examined pathologically. Very large spleens, greater than 400 gm, uniformly do. Splenectomy is often performed at the time of laparotomy in order to determine whether Hodgkin's disease has truly involved the spleen. If it has, there is a 50 percent chance that the liver will also be involved.

Fever, or pleuritic pain secondary to splenic infarction, and heaviness or discomfort in the left upper quadrant are the symptoms associated with splenic enlargement. Patients have been described who have *primary splenic lymphosarcoma*. Such patients have enlarged spleens with pathologic infiltrates of lymphosarcoma, sometimes leading to hypersplenism. They may also have atypical, clefted lymphocytes or *lymphosarcoma cells* in their peripheral blood. These patients often have dramatic remissions following splenectomy, although many of them ultimately develop chronic lymphocytic leukemia.

Mediastinum and Retroperitoneum

Anterior mediastinal and abdominal retroperitoneal lymph nodes are often involved with malignant lymphoma, and further infiltration into adjacent parenchymal organs is also common. Mediastinal lymphadenopathy is detected by routine chest x-rays or with tomograms. Retroperitoneal involvement is demonstrated by the use of a lymphangiogram, intravenous cavagram showing indentation of the vena cava by lymph nodes, intravenous pyelogram showing ureters splayed laterally by enlarged lymph nodes, radioactive gallium scan, or by abdominal ultrasound examination. Pain, evidence of lymphatic or venous obstruction, ureteral obstruction, or vena cava obstruction are common complications of lymphadenopathy in these two areas. If inguinal adenopathy is present, the retroperitoneal lymph nodes are probably also infiltrated. The nodular sclerosis variant of Hodgkin's disease is often associated with mediastinal and retroperitoneal lymph node involvement.

Blood

Many abnormalities in the cellular and liquid components of blood have been described: neutrophilic leukocytosis, eosinophilia, lymphocytopenia (usually carries a poor prognosis in Hodgkin's disease), anemia due to hypersplenism, Coombs' test-positive hemolytic anemia, and thrombocytopenia due to hypersplenism or bone marrow invasion. Autoimmune hemolytic anemia is particularly common in the lymphosarcomas. Bone marrow invasion is seen frequently early in the course of the lymphosarcomas but also occurs in advanced stages of Hodgkin's disease. Transition to chronic lymphocytic leukemia is rare in Hodgkin's disease but common in the lymphosarcomas. Elevated serum alkaline phosphatase levels, hypoalbuminemia, hypoferremia, and low plasma zinc and elevated serum copper levels have all been reported in Hodgkin's disease.

The cytopenias seen in the blood of patients with lymphoma may be due to bone marrow infiltration, hypersplenism, immune phenomena including autoimmune hemolytic anemia and thrombocytopenia, drug or radiation therapy, blood loss, and shortened red blood cell survival secondary to reticuloendothelial hyperplasia (anemia of chronic disease).

Bone Marrow

Because of spotty involvement and the difficulty of finding and recognizing Reed-Sternberg cells, it is often hard to diagnose Hodgkin's disease in bone marrow specimens. Diffuse fibrosis, marrow aplasia, and megakaryocytosis are nonspecific findings in patients with Hodgkin's disease. Less than 10 percent of patients with early stage Hodgkin's disease have definite marrow involvement with lymphoma, whereas as mentioned previously, over 50 percent of patients with non-Hodgkin's lymphoma have infiltrates in their bone marrow at the time of diagnosis.

Lung

The mediastinum, lung parenchyma, or pleura may be involved with malignant lymphoma. Occasionally cavitation and abscess formation are manifestations of pulmonary Hodgkin's disease. Superinfection with bacteria, fungi, toxoplasma, *Pneumocystis carinii,* or cytomegalic inclusion disease may occur, particularly in advanced cases being treated with chemotherapy or radiotherapy. In some cases needle biopsy or open biopsy of the lung is required to distinguish between lymphomatous involvement of the lung and secondary infection. Pleural effusions are common in patients with lymphosarcoma and may be due to direct invasion of the pleura or secondary to venous and lymphatic obstruction in the mediastinum. Unless cytologic examination demonstrates lymphomatous involvement in the pleural stage, x-irradiation to the mediastinum is indicated to relieve the pleural effusion. Similar benefit is often achieved with systemic chemotherapy.

Central Nervous System

Although involvement of the brain is uncommon in the malignant lymphomas, spinal cord involvement is not. An epidural mass may be the first manifestation of a malignant lymphoma, usually as a result of extension from the mediastinal or retroperitoneal lymph nodes. Back pain, bowel and bladder dysfunction, and other signs of cord compression are common. Usually myelography followed by surgical decompression is performed as an emergency procedure. Follow-up treatment consists of radiotherapy to the spinal cord and systemic chemotherapy. There is controversy over whether spinal cord compression should be treated with radiotherapy alone without surgical decompression. Surgical decompression has an advantage in that tissue can be obtained for definitive diagnosis.

Lymphomas are associated with two types of encephalopathy not due to direct infiltration with lymphoma. Dementia, paralyses, and other neurologic findings characterize *progressive multifocal leukoencephalopathy.* Demyelinization is seen pathologically, and a papavovirus etiology is suspected. In *subacute cerebellar degeneration,* the second type, cerebellar symptoms are prominent, along with demyelination of fibers in the cerebellum. No specific treatment is available for either of these encephalopathies.

Skin

Both lymphomatous infiltration of skin and nonlymphomatous lesions are associated with Hodgkin's disease and non-Hodgkin's lymphoma. The lymphomatous skin infiltrates appear as red or purple, well demarcated, nontender, palpable lesions. The nonspecific skin reactions include bullae, eczema, papules, hyperpigmentation, and alopecia. Both types of skin lesions often respond to systemic chemotherapy.

In many patients with Hodgkin's disease and a few with non-Hodgkin's lymphoma, pruritis without skin lesions is a troublesome symptom. It responds to antihistamines, phenothiazines, and systemic chemotherapy.

Localized herpes zoster, which can disseminate to involve large parts of the body, is commonly associated with malignant lymphomas. No known effective treatment is available for localized or generalized herpes zoster, although experimental treatment with hyperimmune globulin and transfer factor have been encouraging. The use of adenosine arabinoside for generalized herpes zoster may prove effective.

Primary skin involvement (mycosis fungoides) is described under Primary Lymphoma of the Skin.

Gastrointestinal Tract

Besides involving the liver, it is not unusual for malignant lymphomas to involve the stomach, small intestine, and occasionally the colon. Obstruction of or bleeding into the gastrointestinal tract are common presenting manifestations. A malabsorption syndrome with steatorrhea has also been described. The diagnosis can be made by abdominal exploration or peroral small intestinal biopsy. Localized, primary, gastrointestinal lymphoma may respond completely to large doses of radiotherapy delivered to the abdomen, particularly in patients who have had the primary site of disease removed surgically. Unfortunately, many patients relapse with systemic disease and require treatment with chemotherapy.

Genitourinary Tract

The kidneys may be directly invaded or infiltrated by lymphomatous tumor masses and the ureters obstructed by abdominal or retroperitoneal lymph nodes. Urinary tract disease usually requires radiotherapy for localized disease or chemotherapy for extensive disease. Uric acid nephropathy and uric acid stones can contribute to renal insufficiency. Occasionally the nephrotic syndrome with or without amyloidosis is a complication.

Fever

Fevers due to late-stage malignant lymphoma are common. *Pel-Ebstein fever,* a rare manifestation of Hodgkin's disease, is a fever spike that is cyclic and recurs every few days or weeks. In patients with lymphomas it is often difficult to decide whether the fever is due to lymphoma or to infectious agents. Treatment with the anti-inflammatory drug Indocin is said to suppress fever due to Hodgkin's disease but not that due to infectious agents. This finding has not been confirmed.

Diseases Related to the Malignant Lymphomas

Certain benign diseases have a lymph node pathologic picture resembling that seen in malignant lymphomas. *Brill-Symmers disease* is a benign condition, closely related to atypical lymph node hyperplasia, that is seen in any chronic infection or inflammatory condition such as severe rheumatoid arthritis. Most pathologists have no difficulty in distinguishing the histologic features of lymphocytic lymphosarcoma from the hyperplastic and inflammatory changes seen in Brill-Symmers disease.

The drug Dilantin (diphenylhydantoin) is also associated with lymph node enlargement, in some cases to a moderate or severe degree. In many Dilantin-caused cases the lymph node shows only reactive hyperplasia with a cellular reaction consistent with chronic inflammatory disease. Abnormal reticulum cells and occasionally cells resembling Reed-Sternberg cells may be seen. These cases are usually recognized by the pathologist and cause no problem to the patient, since the lymph node will shrink upon cessation of Dilantin therapy. On the other hand some of these patients show histopathologic features that meet the criteria for malignant lymphoma. In some cases cessation of the drug results in reversion of the histologic picture to normal, while in others the patients go on to die with lymph nodes that all agree are lymphomatous. In a few cases the histologic findings revert to normal after the drug is stopped, but months or years later the patient develops malignant lymphoma. Although lymph node hyperplasia associated with Dilantin is not uncommon, it must be emphasized that patients with histologic features of frank malignant lymphoma and those who go on to develop malignant lymphoma are extremely rare. Some authors argue that the cases in which true malignant lymphoma occurs in association with Dilantan therapy are coincidental.

One common problem is the interpretation of the histopathologic appearance of lymph nodes that lie in drainage areas of skin disease. *Dermatopathic lymph nodes* enlarged secondary to active acne or other dermatologic conditions may be difficult to distinguish from lymphoma. This lymphadenopathy is due to severe lymph node hyperplasia and is not in any way malignant.

An unusual form of malignant lymphoma is *giant follicular lymphoma*. This disease usually presents with enlarging retroperitoneal lymph nodes. The pathologist diagnoses nodular lymphocytic lymphosarcoma, and the patient is treated with radiotherapy or chemotherapy. Often, after a long period of remission, the patient relapses with a highly malignant reticulum cell sarcoma. Large doses of radiotherapy are frequently used in an attempt to eradicate the disease and prevent this usually fatal transformation into reticulum cell sarcoma (diffuse histiocytic).

Burkitt's lymphoma is a malignant disease that is seen primarily in children in central Africa. Usually the jaw, abdominal organs, bone marrow, or other extranodal sites are the first areas to be involved. Splenomegaly and lymphadenopathy are not unusual. The pathologic picture is characterized by diffuse infiltration with lymphoblasts and is characterized by a starry sky appearance due to the presence of reticulum cells in lacunae. The epidemiology of the lymphoma suggests that it is caused by a virus (Epstein-Barr) carried by an insect vector, such as a mosquito. The EB virus genome has been found by DNA hybridization studies to remain in the cell as part of the cell's genome. EB virus–specific capsid and membrane antibodies are also present in the cells of Burkitt's lymphoma. In its early stages the disease can often be cured with radiotherapy or chemotherapy.

Hairy cell leukemia or *leukemic reticuloendotheliosis* is a rare form of chronic leukemia sometimes associated with a clinical picture of malignant lymphoma. The patients often present with pancytopenia, lymphadenopathy, and splenomegaly. The peripheral blood and bone marrow are massively involved with a leukemic process. The leukemic cells are thought by some to be monocytes and by others lymphocytes. They have hair-like projections that make them different from the usual lymphocytic leukemia cell. The disease often progresses slowly, and corticosteroid treatment, splenectomy, or chemotherapy is often temporarily effective.

Another disease with features of lymphoma is called *histiocytic medullary reticulosis* or *malignant histiocytosis.* Lymph node enlargement and hepatosplenomegaly are quite prominent. The neoplastic cells appear to be reticulum cells that are in the process of phagocytizing red cells (erythrophagocytosis), nuclear debris, lipids, hemosiderin, platelets, and even white cells. It is this histologic feature that sets the disease apart from other lymphomas. The neoplastic reticulum cells are localized within the sinuses of lymph nodes, splenic red pulp, liver, and in the bone marrow, and massively infiltrate the sinusoids of the spleen.

Primary Lymphoma of the Skin

There are two main types of lymphomatous involvement of the skin. In one type the skin is infiltrated by malignant reticulum cells or lymphocytes in a manner similar to the infiltration of other organs by malignant lymphomas. Reticulum cell sarcoma appears to be the most frequently associated with direct infiltration of skin by the malignant cells. The infiltrate is often reddish in color, raised, and nontender, and the diagnosis is confirmed by simple biopsy. The disease responds to treatment with radiotherapy or with systemic chemotherapy.

A more unusual form of involvement is called *mycosis fungoides.* This skin disease has three stages. In the initial stage, *erythroderma,* there may be nonspecific skin eruptions including an overall bright red appearance. Over a period of months or years irregular thickening of the skin, the *plague stage,* develops. At this time characteristic histologic changes are seen in the skin which allow a definitive diagnosis. Finally the patient develops the *tumor stage,* characterized by nodular infiltrates that may ulcerate. Lymph node enlargement, hepatosplenomegaly, and a clinical picture of malignant lymphoma are associated with this stage. Treatment with radiotherapy, chemotherapy, or both is used, but most often the patient dies from complications of the disease.

Sézary's syndrome is a condition characterized by mycosis fungoides-like skin involvement and abnormal circulating lymphocytes that resemble atypical lymphs or lymphosarcoma cells. The abnormal mononuclear cells stain positive with periodic acid–Schiff's (PAS) reagent. In both mycosis fungoides and Sézary's syndrome skin biopsies show focal collections of abnormal mono-nuclear cells in the epidermis, called *Pautrier abscesses*. As with mycosis fungoides, Sézary's syndrome is treated with radio-therapy, chemotherapy, or both.

Approach to the Patient with Malignant Lymphoma

The management of patients with malignant lymphoma is ex-tremely complex. Although it is necessary to individualize the evaluation of each patient, a general approach can be outlined.

The first problem is to establish a pathologic diagnosis. Most often these patients present with enlarged lymph nodes. Three factors usually determine when such enlarged nodes should be biopsied. The physical findings are of primary importance. Lym-phomatous nodes are usually rubbery in consistency, matted together, large, and nontender. On the other hand, lymph nodes due to viral infections, streptococcal infections of the throat, bladder infections, or skin rashes (dermatopathic lymphadeno-pathy) are often tender, discreet, soft, or firm, but not rubbery or hard, and do not usually reach the size of those seen in malignant lymphoma. A second factor that may delay biopsy is the presence of a ready explanation for lymphadenopathy. This may be as sim-ple as a smallpox vaccine with regional lymphadenopathy or as vague as a mild sore throat a few weeks prior to the recognition of lymphadenopathy. If the possibility exists that the lymph nodes are due to a nonmalignant cause, a 4- to 6-week wait before biopsy is reasonable. Finally, if other historical features or physi-cal findings are present that suggest lymphoma, then biopsy should not be delayed.

It is best to biopsy cervical rather than inguinal lymph nodes. Inguinal lymph nodes tend to have areas of hyperplasia secondary to chronic infections or inflammatory disorders of the lower limbs. It may be difficult for the pathologist to diagnose malig-nant lymphoma in the face of lymph node hyperplasia.

After one or more lymph node biopsies have established the diag-nosis of malignant lymphoma, then documentation of the extent of disease spread, i.e., clinical staging, must be undertaken. The data required for staging have been outlined (Clinical and Patho-logic Staging of Malignant Lymphomas). In Hodgkin's disease it is recommended that a lymphangiogram or gallium scan be used to help plan laparotomy, and in non-Hodgkin's lymphoma an early bone marrow biopsy is recommended. Patients with non-Hodgkin's lymphoma and normal marrow need to be staged with abdominal exploration only if their disease is truly localized (Stage I or II) and of the mature, small cell type. Lymphoblastic lymphosarcoma and reticulum cell sarcoma are unlikely to be cured by radiotherapy and therefore are treated with systemic

Approach to patient with Hodgkin's disease and non-Hodgkin's lymphoma

I. History
  A. Symptoms of compression or obstruction by large lymph nodes
  B. Symptoms of spinal cord involvement
  C. Symptoms suggesting involvement by extralymphatic lymphoma (nasopharynx, bone, gastrointestinal tract)
  D. Systemic symptoms: weight loss, night sweats, fever, pruritis
II. Examination
  A. Abdominal masses
  B. Lymph node enlargement
  C. Signs of extralymphatic involvement
  D. Skin infiltration, herpes zoster, bleeding manifestations
  E. Signs of liver disease
  F. Sign of obstruction or pressure by lymph nodes (mediastinal, abdominal, axillary, pelvic or femoral)
  G. Signs of spinal cord involvement
  H. Splenomegaly and hepatomegaly
III. Laboratory Data
  A. Blood counts
  B. Bone marrow examination, including biopsy
  C. Bone scan
  D. Chest x-ray (lung tomograms, if indicated)
  E. Creatinine, serum
  F. Erythrocyte sedimentation rate
  G. Liver function tests
  H. Lymph node biopsy
  I. Peripheral blood smear
  J. Protein electrophoresis, uric acid, Coombs' test
  K. Skeletal x-rays including skull and long bones
IV. Further Procedures to be Considered in Some Patients
  A. Abdominal exploration with splenectomy, biopsy of abdominal lymph nodes, liver biopsy and iliac crest biopsy
  B. Gallium 57 scan for lymphadenopathy
  C. Inferior vena cavagram
  D. Intravenous pyelogram
  E. Liver scan
  F. Lymphangiography
  G. Total body scan (computerized)

chemotherapy without pathologic staging. The rare patient with Stage I or II (PS) lymphocytic lymphosarcoma is usually treated with combined radiotherapy and chemotherapy.

In the case of Hodgkin's disease, patients with clinical stages IA, IB, IIA, IIB, and IIIA can be treated in hopes of obtaining a long remission or cure with radical radiotherapy and should undergo pathologic staging. Those who are in stage IIIB or IV should be treated with systemic chemotherapy, and perhaps radiotherapy to any large masses of tumor tissue, but do not require abdominal exploration. More will be said about the therapy of these diseases, but it is necessary to know this much in order to proceed rationally with the evaluation of these patients.

Patients who have not been excluded from radical radiotherapy for cure by clinical staging (including bone marrow examination) should then be considered for abdominal exploration. The abdominal exploration may be done by a formal laparotomy or by laparoscopy and laparoscope-directed percutaneous biopsies. Most importantly, biopsies of the liver should be obtained to look for lymphomatous involvement, since if such involvement is found, the patient is not curable by radical radiotherapy.

Splenectomy may be performed at laparotomy in order to demonstrate lymphoma in this organ, thereby advancing the pathologic stage, and also to give some indication of the likelihood of liver involvement. Peripheral blood counts may be less depressed by radiotherapy or chemotherapy, if the spleen has been removed. The radiation field for an enlarged spleen is large and entails possible destruction of tissue in the lower lobe of the left lung and in the upper pole of the left kidney. This can be avoided by removal of the enlarged spleen, since the radiation field for treatment of the splenic pedicle left behind after splenectomy is equivalent to that for treatment of a normal-sized spleen. However, in children and young adults under the age of 30, an increased incidence of blood-borne sepsis has been found after splenectomy.

Abdominal exploration can discover lymph node involvement in unusual areas such as the porta hepatis. This allows radiation to be delivered in curative doses to areas that would not routinely be irradiated during radical radiotherapy. Furthermore, exploration of the retroperitoneal area, if negative, may downgrade the patient's pathologic stage as compared to his clinical stage. It must be remembered, however, that it is difficult to explore all the retroperitoneal lymph node–bearing regions. Although the lymphangiogram helps in locating suspicious lymph nodes for biopsy, many lymph nodes are buried beneath the duodenum and stomach and cannot be adequately palpated, visualized, or biopsied.

Therefore a negative retroperitoneal exploration does not mean that the patient does not have small foci of disease in this area.

A large section of iliac bone marrow should be obtained at laparotomy. This is particularly important in the case of patients with clinically advanced Hodgkin's disease or the occasional patient with non-Hodgkin's lymphoma who is undergoing abdominal exploration. This large sample of bone marrow will sometimes show that the patient has pathologic stage IV disease, even though a previous percutaneous marrow biopsy was negative. Finally, during laparotomy the ovaries can be placed behind the uterus or laterally outside the usual radiation field in order to preserve ovarian function in young females.

The mode of radiotherapy used determines to some extent whether Hodgkin's disease patients with Stage IA disease, particularly if they have lymphocytic predominance or nodular sclerosis subtypes, should undergo laparotomy. If total nodal irradiation, that is, delivery of tumoricidal doses of radiotherapy to all lymph node–bearing regions from the occipital to the inguinal, is employed, laparotomy yields few benefits to patients with clinical stage IA and possibly IIA disease with prognostically good histologic types. In these patients it may be possible to eliminate the need for laparotomy.

After clinical and pathologic staging, Hodgkin's disease patients with Stages IA, IB, IIA, IIB, or IIIA should be treated with radical radiotherapy with curative intent. Patients with pathologic Stage IIIB or IV disease should be treated with combination chemotherapy. Some experts recommend the use of combined radiotherapy and chemotherapy in Stages IB, IIB, and IIIA. This carries some risk of irreversible bone marrow depression, with associated infection and bleeding, and perhaps risk of developing second malignant diseases such as leukemias and sarcomas. There is evidence that combined radiotherapy and chemotherapy improves the duration of complete remission, but it is also clear that in comparison to sequential use of radiotherapy and chemotherapy there is no significant change in overall survival. Thus the combined approach may delay the appearance of clinical relapse but not improve the survival of the patient.

Greater attention must be given to the psychological implications of these diagnostic and therapeutic procedures in patients with Hodgkin's disease and lymphosarcoma. Patients with these diseases are often sophisticated and should be told everything about their disease and much about the prognosis. Only by being frank and describing the reasons for and side effects of these various procedures can one obtain complete cooperation from patients and their families. In general, drug therapy for depression or anxiety has not been particularly helpful, but good, close interactions with patients and families has helped a great deal.

Therapy of Malignant Lymphomas

Radiotherapy

Approximately 4,000 rads must be delivered to a lymph node region over a period of 3½ to 4 weeks to ensure eradication of Hodgkin's disease. This treatment requires the use of megavoltage machines, such as the linear accelerator, and the expertise of a well-trained radiotherapist. Lymph node areas must be blocked out properly to avoid excessive exposure to areas such as liver, spinal cord, lung, and bone marrow. Experience has shown that, if these techniques are used correctly, surgical extirpation has no place in the therapy of malignant lymphomas.

Initial good results were obtained by treating Stages IA and IIA Hodgkin's disease with high dose, megavoltage radiotherapy. It was then decided that, if radiotherapy were extended to adjacent or contiguous lymph node groups, even if those were not involved histologically or clinically, all patients in the early stages of Hodgkin's disease could be cured. This *extended field irradiation* and a technique called *total nodal irradiation (TNI)* are now used in most radiotherapy centers. With TNI, all lymph node–bearing areas from the occipital to the inguinal area receive tumoricidal doses of radiotherapy.

TNI was developed as a result of finding that many patients with extended field irradiation, particularly those with prognostically poor histologic types, were relapsing with retroperitoneal lymphoma. Comparison of extended field irradiation with total nodal irradiation showed that retroperitoneal relapses could be significantly decreased. As one might guess, a patient with stage III Hodgkin's disease involving the retroperitoneum, if treated by radiotherapists using extended field irradiation, will receive essentially the same radiation therapy as a patient treated by others with total nodal irradiation. It is only in patients with very limited disease, who have been carefully examined with procedures such as laparotomy, that extended field irradiation may reduce the amount of radiotherapy a patient receives. Because many radiotherapists consider the retroperitoneal area to be contiguous with the neck (cervical) region by way of the thoracic duct, the radiotherapy fields chosen by a proponent of extended field irradiation may again be similar (except for eliminating pelvic node irradiation) to those used by a total nodal irradiation proponent when treating a patient with cervical node Hodgkin's disease.

Complications of radical radiation therapy include bone marrow depression, spinal cord damage — for example, numbness and tingling in the fingers and toes upon flexion of the neck (Lhermitte's sign) — fatal radiation pneumonitis or pericarditis, radiation-induced leukemia and other malignancies, and hypothyroidism.

Results of radical radiotherapy of Hodgkin's disease are difficult to evaluate, because some are reported after 2-year followup and others after 5. Some centers use extended field irradiation and others total nodal irradiation. The aggressiveness with which staging was pursued is another important variable, as is the histologic type treated: for example, excellent results are reported from centers where the nodular sclerosis type of Hodgkin's disease is prevalent.

Stage IA and IIA patients treated with radical radiotherapy with curative intent should expect 70- to 80-percent recurrence-free (*no* *e*vidence of *d*isease or NED) survival at 5 years. A 5-year relapse-free survival of 50 percent should be expected for Stages IB and IIB. Although Stage IIIB patients do poorly after total nodal irradiation (17 percent 5-year NED survival), 40 to 50 percent of patients with Stage IIIA disease will survive free of disease. Radical radiotherapy is not recommended as treatment for Stage IIIB or IV disease.

Palliative radiotherapy — radiation given for relief of symptoms but without curative intent — is useful in all lymphomas for the treatment of obstructing or painful lesions, or for large masses that are causing symptoms. This palliative use of radiation must be distinguished from radical radiotherapy given to many involved and uninvolved lymph node groups in an attempt to eradicate Hodgkin's disease from the patient's body.

In non-Hodgkin's lymphomas, total nodal irradiation for cure has been performed on only a small number of patients. Although the small number of reported cases showed good results, our own experience suggests that in most cases the disease reaches the liver, gastrointestinal tract, or bone marrow early in its course and is therefore incurable. For this reason we recommend total nodal irradiation for cure only in the more benign histologic types and only in pathologic Stages IA or possibly IIA. Certainly in lympho-blastic lymphosarcomas and reticulum cell sarcomas, unless the latter are of extranodal origin, there is no place for aggressive radiotherapy. Even in the more prognostically favorable nodular lymphomas there is little evidence that survival is improved by total nodal irradiation.

Another radiotherapeutic technique, called total *body* irradiation, during which the patient's total body receives 100 to 150 rads, is used for the palliation of non-Hodgkin's lymphomas. It must be distinguished from total *nodal* irradiation, during which certain lymph node groups receive many thousands of rads of radio-therapy with curative intent. Patients with nodular, non-Hodgkin's lymphomas, particularly if their bone marrow is not extensively involved, may have long periods of remission without the need for chemotherapy. Repeated courses of total body irradiation or chemotherapy can be used following initial treatment.

Chemotherapy Given our present knowledge, it appears that the use of multiple drug or combination chemotherapy is the treatment of choice for the palliation, and in some cases the cure, of advanced stages of Hodgkin's disease. Combination chemotherapy also plays a large role in the palliation of non-Hodgkin's lymphoma. Before describing the two most commonly used protocols, one for the treatment of Hodgkin's disease and the other for the treatment of non-Hodgkin's lymphoma, we shall review the clinically important characteristics of the antilymphoma drugs. Some of these drugs are also discussed in Chapter 9. Appropriate references, package inserts and reports of toxic reactions must be consulted before any attempt is made to use these extremely potent drugs.

Vinca Alkaloids. Vinblastine (Velban) is an alkaloid of the peri-winkle plant closely related to vincristine (Chapter 9). In fact these two drugs differ only in one side chain of the parent mole-cule. Vinblastine is used primarily in the treatment of Hodgkin's disease, and vincristine in all types of malignant lymphoma. As an inhibitor of mitosis, vinblastine has been used as a single drug in the treatment of Hodgkin's disease that has become resistant to alkylating agents. With the introduction of combination chemo-therapy, however, its use has been limited. Approximately 90 per-cent of patients with Hodgkin's disease will respond to vinblastine, but remissions usually last about 12 months and are not complete. Vinblastine has sometimes been substituted for vincristine in combination chemotherapy regimens for Hodgkin's disease, but its propensity to cause leukopenia has limited its usefulness. Abdominal pain, neuritic pain, and intestinal ileus occasionally develop with vinblastine, but usually not the severe neurotoxicity seen with vincristine. Precautions must be taken to prevent extra-vasation into tissues at the time of intravenous injections, as this will cause tissue necrosis. An oral preparation is not available.

Procarbazine. Procarbazine (Natulan, methylhydrazine) is used for treating both Hodgkin's disease and non-Hodgkin's lymphoma. Its mode of action is not understood. It is cytotoxic, perhaps because it undergoes auto-oxidation with generation of hydrogen perox-ide. The hydrogen peroxide interacts with DNA, causing an effect similar to that of ionizing radiation. Many other procarbazine-induced derangements of biochemical functions in normal and neoplastic cells have also been described. Although the drug was originally used for treatment of advanced Hodgkin's disease resistant to alkylating agents and vinca alkaloids, it is now used principally as part of combination chemotherapy. Approximately 50 percent of malignant lymphomas give some response, either objectively or subjectively, when treated with procarbazine alone. The duration of the response is usually short, however, less than three months.

The toxic effects of procarbazine are severe and include bone marrow depression, nausea and vomiting, dermatitis, and alopecia. An unusual central nervous system side effect causes drowsiness and potentiation of barbiturates and alcohol. An Antabuse-like reaction to alcohol, with nausea and vomiting, also occurs. Since procarbazine is a weak monoamine oxidase inhibitor, cheese and bananas, which have a high tyramine content, should be avoided, as well as tricyclic antidepressant drugs. Procarbazine can produce Heinz body type hemolytic anemia, so the drug dose should be reduced in patients with impaired hepatic or renal function. When bone marrow suppression occurs, the drug dose should be adjusted downward.

Adriamycin (doxorubicin). Adriamycin is an antibiotic isolated from soil fungi. It differs from daunomycin by only a single hydroxyl group, inhibits DNA synthesis similarly to daunomycin, and is therefore active during S phase. At the cellular level, adriamycin binds to DNA by intercalation between base pairs and inhibits RNA synthesis by template disordering and steric obstruction. Adriamycin has been used alone or in combination with other drugs for treatment of both Hodgkin's disease and non-Hodgkin's lymphoma. The response rate when it is used alone is less than 50 percent. It is employed primarily for patients refractory to other drugs and as part of combination chemotherapy programs. This drug is used for induction of remission and seldom as part of maintenance therapy.

Its toxicity is similar to that of daunomycin, i.e., mouth ulcers, bone marrow depression, alopecia, nausea, and vomiting. Adriamycin is irritating to tissues, if extravasation occurs during intravenous infusion. Cardiotoxicity, manifested by severe and sometimes irreversible congestive heart failure, has been a major limiting factor, particularly in older patients. Most cases of cardiac toxicity occur at a cumulative dose greater than 550 mg per square meter of body surface area, but a few patients may exhibit such toxicity at lower doses.

Nitrosoureas. The nitrosoureas are a unique group of antineoplastic drugs obtained from chemical synthesis. 1,3-bis-(2-chloroethyl)-1-nitrosourea (BCNU) was the first compound investigated. BCNU is available only for intravenous injections. Two other nitrosoureas, CCNU and methyl CCNU, have also been prepared and are available in capsules for oral administration. There is no generally accepted protocol for administering these drugs. They are lipid-soluble and therefore find their way into the central nervous system. The most consistent toxicities are those of delayed bone marrow suppression, leading, usually 4 to 6 weeks after administration, to severe thrombocytopenia. Anemia and leukopenia may also occur. Gastrointestinal toxicity, manifested by severe nausea and vomiting after administration of the drug, is common. This is particularly true in the case of CCNU and methyl CCNU. The nitrosoureas are cytotoxic and have alkylating capability, but their mechanism of action in tissues is unknown. Currently these drugs are used in the treatment of Hodgkin's disease either after failure of combination chemotherapy or for maintenance therapy after induction with combination chemotherapy.

Bleomycin (Blenoxane). Bleomycin is an antibiotic obtained from a strain of soil fungi. A test dose should be given before a full dose is administered, since anaphylactic reactions to the drug have been reported. Its mechanism of action is unknown. Pulmonary infiltrates, decreased vital capacity, and potentially fatal pulmonary insufficiency may occur after large cumulative doses (300 mg or units) or in some cases even after much smaller doses. Side effects also include fever, gastrointestinal upset, mucosal ulcerations, and skin rash, particularly on the hands and elbows, characterized by erythemia or hyperkeratosis.

The drug is particularly effective against Hodgkin's disease and to a lesser extent against other lymphomas. Because it has little bone marrow toxicity, it is prescribed for patients who have previously received marrow suppressive drugs. Again because of its lack of toxicity to bone marrow it is combined into multiple drug protocols.

Combination Chemotherapy of Hodgkin's Disease

The standard chemotherapy for Hodgkin's disease is now a combination of four drugs, nitrogen mustard (or sometimes cyclophosphamide), procarbazine, vincristine, and an adrenal corticosteroid such as prednisone. This has been termed MOPP therapy (M for Mustargen, O for Oncovin or vincristine, P for procarbazine, P for prednisone). Six or more cycles, each of 28 days' duration, are given as initial treatment. On days 1 and 7 of each of these cycles nitrogen mustard is given intravenously along with vincristine. On days 1 through 14 the patient receives procarbazine and — either in cycles one and four only or else in all cycles — prednisone orally. On days 15 through 28 no therapy is given. With this protocol approximately 70 percent of patients go into complete remission, and 50 percent of these remain continuously free of disease for at least two years. There is debate over whether a patient who has gone into complete remission should be given maintenance therapy, for example, three cycles per year of MOPP therapy for two years. Although the available data are in conflict, maintenance therapy following induction of remission in Hodgkin's disease is often recommended. A similar MOPP program has been used for treatment of patients with non-Hodgkin's lymphoma.

Combination Chemotherapy of non-Hodgkin's Lymphoma

Like the MOPP therapy used to treat Hodgkin's disease, combination chemotherapy is now considered standard therapy for non-Hodgkin's lymphoma. Several protocols exist for giving cyclophosphamide, vincristine, and prednisone (*C*ytoxan, *On*covin, *p*rednisone, or COP). Some use a reduced dose of cyclophosphamide, if the patient has been previously treated with radiotherapy or chemotherapy, or if he or she has significant bone marrow involvement. In one of the protocols cyclophosphamide and vincristine are administered intravenously every two weeks. A five-day course of oral prednisone follows the intravenous injections. These cycles are continued, sometimes at a reduced dosage if bone marrow suppression intervenes, until the patient relapses. The addition of bleomycin or adriamycin or both to each of the cycles has also been tried in hopes of increasing the number of remissions and perhaps prolonging the duration of these remissions. The remission rate for COP therapy is approximately 60 percent, but most remissions are not complete, and evidence of the disease often is found on physical examination or on examination of the peripheral blood or bone marrow. However, the patients are able to function normally or almost normally. These remissions last for months in the case of lymphosarcoma and even years, if the lymphoma is nodular.

For patients who cannot tolerate combination chemotherapy because of severe bone marrow suppression from previous therapy, advanced age, or concurrent diseases, single- or double-drug chemotherapy may be considered. When the patient relapses, another single agent is prescribed. In sequential, single-drug therapy, an alkylating agent such as cyclophosphamide is used first, and then either vincristine or prednisone is substituted for it after relapse. Prednisone is particularly useful if the patient has bone marrow suppression, hypersplenism, or one of the autoimmune phenomena that causes thrombocytopenia or anemia. After cyclophosphamide, vincristine, and prednisone have been given, drugs such as the nitrosoureas, procarbazine, adriamycin, or even bleomycin can be considered. These last give partial short-duration remissions, particularly in the case of reticulum cell sarcoma. Recent data suggest that nodular lymphosarcomas with a prognostically good histologic picture respond as well to a single alkalyzing agent as to COP chemotherapy.

INFECTIOUS MONONU- CLEOSIS

Infectious mononucleosis is a transmissible, self-limited disease that has some histologic and virologic similarities to malignant lymphoma. Because of the blood abnormalities and prominent lymphadenopathy associated with this disease, many cases are referred to hematologists.

The etiology of infectious mononucleosis has been shown by virus isolation and antibody studies to be the Epstein-Barr, or EB, virus. It is interesting that the EB virus has also been associated with Burkitt's lymphoma, nasopharyngeal carcinoma, chronic lymphocytic leukemia, certain poorly differentiated lymphomas, Hodgkin's sarcoma, and sarcoidosis. It is possible that abnormal lymph nodes involved with inflammatory or malignant diseases serve as a site of proliferation for a potentially latent virus such as EB. The virus infects B lymphocytes, and this results in the production of atypical lymphocytes that have been typed as T cells.

Infectious mononucleosis usually occurs between ages 15 and 25. It is characterized by a remittent fever, particularly severe in the afternoon and evening, usually accompanied by drenching night sweats. Headache, dysphagia, pharyngitis, jaundice, polyneuritis, and central nervous system abnormalities may all be part of the syndrome. Particularly prominent physical findings are diffuse lymphadenopathy, pharyngitis, and splenomegaly. A petechial rash on the palate and puffiness about the eyes are other early manifestations. Evidence of hepatitis and jaundice and elevated transaminase and alkaline phosphatase levels are commonly found. The liver disease rarely progresses to hepatic failure, and healing in almost all cases is complete. Complications include acute meningitis or encephalitis, thrombocytopenia, and hemolytic anemia associated with an anti-i antibody and positive results to the direct Coombs' test.

Lymph node enlargement is a prominent feature, so sometimes a lymph node biopsy is performed. This should not happen if this disease is suspected, as serologic tests can confirm the diagnosis. The histopathologic features include subtotal destruction of lymph node architecture with lymphocyte proliferation. There may be infiltration of sinuses, capsule, and perinodal tissues. Occasionally a very immature lymphocyte or reticulum cell simu- lates the appearance of a Reed-Sternberg cell. The pathologic picture is very similar to that of postvaccinial nodes draining the site of vaccination. In most cases an alert pathologist can distinguish the nodal appearance from that of Hodgkin's disease. The peripheral blood findings are striking; there is an absolute lymphocytosis (greater than 4.5×10^9 per liter) and many (greater than 1.0×10^9 per liter) of the lymphocytes are atypical in appearance.

Some atypical lymphocytes have cytoplasm with the usual ground-glass blue color but abnormally vacuolated (Plate 49). Other lymphocytes have nuclei lobulated like those of a monocyte (Plate 50). Finally, some appear to be lymphoblastoid like those seen after transformation with phytohemagglutinin (Plate 51). These cells can usually be differentiated from lymphosarcoma cells by their comparatively larger amount of cytoplasm and the presence of other atypical lymphocytes with vacuolization and monocytoid nuclei. Red cells appear to indent the cytoplasm of the atypical lymphocytes. Such *indentocytes* are seen not only in infectious mononucleosis but also in infectious hepatitis and many other viral infections. The atypical lymph appears in many respects to be a transformed lymphocyte, and therefore it is not surprising to find it in viral infections, drug hypersensitivity reactions (PAS, Dilantin, Mesantoin), and graft-versus-host reactions.

Many immunologic changes can be detected in the serum of patients with infectious mononucleosis. Antibody to EB virus is absent in serum obtained before infectious mononucleosis develops, is consistently present in rising titer during the disease, and then persists for years. Therefore EB virus titers are useful for diagnosis only in rare cases when a distinct rise is detected in specimens obtained early in the illness.

A macroglobulin called the *heterophil antibody* appears in the serum. It agglutinates sheep red cells and can be absorbed completely from the serum by preincubation with beef red cells but not with guinea pig kidney tissue. This is the basis of the absorbed *heterophil test,* which, when performed with tube dilutions, used to be standard for the diagnosis of infectious mononucleosis. The heterophil antibody test usually becomes positive within three weeks after the initial symptoms.

A simpler procedure has replaced the heterophil test. Finely ground guinea pig kidney or beef red cell stroma, followed by a drop of horse cells, is added to aliquots of serum on a slide. Horse cell agglutination is more specific for the diagnosis of infectious mononucleosis than is sheep cell agglutination. This test is made even more specific by added absorption with guinea pig or beef tissues (see Table 10-2). Results are considered positive if agglutination occurs in the presence of guinea pig tissue but not with beef erythrocytes. This *Monospot test,* or horse cell agglutination with absorption, has approximately 3 percent false positive and 3 percent false negative results as compared to standard absorbed heterophil tests. Many of these false positives occur in the testing of patients with malignant lymphoma. It should be emphasized that the Monospot test agglutination must appear within 1 minute

Table 10-2 : Results of Absorbed Heterophil Test in Infectious
Mononucleosis, Lymphoma, and Serum Sickness

| | Result with and without Absorption | | |
Disease	Without	Guinea Pig Kidney	Beef Red Cell
Mononucleosis (IM)	+	+	–
Lymphoma and other non-IM diseases	+	–	+ or –
Serum sickness	+	–	–

of mixing the reagents together. If it appears after 1 minute, it is probably a nonspecific reaction, and the test should be considered negative.

Serum sickness, a disease characterized by lymphadenopathy following injection of nonhuman serum, is associated with a positive heterophil test. It reverts to negative with guinea pig or beef tissue preabsorption.

Other unusual antibodies seen in patients with infectious mononucleosis include antibodies that give false positive results for syphilis, antinuclear antibodies, cold-reacting rheumatoid factor, Donath-Landsteiner cold hemolysins, lymphocytotoxins, and antibodies against T and B lymphocytes. An interesting antibody is the anti-i seen in association with acquired hemolytic anemia following infectious mononucleosis. It appears that in acquired hemolytic anemia the i antigen, a fetal antigen, is unmasked on the red cell, and an immune reaction results. Antibodies may also be involved in the neutropenia and thrombocytopenia sometimes seen with this disease.

A syndrome known as heterophil-negative mononucleosis has been described. In this disease fever, lymphadenopathy, and other manifestations of infectious mononucleosis are present, but the heterophil test is negative even weeks after the onset of symptoms. It has been found that various agents may cause this syndrome, including cytomegalic virus and toxoplasmosis. In the cytomegalic virus–caused form cervical lymphadenopathy and sore throat are rarely present. Cytomegalic mononucleosis often follows open heart surgery, organ transplantation, and blood transfusion. Adenovirus, rubella virus, and herpes simplex are other candidate viruses for causing heterophil-negative mononucleosis.

Infectious hepatitis and infectious lymphocytosis must also be distinguished from infectious mononucleosis. *Infectious lymphocytosis* usually occurs as an epidemic in the pediatric age group, with white cell counts ranging from 20 to 100 $\times$ 10^9 cells per liter. Respiratory distress, diarrhea, and aseptic meningitis are some of its complications. The absolute lymphocyte count is elevated, with many small lymphocytes present. Serologic testing for the heterophil antibody usually separates infectious mononucleosis from infectious hepatitis, lymphocytic leukemoid reactions, infectious lymphocytosis, and serum sickness.

There is no specific therapy for infectious mononucleosis. Antibiotics, γ-globulin, and corticosteroids are ineffective. Patients who are severely infected, particularly with exudative pharyngitis, are given corticosteroids, but there is no definite evidence that they are of value. Only in the case of life-threatening complications should they be used in large doses for any length of time. Fatal infections are extremely rare, and patients recover without sequelae.

Approach to Patient with Lymphadenopathy or Splenomegaly

The evaluation and treatment of patients who present with lymphadenopathy or splenomegaly must be individualized, but the following should serve as a useful approach (and see p. 366). First, symptoms suggestive of malignant lymphoma, infectious mononucleosis, or one of the diseaes that cause heterophil-negative infectious mononucleosis are elicited. Physical examination will detect the presence of fever, weight loss, skin rashes, and signs of hepatitis. A search for infected teeth, skin, nail, or bladder infections that might cause enlarged lymph nodes may uncover the etiology for enlargement of lymph nodes. Chest x-rays will detect hilar or mediastinal adenopathy. The peripheral blood should be examined for evidence of cytopenias, atypical lymphocytosis, and lymphocytes associated with lymphosarcoma or chronic lymphocytic leukemia. A bone marrow examination may help decide whether the patient has malignant lymphoma or leukemia. Serologic tests for mononucleosis (e.g., Monospot test) are readily available and should be performed. If these initial screening tests do not suggest the diagnosis of lymphocytic leukemia or malignant lymphoma, then the patient may be observed for a period of weeks. If lymph nodes continue to enlarge or do not regress completely, lymph node biopsy must be performed.

If the patient has persistent fevers, weight loss, and lymph nodes that are rubbery and matted together rather than soft and discreet, or if physical examination and blood studies indicate the presence of hypersplenism, then biopsy or other surgical diagnostic procedures are indicated. In some patients with splenomegaly, the etiology is not clear, but the patient has no symptoms, signs, or laboratory tests suggestive of serious disease. These patients are often observed for awhile before a splenectomy is performed.

Diseases causing lymphadenopathy, splenomegaly, or both

I. Causes of Lymphadenopathy
   A. Acute infections (bacterial, viral, fungal, etc.)
   B. Brucellosis
   C. Cat scratch fever
   D. Collagen diseases, for example, lupus erythematosus or rheumatoid arthritis
   E. Cytomegalic virus inclusion disease
   F. Drug reactions
   G. Infectious mononucleosis
   H. Leukemia
   I. Malignant lymphoma
   J. Metastatic epithelial neoplasms
   K. Sarcoidosis
   L. Serum sickness
   M. Tuberculosis

II. Causes of Splenomegaly
   A. Chronic infections (tuberculosis, brucellosis, subacute bacterial endocarditis)
   B. Chronic malaria
   C. Felty's syndrome
   D. Hemolytic anemia
   E. Kala azar
   F. Lipid storage diseases (Gaucher's disease) and other storage diseases
   G. Liver disease (portal hypertension with congestive splenomegaly)
   H. Lupus erythematosus
   I. Malignant lymphoma
   J. Myeloproliferative diseases
   K. Primary idiopathy
   L. Sarcoidosis
   M. Spleen cyst
   N. Thalassemia

Case Development Problems: Malignant Lymphoma

Patient History No. 1

A 25-year-old woman complains of fever, night sweats, and unexplained itching. On physical examination, a mass of lymph nodes is found on the left side of her neck. They are firm and appear matted together. A complete blood count and peripheral blood smear are normal. Chest x-ray shows an anterior mediastinal mass and hilar adenopathy.

1. What further information would you require in order to complete the evaluation of this patient?

Obviously the diagnosis of a malignant lymphoma, such as Hodgkin's disease, should be considered. Biopsy of the lymph node mass should be done concurrently with such simple procedures as physical examination to determine the size of the liver, spleen, and other lymph nodes, and blood chemistry evaluation including liver function tests, uric acid levels, erythrocyte sedimentation rate, and serum calcium levels. Special lung x-rays necessary to determine whether there is parenchymal involvement by the mediastinal and hilar masses should also be considered. If the diagnosis of malignant lymphoma, Hodgkin's type, is made by biopsy, then bone marrow biopsy, lymphangiogram, intravenous pyelogram, inferior vena cavagram, gallium scan, or abdominal ultrasonic testing should be considered. Skin tests for tuberculosis and for common antigens to determine whether anergy is present are sometimes helpful.

Lymph node biopsy shows Hodgkin's disease, nodular sclerosis type. Lung x-rays show involvement of lung parenchyma bordering on the mediastinum. The spleen is not palpated in the left upper quadrant. Alkaline phosphatase and transaminase levels (liver function tests) are normal. A bone marrow biopsy and lymphangiogram are negative.

2. What is the clinical stage of this patient?

Stage II_EB. Lymphomatous nodes on one side of the diaphragm and extranodal disease in the lung parenchyma bordering the mediastinal lymph nodes place the patient in stage II_E. The E indicates that she has extranodal disease. The B indicates that she has systemic symptoms, fever, and night sweats. Pruritis is not considered a B symptom.

3. How would you now proceed?

A laparotomy or at least an abdominal exploration with laparoscopy and percutaneous biopsy of suspicious sites should be performed. Abdominal exploration is needed to detect liver involvement by Hodgkin's disease. A splenectomy with all its benefits and possible complications and placement of the ovaries outside the radiation field should also be performed. The abdominal exploration may also locate disease outside the fields treated by routine radiotherapy.

A laparotomy is undertaken. The spleen is removed and found to be involved by Hodgkin's disease. The liver shows small infiltrates with mononuclear cells but no Reed-Sternberg cells. A few granulomata are also found in the liver and spleen. The retroperitoneal lymph nodes are negative for Hodgkin's disease as determined by biopsy.

4. What is the pathologic stage of this patient?

Nonspecific infiltrates and granuloma are not enough to make the diagnosis of Hodgkin's disease of the liver. However, with splenic involvement, there is a good possibility that the liver is also involved, although this was not proved by biopsy. Small foci of Hodgkin's disease can easily be missed by the biopsy procedures used at the time of laparotomy. Despite these possibilities, the patient is staged as PS (pathological stage) $III_{SE}B$ and not Stage IV.

5. How would you treat this patient?

As a patient with Stage IIIB Hodgkin's disease, she should be treated with combination chemotherapy.

Many therapists believe that radiation should also be given to large masses of lymphoma to prevent subsequent relapse in these areas. For this reason the patient was given high dose radiotherapy to the mantle region, which includes the neck, axillary, and mediastinal lymph nodes, after MOPP chemotherapy had been completed.

6. What side effects can occur from radiation of the mantle region?

Hypothyroidism due to radiation of the thyroid and bone marrow suppression due to sternal marrow irradiation are relatively common problems. Usually the patient's blood counts recover several months after treatment. In some cases bone fractures with fibrous nonunion, pericarditis and myocarditis, inflammation of the mucous membrane in the radiated field, and nausea and vomiting complicate this radiotherapy.

The patient receives six cycles of MOPP therapy and mantle radiotherapy, and all clinically detectable disease disappears. The spleen becomes normal in size, and liver function tests normalize. The patient is in complete remission for 2 years but then suffers a relapse, with growth of lymph nodes in the abdominal area.

7. What therapy can now be offered to this patient?

MOPP chemotherapy may be reintroduced or irradiation to the abdominal lymph nodes tried, or both. Often such patients will go back into remission for significantly long periods of time. Chemotherapy with bleomycin, nitrosoureas, or adriamycin can also be considered. Combinations of these drugs are being worked out for retreatment of patients relapsing following chemotherapy or radiotherapy for Hodgkin's disease.

*Patient History
No. 2*

An asymptomatic man, age 60, presents with enlarged lymph nodes throughout his body. Those about his neck, axillae, and groin are particularly enlarged. A lymph node biopsy reveals malignant lymphoma characterized by sheets of mature lymphocytes replacing the normal lymph node architecture. Nodules of lymphocytes are present, but no Reed-Sternberg cells. On examination, the patient's spleen is enlarged. Anemia, leukopenia, and thrombocytopenia are discovered. Examination of the peripheral blood smear shows no abnormalities, except a few atypical lymphocytes. The Coombs' test is negative.

1. What is the diagnosis, and what would you do to evaluate this patient further?

The patient has non-Hodgkin's lymphoma of the nodular, lymphocytic, or well-differentiated type. Studies should be done to further document the extent of disease. A bone marrow biopsy is necessary, since 80 percent of patients with non-Hodgkin's lymphoma will have marrow involvement. An intravenous pyelogram or cavagram will help determine whether the retroperitoneal area is involved. The consequences of malignant lymphoma should be investigated by measurement of serum uric acid levels and renal and liver function tests.

2. Prior to performing the bone marrow biopsy, what do you give as the clinical stage? (All chemical tests and x-rays are normal.)

Since the patient has lymph node disease on both sides of the diaphragm, and the spleen is involved, the patient is staged as III_SA.

Bone marrow examination reveals scattered, large nodules of lymphocytes infiltrating the bone marrow.

3. What is the stage now?

Bone marrow involvement advances the stage to IV. This is commonly the case in non-Hodgkin's lymphoma and is the reason why radical radiotherapy for cure is seldom considered.

4. What is the likely cause for pancytopenia in this patient?

The pancytopenia is probably due to two factors: (1) the replacement of the bone marrow by lymphoma and (2) hypersplenism due to infiltration of the spleen by lymphomatous tissue.

5. How would you consider treating this patient?

Two possible modes of therapy should be considered. Total body irradiation has been used to treat patients with nodular lymphocytic lymphosarcoma, even with bone marrow involvement. If total body irradiation cannot be administered, an alternative is to treat with combination chemotherapy, cyclophosphamide and prednisone. Prednisone would be particularly useful, since he suffers from hypersplenism. If cytotoxic agents alone are used, bone marrow production is often suppressed, and pancytopenia worsens before any beneficial effect of cytotoxic agents becomes evident.

6. What histopathologic features in the lymph node biopsy will determine the prognosis and the likelihood of response to therapy?

The presence of a nodular lymphoma is associated with a particularly good prognosis, both with total body irradiation and with chemotherapy. The mature lymphocyte infiltrate also carries a better prognosis than do lymphoblastic or reticulum cells.

The patient is treated with chemotherapy, and all evidence of disease disappears. One year later, however, rapidly enlarging nodes are found in his neck.

7. What procedures would you consider now?

Rapidly enlarging nodes in a patient with nodular lymphocytic lymphosarcoma suggest that the disease has been transformed into a more malignant form of lymphoma, that is, reticulum cell sarcoma (DH). A repeat biopsy should be done to confirm or deny this possibility.

Reticulum cell sarcoma is found in the lymph nodes, and the disease progresses rapidly, with more lymph nodes appearing weekly in all areas; the neck nodes are particularly large.

8. What therapy would you consider?

Treatment with palliative radiotherapy to the enlarging neck lymph nodes probably holds the best promise of slowing the disease. Multiple drug therapy with procarbazine, nitrosoureas, bleomycin or adriamycin can be tried, but these drugs are often ineffective against this highly malignant disease.

At this time atypical lymphocytes with large clefted nuclei and nucleoli are found in the patient's peripheral blood. The total white count rises to 40×10^9 per liter and is made up of 90 percent of these atypical lymphocytes.

9. What is the likely diagnosis, and how does it affect prognosis or therapy?

Most likely the patient's lymphoma has developed a leukemic phase. Prognosis and treatment are not changed by the development of this leukemic phase.

MULTIPLE MYELOMA AND WALDENSTRÖM'S MACROGLOBULINEMIA

Multiple myeloma and a closely related disease, Waldenström's macroglobulinemia, are B lymphocyte diseases. Multiple myeloma is characterized by painful bone lesions, proliferation of plasma cells in the marrow, and the presence of an abnormal, monoclonal, 7S immunoglobulin in serum or urine. Waldenström's macroglobulinemia on the other hand has a clinical picture similar to that of non-Hodgkin's lymphoma but is associated with a monoclonal immunoglobulin with characteristics of a macroglobulin. Before describing these diseases we shall review how proteins, in particular immunoglobulins, are characterized.

Characterization of Immunoglobulins

When serum is electrophoresed on a supporting medium such as cellulose acetate or agarose, distinct bands of proteins are produced. Serum albumin is identified at the anodal end of the supporting medium, while immunoglobulin bands are seen near the cathode. The major bands are albumin and the α_1-, α_2-, β-, and γ-globulins. Proteins that participate in immunological reactions, so-called antibodies, are immunoglobulins. They are usually found in the β-globulin or γ-globulin regions, although some travel more anodally.

Immunoglobulins help protect individuals from infections and are part of the immune defense mechanism. They are produced by B lymphocytes that have been transformed into morphologically recognizable plasma cells. Plasma cells are normally found in all tissues but are recognized in bone marrow preparations as large cells with dark purple cytoplasm (Plate 65). Their nuclei are usually single, eccentric, and separated from the cytoplasm by a perinuclear clear zone.

Five antigenic types of immunoglobulins have been described. They can be identified by a reagent that is created when antibodies are raised against a known type; the reagent is used as a typing serum. The five types are called IgG, IgA, IgM, IgD, and IgE. An anti-IgG typing serum will react with IgG immunoglobulins. Immunoglobulins themselves are antibodies and will react specifically against antigens such as bacterial cell walls and viral coat proteins. The IgG, IgA, and IgD types are of small molecular weight, approximately 150,000, as compared to IgM, whose molecular weight is approximately one million. At ultracentrifuge speeds the smaller molecular weight immunoglobulins sediment at 7S (Svedberg units) and the IgM at 19S. IgE is intermediate at 8.2S and has a molecular weight of about 196,000.

A technique called immunoelectrophoresis uses the differences both in electrophoretic mobility and antigenic characteristics to separate the five immunoglobulin classes (see Table 10-3). It is performed by first electrophoresing a patient's sera and then cutting a trough parallel to protein bands. An antiserum raised against normal human serum is placed in the trough. As a result of the serum proteins diffusing toward the antibodies in the trough, precipitin lines appear in the supporting agar medium. These precipitin lines are then characterized according to their shape, size, and location. They can further be characterized by adding specific antisera to the trough — for example, anti-IgG serum, which will precipitate only the IgG immunoglobulins. When such monospecific antisera are used, all the bands seen with antinormal whole human serum can be identified. With experience monospecific antisera may not be required to identify some of the larger bands, such as IgG, IgA, and IgM. The quantities of IgD and IgE are usually too small to detect by this procedure. The presence of a monoclonal immunoglobulin, that is, an immunoglobulin produced by one clone of plasma cells with each molecule more or less identical with the next, is detected on immunoelectrophoresis by a thickening and distortion of the normal precipitin line. When simple electrophoresis on cellulose acetate or agarose gel is performed, the monoclonal immunoglobulin appears as a large band in the α_2- to γ-mobility regions.

The quantity of each serum immunoglobulin can be determined by radial immunodiffusion. Antibody is mixed with agar and then placed in a Petri dish. Wells are cut in the Petri dish, and several known concentrations of the immunoglobulin to be assayed are each placed in a well. As the material in each well diffuses through the antibody-containing agar, precipitin lines appear as a circle around the well. The higher the concentration of immunoglobulin in the wells, the greater the diameter of the circle. Unknown samples can be introduced into other wells and their concentration estimated on the basis of the diameter of the circles produced. Using a different Petri dish for each immunoglobulin class, it is possible to determine the concentration of each of the five im-

Table 10-3 : Characteristics of Serum Immunoglobulins

	IgG	IgA	IgM	IgD	IgE
Molecular weight (daltons)	160,000	170,000	1,000,000	180,000	196,000
Sedimentation constant (S)	6.6	6.85*	19.0	7.0	8.0
Quantity per 100 ml serum in grams	1.2	0.2	0.1	0.003	0.00003
Half-life (days)[†]	20-30	6-7	5-10	3	2

*Secretory IgA with transport piece 11.4S; molecular weight 360,000-560,000.
[†]Bence Jones protein has half life of 24 hours.
Adapted from Snapper, I., and Kahn, A., *Myelomatosis: Fundamentals and Clinical Features.* Baltimore: University Park Press, 1971, p. 31.

munoglobulin classes. Also, if a monoclonal spike is seen on cellulose acetate or agarose electrophoresis, the concentration of each immunoglobulin can be determined by radial immunodiffusion, and the one present in highest concentration is presumably responsible for the monoclonal spike. By addition of electrophoretic techniques to the radial immunodiffusion procedure, it is possible to shorten the procedure to only a few hours. Concentration of immunoglobulins can also be assayed automatically by the use of precipitating antibodies against each of the five immunoglobulin classes and subsequent measurement of the turbidity produced when these antibodies react with their complementary immunoglobulins.

Thus an immunoglobulin can be characterized by its sedimentation velocity, immunologic reactions with five typing sera, and electrophoretic mobility. Finally, it can be characterized by subtyping the amino acid chains that make up the immunoglobulin molecule. All 7S immunoglobulins are made up of four polypeptide chains bound together by disulfide bridges. The interchain bonds can be broken, producing four polypeptides: one pair of identical heavy chains (H chains) and one pair of identical light chains (L chains). The heavy chains are identified by Greek letters: the H chain of IgG is γ; that of IgA, α; IgM, μ; IgD, δ; and IgE, ϵ. Heavy chains contain the antigenic groups that immunologically differentiate the five immunoglobulin classes. The light chains are identical to the Bence Jones proteins found in the urine of some myeloma patients (see Immunoglobulins in Multiple Myeloma). Both the light and the heavy chains may serve as antigens. Antibodies raised against light chains are used to differentiate at least two different antigenic subtypes, designated by the letters κ and λ. Thus, an immunoglobulin molecule is characterized by light chain subtype and by heavy chain antigenic class. It is believed that a plasma cell produces both the heavy and light chains of one of the ten possible immunoglobulin types (for example an IgG immunoglobulin may have either a kappa or lambda light chain).

Clinical Findings in Multiple Myeloma

Patients with multiple myeloma present in their fifth decade or beyond with anemia, pancytopenia, or bone pain. On investigation they are often found to have osteolytic defects of the ribs or skull and osteoporesis of the spine, along with fractures and wedging of vertebral bodies. Examination of bone marrow specimens (Plate 65) shows replacement of normal hematopoietic elements with sheets of plasma cells or nucleolated plasma cells called *plasmablasts*. Some of the plasma cells are binucleated or trinucleated; others resemble reticulum cells. Monoclonal immunoglobulins are found in either serum, urine, or both. Almost always the concentrations of the normal serum immunoglobulins are decreased. Renal failure and amyloidosis often complicate the clinical picture. Amyloid is a substance found in various tissues and is made up in part of immunoglobulins deposited in parenchymal tissues. As a result of this deposition, enlargement and dysfunction of organs such as the kidneys and liver may occur. The material is identified by staining with Congo red and looking for birefringence with a polarizing microscope.

Multiple myeloma should be suspected when elderly patients present with unexplained anemias or persistent, unexplained, low back pain. Early disease is often overlooked because the peripheral blood examination and routine blood chemistries are usually normal, with the exception of the protein electrophoretic pattern. The blood picture may be normal except for a normochromic, normocytic anemia and rouleaux. *Rouleaux* (Plate 66) refers to the stacking of red cells one upon the other, usually due to abnormalities in immunoglobulins or other plasma proteins such as fibrinogen. Probably related to rouleaux formation is the difficulty of obtaining blood from myeloma patients by finger stick. The erythrocyte sedimentation rate is rapid, usually over 100 millimeters per hour, again as a result of abnormalities in immunoglobulins and fibrinogen.

Unless the patient develops the rare leukemic form of myeloma called plasma cell leukemia, plasma cells are seen only in small numbers or not at all in the peripheral blood. Probably as a result of bone involvement, the serum calcium level is elevated, and hypercalcemia with its complications may be a presenting problem. Because of the increased turnover of plasma cells, uric acid levels are also high. The hypercalcemia and hyperuricemia may be contributing factors to the development of renal failure often associated with multiple myeloma. Infiltration of the kidney by plasma cells, development of amyloidosis, and precipitation of immunoglobulins in the renal tubules, particularly Bence Jones (light chain component of immunoglobulins) proteins, also contribute to the renal insufficiency. Even if renal function tests are normal, patients with myeloma can go into renal failure if dehydrated. This often happens in undiagnosed myeloma patients who are dehydrated in preparation for intravenous pyelography.

The prognosis of myeloma with or without treatment is related to the presence or absence of renal insufficiency. Patients who have renal disease from the onset will have more complications and succumb to the disease sooner than those without. Recently, chronic renal dialysis has helped patients maintain useful lives in spite of little or no renal function secondary to multiple myeloma.

It is usual for patients with myeloma to have bone disease. Perhaps less than 5 percent have normal x-rays. The most common abnormality is osteoporosis, or decreased density of the vertebral column. Osteolytic lesions in the skull, ribs, pelvis, or vertebral column, when present along with osteoporosis, should make the radiologist strongly suspect multiple myeloma. The osteolytic lesions in the myelomatous skull must be distinguished by x-ray features, by associated blood and bone marrow findings, or, rarely, by biopsy of the osteolytic areas from metastatic carcinoma and normal venous lakes. Only occasionally are osteoblastic bone lesions seen.

Rarely, a plasmacytoma, or localized collection of plasma cells, will cause osteolysis and, sometimes, monoclonal protein production. Plasmacytomas, whether single or multiple, represent the earliest stage in the development of some cases of multiple myeloma.

Immunoglobulins in Multiple Myeloma

The immunoglobulin abnormalities of multiple myeloma include suppression of normal immunoglobulin synthesis and presence in the serum or urine of monoclonal protein(s), which may be complete immunoglobulins or parts of immunoglobulins, such as light or heavy chains. They appear as "M" (myeloma or monoclonal) spikes or peaks on simple electrophoresis after scanning with a densitometer. Monoclonal spikes of γ-mobility have a 4:1 height–to–base-width ratio; the ratio is 3:1 for proteins in the more anodal regions. Immunoelectrophoresis or determination of L chain subtype helps decide whether a peak on electrophoresis is due to a monoclonal protein. If only κ or only λ L chains are present, the immunoglobulin is probably monoclonal. In approximately 50 percent of myeloma patients an M spike is seen only in the serum. In 20 to 30 percent of patients the normal immunoglobulins are depressed in the serum, but no *serum* M component is detected. In the urine, however, L chains or Bence Jones proteins are present. In another 20 percent an abnormal M component is found in both serum and urine. In only 2 percent of patients are M components lacking in both serum and urine. In most of these patients the normal serum immunoglobulins are depressed, but in very rare individuals, perhaps those early in the course of their disease, normal concentrations of immunoglobulins are present.

Eighty percent of M components are in the IgG class and about twenty percent in the IgA class. IgM myeloma proteins are rare and usually associated with the clinical picture of Waldenström's macroglobulinemia (discussed later in this chapter). The antibody functions of myeloma, monoclonal, immunoglobulins are usually unknown, but it is clear that at least some monoclonal myeloma proteins are antibodies directed against specific antigens.

Bence Jones proteins, or L chains, precipitate when heated to $56°C$, dissolve when heated to boiling, and reprecipitate with cooling. This test is technically difficult to do, and false positives are likely. For this reason, protein electrophoresis of a concentrated, random specimen of urine is a better screening test for Bence Jones proteinuria. A monoclonal protein running in the β or γ region of a urine electrophoresis is most likely an L chain protein. Incidentally the plastic, chemically impregnated sticks (Lab Stix) now used for routine urine protein testing are insensitive to Bence Jones proteinuria.

Unusual proteins such as *pyroglobulins,* which irreversibly gel at $56°C$, and *cryoglobulins,* which reversibly precipitate when exposed to low temperatures $(4°C)$, are sometimes found in serum or plasma from patients with multiple myeloma. Most of the cryoglobulins found in myeloma patients are IgG or IgM paraproteins or mixtures of both. These cryoglobulins may cause pain, blanching, and cyanosis in fingertips or toes after exposure to cold temperatures. This *Raynaud's phenomenon* may also occur in the presence of high titers of cold agglutinins, such as are found in idiopathic cold hemagglutinin disease or Waldenström's macroglobulinemia.

Not all M spikes are due to multiple myeloma; in some cases they are not monoclonal but, rather, made up of proteins containing more than one type of light chain or, less likely, more than one H chain type. M spikes have been detected in diseases such as chronic infections (e.g., cholecystitis), malignant lymphoma, hepatoma, pernicious anemia, Gaucher's disease, thymomas, sarcoidosis, autoimmune diseases, cirrhosis, carcinomas — as of the lung and rectum — and Kaposi's sarcoma. In a few patients a serum M spike will precede the detection of myelomatous skeletal or bone marrow abnormalities by months or years. Some elderly individuals have M spikes but do not develop myeloma. These conditions have been referred to as *premyeloma* and *benign monoclonal gammopathy,* respectively.

Bone Marrow in Multiple Myeloma

The bone marrow findings of multiple myeloma are usually easily recognized. There are plasma cells, some multinucleated, and plasmablasts, often appearing to replace normal marrow elements. *Grape cells,* or large plasma cells with many large, blue, cytoplasmic vacuoles, and *flame cells,* or *thesaurocytes,* containing bright red material in the cytoplasm, have also been described. The latter are associated with IgA myeloma proteins. The plasma cells can appear relatively normal and therefore can be difficult to distinguish from reactive plasmacytosis seen in inflammatory or malignant, nonmyelomatous diseases. Metastatic carcinomas with involvement of the liver in particular may give rise to an intense marrow plasmacytosis. In a few cases the marrow does not show typical plasma cells but, rather, a cell that resembles a reticulum cell. In rare cases the diagnosis of reticulum cell sarcoma has been made on microscopic examination of bone marrow from patients with the clinical picture of multiple myeloma.

Myeloma-Related Diseases

Franklin's Disease

Rare patients with a clinical picture of malignant lymphoma, including lymphadenopathy, splenomegaly, palatal edema, and no osteolytic lesions, have γ, heavy chain fragments in their sera and urine (Franklin's disease). One such fragment is the *Fc piece,* which is one of three pieces into which papain splits 7S immunoglobulins. The two other pieces each contain half of one heavy chain and one whole light chain and are called the *Fab fragments.* The Fab fragment determines the specificity of the antibody molecule. The Fc fragment consists of the remaining halves of two heavy chains still connected by a disulfide bridge. Excretion of Fc fragments should be suspected if the serum and urine monoclonal spike migrate together electrophoretically. This is in contrast to the electrophoretic findings in multiple myeloma where the large myeloma protein migrates differently from the smaller L chain (Bence Jones) protein in the urine.

Heavy Chain Disease

Unusual patients with a clinical picture similar to that of malignant lymphoma produce monoclonal, α, heavy chains (part of IgA immunoglobulin). The disease is called α *heavy chain disease* or *Mediterranean lymphoma* and is associated with intestinal malabsorption. It is interesting that the IgA molecule is normally secreted in the intestine.

Heavy chains of IgM macroglobulins (μ-chains) are excreted in rare patients with a clinical picture of chronic lymphatic leukemia.

Kaposi's Sarcoma

Kaposi's sarcoma is characterized by dermatologic lesions found on the extremities, in the abdomen, and in other locations. The lesions appear as small, multiple, firm, purple papules that grow to several centimeters in size. Histologically, spindle cells are prominent; these are thought to be derived from reticulum cells or cells of the adventitia of small blood vessels. Malignant lymphoma often is present in lymph nodes from patients with advanced Kaposi's sarcoma, and the disease may terminate in a clinical picture similar to that of non-Hodgkin's lymphoma or, in a few cases, multiple myeloma. The skin lesions respond to radiotherapy and to chemotherapy similar to that used for malignant lymphomas.

Myeloma Skin Disease

A very rare skin disorder, *lichen myxedematosus,* characterized by the progressive accumulation of proteinaceous infiltrates in the dermal layers of the skin of the head, trunk, and extremities, is associated with plasmacytosis in the bone marrow and a monoclonal M spike in the serum but without skeletal lesions. These patients may respond to treatment with phenylalanine mustard, a drug used to treat multiple myeloma.

Treatment of Multiple Myeloma and Related Plasma Cell Dyscrasias

The alkylating agent phenylalanine mustard (Alkeran) is considered the drug of choice for patients with multiple myeloma and related diseases. It has many of the usual toxicities of alkylating agents, namely nausea, vomiting, and bone marrow depression. The bone marrow depression is often delayed, appearing one or more weeks after exposure to the drug. This delayed bone marrow toxicity must be considered in adjusting dosage. Once it has taken place, severe bone marrow depression can last for weeks or even months. A number of cases of myeloma terminating in acute myelocytic, myelomonocytic, or other variants of myelocytic leukemia have been reported after treatment with phenylalanine mustard.

At least three different programs that use phenylalanine mustard are available for treatment of multiple myeloma. In one combination chemotherapy program, large daily doses are given on 4 consecutive days, along with prednisone. This 4-day regimen is repeated every 6 weeks. Another regimen consists of administering a large quantity of phenylalanine mustard in divided doses over a period of 10 days. Once this loading dose has been given, then lower dose, maintenance therapy is started immediately or after a short wait to allow recovery of blood counts. A third treatment schedule calls for small doses of phenylalanine mustard each day, depending on blood counts done weekly or biweekly. Approximately 50 percent of myeloma patients will respond to treatment with Alkeran and those that respond will live approximately two years longer than nonresponders.

Cyclophosphamide is probably an equally effective treatment for multiple myeloma. Because of the good results reported with phenylalanine mustard, cyclophosphamide therapy is often used only after Alkeran therapy has failed. Radiotherapy is sometimes required to control pain from vertebral or rib fractures.

The long-term prognosis of multiple myeloma is not particularly good, with or without treatment. Patients who do not respond or are not treated usually die within a year or two, and even those who have a good response to therapy die within four years. Occasional patients live for many years on maintenance doses of cyclophosphamide or phenylalanine mustard.

The hypercalcemia seen in multiple myeloma may be treated with saline- and diuretic-induced diuresis, adrenal corticosteroid therapy, or with the antibiotic mithyramycin. The latter is given as a rapid intravenous infusion that lowers serum calcium, usually for a period of days. Repeated doses may be administered, since it has little effect on bone marrow and, if given properly, little in the way of toxicity. The calcium lowering effect has not been adequately explained, but calcium does appear to be deposited back into bone.

If a patient becomes resistant to either cyclophosphamide or phenylalanine mustard therapy, then the other drug is used. If he is resistant to both, then consideration should be given to nitrosoureas, high dose corticosteroid therapy, or to agents such as adriamycin. Urethane or fluoride for bone pain are no longer considered helpful. Allopurinol is used to treat hyperuricemia.

Since the plasma cell infiltration of the bone marrow usually persists despite treatment, other indicators of response must be used. Reduction in serum or urine myeloma protein concentration is a good indicator of response, as is improvement in anemia and serum albumin level, alleviation of hypercalcemia and hyperuricemia, and regression of measurable lesions.

Waldenström's Macroglobulinemia

Waldenström's macroglobulinemia is a disease of the elderly and is manifested by a clinical picture similar to that of malignant lymphoma, including lymphadenopathy and hepatosplenomegaly. A hemorrhagic tendency, recurring infections, visual disturbances, polyneuritis, and Raynaud's phenomenon are possible complications. Osteolytic lesions and renal failure, except when due to amyloidosis, are rare. The serum has a high concentration of monoclonal macroglobulins, which can cause a *hyperviscosity syndrome* with coma, dilation of retinal veins, and other central nervous system symptoms. Rising serum viscosity levels are often associated with a worsening clinical course. Macroglobulins cause the hemorrhagic tendency by coating platelets and interfering with their function. Therefore bleeding from small blood vessels, mucosa, and skin is not uncommon. Bence Jones protein rarely is found in macroglobulinemia.

Except for rouleaux formation, the peripheral blood from patients with macroglobulinemia is unremarkable. The bone marrow and lymph nodes show infiltration by cells having morphologic characteristics of both plasma cells and lymphocytes, so-called *plymphocytes* (Plate 67). In Wright-stained marrow preparations, they have the ground-glass blue cytoplasm of the lymphocyte but the nuclear characteristics of a plasma cell. They may represent transition forms between B lymphocytes and plasma cells. Intranuclear inclusions can be demonstrated by the use of the PAS stain, but their significance is unknown.

Waldenström's macroglobulinemia is treated with alkylating agents such as cyclophosphamide or chlorambucil. Patients do not respond dramatically, but hepatosplenomegaly and lymphadenopathy improve, and IgM macroglobulin concentration slowly falls. The hyperviscosity syndrome can be treated in an emergency by *plasmaphoresis,* that is, removal of the patient's plasma and replacement by normal plasma. This is possible because the large size of the IgM molecule prevents its escape from the intravascular space. In contrast, the 7S immunoglobulins of myeloma are distributed throughout the extravascular space, and their removal by plasmaphoresis results in mobilization of extravascular immunoglobulins into plasma. Attempts to dissociate IgM molecules into their smaller constituents by use of penicillamine and mercaptoethanol have not been successful. Rarely, the hyperviscosity syndrome is caused by aggregation of IgA or IgG monoclonal immunoglobulins and therefore arises in patients with multiple myeloma.

Case Development Problem: Multiple Myeloma and Macroglobulinemia

As part of an evaluation for anemia in a 70-year-old man, a serum protein electrophoresis pattern is obtained that shows a tall, thin spike at the most cathodal end of the pattern. Normal immunoglobulins appear to be depressed. On immunoelectrophoresis a thickening and distortion of the IgM precipitin band is seen. The immunoelectrophoretic pattern when anti-κ and anti-λ typing serum are used shows only λ-chains. Radial diffusion immunoassay reveals five times the normal amount of IgM and decreased quantities of IgG and IgA.

1. Using these data, characterize the abnormal protein spike.

This patient has a monoclonal IgM macroglobulin with λ L chains and of γ-mobility on electrophoresis.

2. What studies would you do to determine whether the patient has malignant lymphoma, multiple myeloma, or Waldenström's macroglobulinemia?

Bone marrow or lymph node examination should be most helpful. A finding of infiltrates of lymphocytes would favor malignant lymphoma; plymphocytes would suggest macroglobulinemia, especially if they have PAS-positive intranuclear inclusions; and plasmacytosis, particularly with abnormal or nucleolated forms, would suggest multiple myeloma. A skeletal survey is helpful, because the typical osteolytic lesions of myeloma are infrequently or rarely seen in malignant lymphoma or Waldenström's macroglobulinemia. Lymphadenopathy and hepatosplenomegaly associated with an IgM monoclonal spike is evidence for Waldenström's macroglobulinemia.

3. List the factors that lead to renal insufficiency in patients with Waldenström's macroglobulinemia or multiple myeloma.

   a. Direct infiltration of kidney with lymphomatous or myelomatous tumor
   b. Hypercalcemia
   c. Hyperuricemia with uric acid nephropathy, uric acid stones, and obstructive uropathy
   d. Precipitation of Bence Jones protein in renal tubules
   e. Development of amyloidosis
   f. Susceptibility to chronic, recurrent renal infections due to immune system dysfunction
   g. Renal tubular abnormalities due to filtration of immunoglobulins (mechanism unknown)
   h. Dehydration secondary to nausea, vomiting, or preparation for intravenous pyelography

4. Your patient develops bleeding from the nose and gums. What mechanisms could cause this abnormal bleeding tendency?

   a. Interference with the last stages of clotting, due to the presence of the abnormal immunoglobulin
   b. Thrombocytopenia due to infiltration of the bone marrow
   c. Hypersplenism, if splenomegaly is present, leading to thrombocytopenia
   d. Coating of platelets with immunoglobulin, thereby interfering with function
   e. Bone marrow suppression and thrombocytopenia secondary to drug therapy

The patient's skeletal survey is negative, and his bone marrow shows plasmacytoid lymphocytes.

5. What is the most likely diagnosis, and how would you treat this patient?

The most likely diagnosis is Waldenström's macroglobulinemia. Treatment should be instituted with plasmaphoresis to lower the plasma IgM concentration and thereby ameliorate the bleeding tendency. Chemotherapy with an alkylating agent, such as cyclophosphamide or chlorambucil should also be begun, as well as treatment of dehydration, hypercalcemia, hyperuricemia, and renal failure, if present.

Before treatment is instituted, the patient is noted to have Raynaud's phenomenon, with blanching and pain in his fingertips following exposure to cold.

6. What are the probable mechanisms for this phenomenon?

Hyperviscosity and sludging of blood in small vessels, due to macroglobulinemia; cryoglobulins that precipitate from the plasma at low temperature, thereby plugging small capillaries and causing tissue anoxia; or a high titer of cold agglutinins, proteins that agglutinate red cells at low temperatures and plug blood vessels in a manner analogous to cryoglobulins, are all possible mechanisms of Raynaud's phenomenon.

TOPICS FOR DISCUSSION

Etiology of malignant lymphoma

Immunologic classifications of malignant lymphoma

Clinical classifications of malignant lymphoma

Staging and staging procedures in Hodgkin's disease and non-Hodgkin's lymphoma

Approach to the patient with lymphadenopathy

Nervous system manifestations of malignant lymphoma

The skin and malignant lymphomas

Pathology of malignant lymphomas

Bone marrow and malignant lymphomas

Radiotherapy of malignant lymphomas

Chemotherapy of malignant lymphomas

Surgery and malignant lymphomas

Methods of evaluation of response to therapy

Pharmacology of antilymphoma drugs

Etiology of Hodgkin's disease

Combination chemotherapy of malignant lymphoma

The nature of the Reed-Sternberg cell

Characteristics of the reticulum cells seen in malignant lymphomas

Complications of malignant lymphomas

Characterization of monoclonal proteins

Therapy of multiple myeloma

Evaluation of response to therapy in multiple myeloma

Hyperviscosity syndrome

Macroglobulins — structure, function, and pathology

Cryoproteins — structure, function, and abnormalities

Raynaud's phenomenon and syndrome

Exotic infections in advanced lymphomas

The immune system and lymphomas

Leukemic phase of malignant lymphomas — morphology and clinical correlates

Heavy chain diseases

Immunologic and structural characterization of immunoglobulins

Physical chemistry and physiology of immunoglobulins

IgD and IgE myeloma

Myeloma kidney

Primary and secondary amyloidosis

Therapy of amyloidosis

Plasma cell leukemia

Histiocytic medullary reticuloendotheliosis or malignant histiocytosis

Hairy cell leukemia

Immunoblastic lymphadenopathy and sarcoma

Leukemic and other malignancies as a consequence of chemotherapy and radiotherapy

SELECTED REFERENCES

Lymphoma — General Considerations

Bakemeier, R. F. Therapy of the Malignant Lymphomas and Chronic Lymphocytic Leukemia. In R. I. Weed (ed.), *Hematology for Internists.* Boston: Little, Brown, 1971.

Banks, P. M. and Berard, C. W. Chapter 116, Histopathology of the Malignant Lymphomas. In W. J. Williams, E. Beutler, A. J. Erslev, and R. W. Rundles (eds.)., *Hematology* (2nd ed.). New York: McGraw-Hill, 1977.

Bennett, J. M. The Classification and Staging of Malignant Lymphomas. In R. I. Weed (ed.), *Hematology for Internists.* Boston: Little, Brown, 1971.

Luce, J. K., and Frei, E., III. Lymphomas. In C. E. Mengel, et al (eds.), *Hematology: Principles and Practices.* Chicago: Year Book, 1972.

Membrane markers in lymphoproliferative disorders (editorial). *Lancet* 1:670, 1975.

Rundles, R. W. Chapter 117, Hodgkin's Disease; Chapter 118, Lymphocytic Lymphomas; Chapter 119, Histiocytic Lymphoma. In W. J. Williams, E. Beutler, A. J. Erslev, and R. W. Rundles (eds.), *Hematology* (2nd ed.). New York: McGraw-Hill, 1977.

Weinstein, I. M. Chapter 107, Lymph Node Enlargement and Splenomegaly. In W. J. Williams, E. Beutler, A. J. Erslev, and R. W. Rundles (eds.), *Hematology* (2nd ed.). New York: McGraw-Hill, 1977.

Ziegler, J. L., Magrath, I. T., and Gerber, P., et al Epstein-Barr virus and human malignancy. *Ann. Intern. Med.* 86:323, 1977.

Hodgkin's Disease

Goldsmith, M. A., and Carter S. K. Combination chemotherapy of advanced Hodgkin's disease. *Cancer* 33:1, 1974.

Kaplan, H. S. *Hodgkin's Disease.* Cambridge: Harvard University Press, 1972.

Kaplan, H. S., and Rosenberg, S. A. Hodgkin's disease: Current recommendations for management. *CA* 25:306, 1975.

Kaplan, H. S., and Rosenberg, S. A. The management of Hodgkin's disease. *Cancer* 36:796, 1975.

Rosenberg, S. A., and Kaplan, H. S. The management of stages I, II, III Hodgkin's disease with combined radiotherapy and chemotherapy. *Cancer* 35:55, 1975.

Ultmann, J. E., and Moran, E. M. Clinical course and complications associated with Hodgkin's diseases. *Arch. Intern. Med.* 131: 332, 1973.

Wintrobe, M. M., et al Hodgkin's Disease; Lymphomas Other than Hodgkin's Disease. In M. M. Wintrobe, et al (eds.), *Clinical Hematology* (7th ed.). Philadelphia: Lea & Febiger, 1974.

Non-Hodgkin's Lymphomas

Hellman, S., Rosenthal, D. S., and Moloney, W. C., et al The treatment of non-Hodgkin's lymphoma. *Cancer* 36:804, 1975.

Johnson, R. E., Chretien, P. B., and O'Conor, G. T., et al Radiotherapeutic implications of prospective staging in non-Hodgkin's lymphoma. *Radiology* 110:655, 1974.

Levi, J. A., and Wiernik, P. H. Management of mycosis fungoides — current status and future prospects. *Medicine* (Baltimore) 54:73, 1975.

McElwain, G. J. Chemotherapy of the lymphomas. *Semin. Hematol.* 11:59, 1974.

Peckman, M. J. Radiation therapy of non-Hodgkin's lymphomas. *Semin. Hematol.* 11:41, 1974.

Portlock, C., Rosenberg, S. A., Glatstein, E., and Kaplan, H. Treatment of advanced non-Hodgkin's lymphomas with favorable histologies: Preliminary results of a prospective trial. *Blood* 47:747, 1976.

Ultmann, J. E., and Stein, R. S. Non-Hodgkin's lymphoma. An approach to staging and therapy. *CA* 25:320, 1975.

Myeloma and Immunoglobulins

Alexanian, R. Multiple Myeloma and Related Disorders. In C. E. Mengel, et al (eds.), *Hematology: Principles and Practice.* Chicago: Year Book, 1972.

Bergsagel, D. E. and Franklin, E. C. Section Twenty, Lymphoreticular Disorders — Malignant Proliferative Response and/or Abnormal Immunoglobulin Synthesis-Plasma Cell Dyscrasias. In W. J. Williams, E. Beutler, A. J. Erslev, and R. W. Rundles (eds.), *Hematology* (2nd ed.). New York: McGraw-Hill, 1977.

Davies, D. R., Padlan, E. A., and Segal, D. M. Three dimensional structure of immunoglobulins. *Annu. Rev. Biochem.* 44:639, 1975.

Hill, R. S. Multiple Myeloma and Dysproteinemic States. In R. I. Weed (ed.), *Hematology for Internists.* Boston: Little, Brown, 1971.

Levin, W. C., and Ritzmann, S. E. The Immunoglobulins. In C. E. Mengel, et al (eds.), *Hematology: Principles and Practice.* Chicago: Year Book, 1972.

Salmon, S. E. Immunoglobulin synthesis and tumor kinetics of multiple myeloma. *Semin. Hematol.* 10:135, 1973.

Schwartz, R. S. (ed.) *Progress in Clinical Immunology.* New York: Grune & Stratton, 1974. Vol. II.

Snapper, I., and Kahn, A. *Myelomatosis Fundamentals and Clinical Features.* Baltimore: University Park Press, 1971.

Waldenstrom, J. *Diagnosis and Treatment of Multiple Myeloma.* New York: Grune & Stratton, 1970.

Wells, J. V., and Fridenberg, H. H. Paraproteinenias. *DM:* 1, 1974.

Wintrobe, M. M., et al Plasma Cell Dyscrasias, Multiple Myeloma; Macroglobulinemia, Heavy Chain Diseases, and other Lymphocyte and Plasma Cell Dyscrasias. In M. M. Wintrobe, et al (eds.), *Clinical Hematology* (7th ed.). Philadelphia: Lea & Febiger, 1974.

Infectious Mononucleosis

Evans, A. S. Chapter 107, Infectious Mononucleosis. In W. J. Williams, E. Beutler, A. J. Erslev, and R. W. Rundles (eds.), *Hematology* (2nd ed.). New York: McGraw-Hill, 1977.

Hoaglin, R. J. *Infectious Mononucleosis.* New York: Grune & Stratton, 1967.

Metz, E. N. Infectious Mononucleosis. In C. E. Mengel, et al (eds.), *Hematology: Principles and Practice.* Chicago: New York, 1972.

Stites, D. P., and Leikola, J. Infectious mononucleosis. *Semin. Hematol.* 8:243, 1971.

Wintrobe, M. M., et al Infectious Mononucleosis. In M. M. Wintrobe, et al (eds.), *Clinical Hematology* (7th ed.). Philadelphia: Lea & Febiger, 1974.

11 : Hemostasis

NORMAL HEMOSTASIS

Hemostasis is initiated by vascular injury and culminates in the formation of a firm mechanical barrier that prevents the free escape of blood from the damaged vessel. Three groups of reactions must occur in a concerted fashion to effect hemostasis (Fig. 12). Each alone is insufficient to prevent bleeding. The first series of reactions leads to the building up at the site of vascular injury of a mechanical plug composed of platelets. Second, the platelet plug is stabilized by the activation of the coagulation mechanism, which generates thrombin, leading to the deposition of fibrin that strengthens the friable platelet plug. Finally, a series of limiting reactions prevents the unchecked evolution of thrombin and confines the hemostatic process to the site of vascular injury. The hemostatic mechanism can be effective only in constricted blood vessels, since the full axial force of an unhampered blood flow would disrupt the forming plug.

Primary Hemostasis

Primary hemostasis is initiated when vascular injury disrupts the endothelium, exposing subendothelial connective tissue to the flowing blood (Fig. 13). Platelets are attracted to subendothelial collagen and adhere to the collagen fibers. As platelets adhere, they undergo a series of alterations collectively termed the *release reaction*. A marginal band of circumferential microtubules contracts, forcing the contents of storage granules into an open canalicular system that extends to the surface of the platelet. Among the components extruded from the platelet are calcium, serotonin, proteolytic enzymes, cationic proteins, and the nucleotide adenosine diphosphate (ADP). ADP itself has a marked effect on platelets. It causes them to swell, and it causes the platelet membranes to become "sticky," so that platelets adhere to each other. As they do so, they undergo the release reaction, liberating more ADP. Therefore ADP serves as a chemical mediator and amplifier of the initial stimulus triggered by vascular injury. If the platelets are normal in number and function, the self-perpetuating process of ADP-mediated platelet accumulation results in the formation of large platelet aggregates that cap the area of endothelial injury.

A second chemical mediator may also participate in the buildup of the platelet plug. As the platelets adhere to collagen, membrane phospholipases are activated, cleaving arachidonic acid, a

Fig. 12 : The normal hemostatic sequence

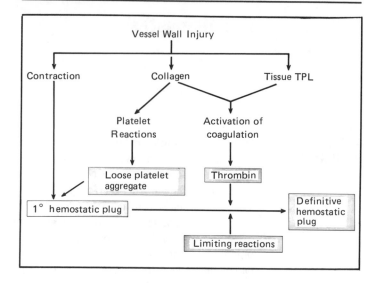

long-chain unsaturated fatty acid, from platelet phospholipids. A second platelet enzyme, cyclo-oxygenase, transforms the arachidonic acid into a cyclic endoperoxide, and a third platelet enzyme, thromboxane synthetase, further transforms the endoperoxide into a labile substance called thromboxane A_2, which is liberated from the platelet. Like ADP, thromboxane A_2 is a potent platelet aggregating agent, but in addition it is a powerful vasoconstrictor, perhaps maintaining the vessel constriction necessary for normal hemostasis. The relative roles of ADP and thromboxane A_2 in normal hemostasis are not yet clear, but both appear to be important.

The formation of the primary hemostatic plug is critically dependent on platelet number and function and on the ability of blood vessels to constrict. Primary hemostasis is independent of the coagulation mechanism. *The integrity of the primary hemostatic sequence is measured by the bleeding time;* coagulation tests do not measure the formation of the primary hemostatic plug.

Coagulation Mechanism

The primary hemostatic mechanism is sufficient to produce temporary cessation of bleeding, but definitive hemostasis requires the participation of the clotting mechanism to stabilize the hemostatic plug.

The central reaction in the coagulation mechanism is the conversion of prothrombin to thrombin, a proteolytic enzyme that cleaves fibrinogen to form fibrin (Figure 14). Two pathways lead to the conversion of prothrombin to thrombin. Both pathways are composed of linked proteolytic enzymes which serve first as substrates and then as active enzymes. Since both culminate in

Fig. 13 : Primary hemostasis. Platelets adhere to subendothelial collagen (1). They release ADP and liberate thromboxanes (2). They aggregate (3) in response to ADP and thromboxanes, causing further aggregation. As they aggregate, platelets change shape, making phospholipids (PF$_3$) available on their membrane. A component of Factor VIII (the von Willebrand factor, VWF) is required for adherence of platelet masses to connective tissue.

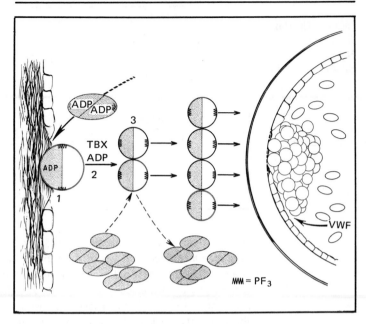

the activation of prothrombin, and since prothrombin itself has been extensively characterized, a detailed consideration of its biochemistry will serve as a model for many of the reactions of the other clotting proteins. In this discussion the active form of a clotting protein is indicated by the letter a.

Prothrombin. Prothrombin is a glycoprotein with an approximate molecular weight of 70,000 daltons. The concentration of prothrombin in blood is about 70 μg per milliliter, or I μM. In its intact, or zymogen form, prothrombin is a single chain with several internal loops formed by disulfide bonds. The active form of the enzyme, thrombin, has a molecular weight of approximately 35,000. The sequence of reactions that leads to the splitting of prothrombin by activated factor X (Xa) has been reviewed in detail in recent articles included in the references to this chapter. Factor Xa cleaves prothrombin at two sites. The first cleavage splits prothrombin into two pieces of approximately equal size, fragment 1.2 and prethrombin. The second scission occurs within prethrombin to produce thrombin, a two-chain enzyme, whose chains are linked by a disulfide bridge.

The rate of conversion of prothrombin to thrombin by Xa, however, is exceedingly slow in the absence of three cofactors: Ca^{2+}, phospholipid, and another clotting protein, Factor V. Prothrombin is linked to the phospholipid surface by ionized calcium, which binds both to the lipid and to the fragment 1 region of prothrombin. Factor Xa is also bound to the phospholipid by

Fig 14 : The clotting mechanism. Factors in boxes require Vitamin K for their complete synthesis. Reactions requiring Ca^{++} are included in the inner rectangle.

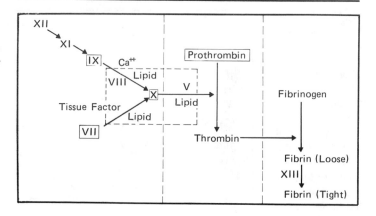

calcium. Factor V associates with lipid directly in the absence of calcium. Once trace amounts of thrombin are generated, Factor V is altered so that it, too, binds to prothrombin at the fragment 2 region. The mutual association of factor Xa, altered factor V, and prothrombin on the lipid surface provides a mechanism by which the reactants are brought close to each other in a critical configuration. It has been estimated that the cumulative effect of the accessory factors increases the rate of thrombin generation from prothrombin by as much as 20,000 times that observed for factor Xa alone; that is, in the presence of cofactors, as much thrombin is generated in 1 minute as would be generated in 2 weeks by factor Xa alone.

Although the primary target of thrombin is fibrinogen, thrombin exerts a "feedback" influence on its own generation. In trace amounts thrombin alters Factor V, potentiating its binding to prothrombin and accelerating thrombin generation, but as the concentration of thrombin increases, thrombin digests Factor V and renders it inactive. Similarly thrombin itself may cleave prethrombin, yielding more thrombin, but it may also cleave the fragment 1.2 peptide of prothrombin, preventing the binding of prothrombin to lipid, since the binding sites would be lost from the molecule. Therefore thrombin exerts an initial positive feedback on its own generation, but at higher concentration thrombin damps the rate of its own elaboration.

The reactions among Factor Xa, prothrombin, Factor V, phospholipid, and Ca^{2+} may be summarized as follows:

1. Initial orientation of reactants: Factor Xa, prothrombin, Factor V bound to phospholipid surface by Ca^{2+} (except for V)

2. First Xa cleavage (slow reaction):

$$\text{Prothrombin} \xrightarrow[\text{Ca^{2+}, V, lipid}]{\text{Xa}} \text{Fragment 1.2 + prethrombin}$$

3. Second Xa cleavage (slow reaction):

$$\text{Prethrombin} \xrightarrow[\text{Ca}^{2+},\ \text{V, Lipid}]{\text{Xa}} \text{thrombin}$$

4. Factor V $\xrightarrow{\text{thrombin}}$ Factor Va

5. Accelerated reaction:

$$\text{Prothrombin} \xrightarrow[\text{Ca}^{2+},\ \text{Va, lipid}]{\text{Xa}} \left\{ \frac{\text{prethrombin}}{\text{fragment 1.2}} \right\} \longrightarrow \text{thrombin}$$

6. Further thrombin reactions: potentiation and damping.

From the foregoing summary it is clear that the binding of calcium to the fragment 1 region of prothrombin is critical for optimum thrombin generation. The specific binding sites for calcium have now been identified. Fragment 1 contains 10 glutamic acid residues that are modified by the carboxylation of the γ-carbon to form γ-carboxyglutamic acid. These modified amino acids are the binding sites for calcium. The γ-carboxylation of prothrombin is a posttranslational event; the primary sequence of prothrombin is completed before the carboxylation reaction takes place. One of the most important recent advances in our understanding of the biochemistry of the coagulation proteins is the discovery that vitamin K, a fat-soluble vitamin long known to be required for normal hemostasis, is needed for the carboxylation of specific glutamic acid residues in prothrombin and in Factors VII, IX, and X as well (see Figure 14). In the absence of vitamin K no carboxylation of the glutamic acid residues in fragment 1 occurs; calcium is not bound; neither prothrombin nor Factor X is linked to phospholipids; the critical orientation of the reactants does not take place; and the rate of prothrombin conversion to thrombin is minimal.

The reactions involving the activation of prothrombin exemplify many of the characteristics of the coagulation mechanism that distinguish it from other proteolytic systems:

1. Linked conversion of inert zymogens to active serine proteases
2. Localization of reactants at surfaces
3. Participation of cofactors that facilitate localization and that also serve as sites for autoregulation of the kinetics of coagulation.

Intrinsic Pathway. Having considered prothrombin in detail, we can now examine the pathways that lead to its activation. The first of these is the *intrinsic blood clotting system,* so named because all its components normally circulate in blood. The intrinsic pathway is activated by vascular injury, which exposes subendothelial tissue to blood. The first component of the pathway is Factor XII, or Hageman factor. Factor XII, a protein of approximately 80,000 daltons, is bound to the exposed subendothelial surface, where it undergoes a limited conformational change that allows it to react with another plasma protein, prekallikrein, converting it to the active proteolytic enzyme, kallikrein. The reaction between surface-bound Factor XII and prekallikrein requires the presence of a cofactor, high molecular weight (HMW) kininogen, which circulates in a complex with prekallikrein. Kallikrein, the active proteolytic enzyme, feeds back on surface-bound Factor XII, cleaving the zymogen into two portions, a fragment of 28,000 daltons that contains a fully active serine protease site and is thus called XIIa, and an inert fragment of 52,000 daltons. The reaction between kallikrein and XII also requires HMW kininogen. Factor XIIa then attacks the next coagulation zymogen, Factor XI, or PTA. Recent evidence suggests that factor XI also circulates bound as a complex with HMW kininogen and that its activation by XIIa is also augmented by HMW kininogen. In these reactions, the surface appears to play a passive role upon which bound factor XII and the prekallikrein–HMW kininogen complex and the Factor XI–HMW kininogen complex can interact.

In addition to the activation of Factor XI, two other reactions occur as coagulation is initiated. Factor XIIa directly activates the fibrinolytic system by cleaving precursors of plasmin, the active fibrinolytic enzyme. Furthermore, kallikrein cleaves the HMW kininogen with which it is associated to yield bradykinin. Therefore we may summarize the initial reactions in the intrinsic coagulation pathway as follows:

1. Initial orientation of reactants: Factor XII and the HMW kininogen–prekallikrein complex and the HMW kininogen–Factor XI complex bind to subendothelial connective tissue exposed by vascular injury;

2. First factor XII reaction (limited)

$$\text{Prekallikrein} \xrightarrow[\text{HMW kininogen}]{\text{XII}} \text{kallikrein}$$

3. Factor XII cleavage

$$\text{Factor XII} \xrightarrow[\text{HMW kininogen}]{\text{kallikrein}} \text{XIIa + fragments}$$

4. Factor XI activation

$$\text{Factor XI} \xrightarrow[\text{HMW kininogen}]{\text{XIIa}} \text{XIa}$$

5. Other reactions

$$\text{Plasminogen precursors} \xrightarrow{\text{XIIa}} \text{plasmin}$$
$$\text{HMW kininogen} \xrightarrow{\text{kallikrein}} \text{bradykinin}$$

Factor XIa, which is surface-bound, activates factor IX (PTC, or

Christmas factor) in a two-step reaction that requires calcium. First, single-chain Factor IX (MW $\sim$ 60,000) is cleaved to form a two-chain intermediate. A peptide is then cleaved from the heavy chain, exposing the active serine-protease site. The next reaction, that between IXa and X, requires calcium, phospholipid, and a cofactor, Factor VIII (antihemophilic factor). These reactions are analogous to those leading to the generation of thrombin. Both Factors IX and X are vitamin K-dependent, in that they contain γ-carboxyglutamic acid residues that bind calcium and thereby link them to phospholipid surfaces. The mechanism by which Factor VIII serves as a cofactor is not understood. Factor VIII is an enormous protein with a molecular weight of at least 1.5 to 2×10^6 daltons. It is composed of repeating identical subunits (MW $\sim$ 200,000 daltons), but the portion of the molecule responsible for its procoagulant activity has not been isolated. The procoagulant activity of Factor VIII, like that of Factor V, is affected by thrombin. Thrombin initially potentiates the action of Factor VIII and then, on prolonged exposure, inactivates Factor VIII. In the presence of Factor VIII, Factor IXa cleaves Factor X. Factor X, a glycoprotein with a molecular weight of 55,000 daltons, has two chains: a heavy chain with a molecular weight of $\sim$ 30,000 daltons and a light chain with a molecular weight of $\sim$ 19,000 daltons. Its activation by Factor IXa results in the release of a glycopeptide from the heavy chain, exposing the active serine protease site. A further small fragment of Xa may be released autocatalytically. Factor Xa is then bound to the lipid surface and is thereby oriented to participate in the subsequent reactions with prothrombin and factor V. We may summarize the reactions leading to the activation of factor X as follows:

1. Activation of Factor IX

$$\text{IX} \xrightarrow[\text{Ca}^{2+}]{\text{XIa}} \text{IXa}$$

2. "Activation" of Factor VIII

$$\text{VIII} \xrightarrow{\text{thrombin}} \text{"activated" factor VIII}$$

3. Orientation of reactants

$$\text{IXa, VIII} \xrightarrow[\text{phospholipid}]{\text{Ca}^{2+}} \text{lipid-bound IXa, VIII}$$

4. Activation of Factor X

$$\text{X} \xrightarrow[\text{VIII, lipid Ca}^{2+}]{\text{IXa}} \text{Xa (lipid-bound)}$$

5. Other reactions

$$\text{"activated" VIII} \xrightarrow{\text{thrombin}} \text{Inactive VIII}$$

In the reactions that constitute the intrinsic clotting pathway the phospholipid surface required for the reactions among Factors IXa, VIII, and X and those among Xa, V, and prothrombin is provided by the platelet surface membrane. Circulating intact platelets do not have the appropriate membrane configuration, but when they undergo the change in shape that follows adherence and aggregation, platelet membranes then provide the appropriate phospholipid configuration to promote the interaction of clotting proteins. The platelet membrane phospholipid is termed *platelet factor three* (PF$_3$).

Extrinsic Pathway. A second pathway, *the extrinsic clotting mechanism,* also leads to the activation of Factor X. A circulating clotting factor, Factor VII, can directly cleave Factor X, but it must first interact with *tissue factor,* a protein released from endothelial cells and other tissues (brain, lung, uterus) by injury. Factor VII is a glycoprotein with a molecular weight of $\sim$ 60,000 daltons. It circulates as a single-chain glycoprotein within which are several residues of γ-carboxyglutamic acid, whose formation requires vitamin K. Upon activation it is converted to a two-chain structure with full coagulant activity, reflecting exposure of an active serine site. Tissue factor must be complexed to phospholipid to serve as a cofactor for Factor VII. Presumably Factor VII forms a complex with tissue factor and phospholipid through the γ-carboxyglutamic acid calcium-binding mechanism.

The exact mechanism by which Factor VII is activated is not fully understood. Several active clotting enzymes including XIIa, kallikrein, plasmin, IXa, and Xa activate Factor VII, but which is primary is not certain. One of the unusual features of Factor VII is that it possesses inherent but limited clotting activity in its single-chain form. When Factor VII is fully activated, it cleaves Factor X at sites that are the same as those split by Factor IXa. Therefore activated Factor VII in the presence of tissue factor bypasses the intrinsic system and provides an alternative mechanism for the activation of X. The interaction between Factor VII and X provides an additional example of autoregulation of coagulation. Two-chain factor VII cleaves Factor X. Factor Xa cleaves single-chain Factor VII to produce two-chain Factor VII. Prolonged incubation of Factor VII with Factor Xa inactivates Factor VII.

The reactions of the intrinsic system are not easily summarized, since the exact mechanism and order of reactions are not yet precisely known, but one formulation is as follows:

1. Intact tissue $\xrightarrow{\text{injury}}$ exposed tissue factor–phospholipid complex

2. Single-chain VII $\xrightarrow[\text{lipid complex}]{\text{tissue factor}}$ Single-chain VII-tissue factor- lipid complex

3. X $\xrightarrow[\text{tissue factor – lipid complex}]{\text{single chain VII}}$ Xa (limited reaction)

4. Single-chain VII $\xrightarrow{\text{Xa}}$ Two-chain VII

5. X $\xrightarrow[\text{Tissue factor-lipid}]{\text{Two-chain VII}}$ Xa (rapid reaction)

Other reactions

Two-chain VII $\xrightarrow{\text{Xa}}$ Inactive VII

Single-chain VII $\xrightarrow[\text{kallikrein, plasmin}]{\text{IXa, XIIa}}$ Two-chain VII

Since both XIIa and IXa can activate VII, the distinction between the two pathways may seem blurred, but physiologically they function as independent mechanisms. Patients with hereditary deficiencies of components of the intrinsic system bleed, although they have normal levels of Factor VII. Conversely, patients with hereditary Factor VII deficiency bleed, although their intrinsic system is intact. Both systems are required for optimal activation of factor X and subsequent conversion of prothrombin to thrombin.

Fibrin. Once thrombin is formed from prothrombin, it reacts with fibrinogen. Fibrinogen is a molecule composed of three pairs of chains, termed Aα, Bβ, and γ. Thrombin cleaves peptide bonds in the Aα and Bβ chains, releasing peptide fragments A and B. The resulting protein *fibrin* now consists of three pairs of chains α, β, and γ.

Fibrin monomer polymerizes with itself in end-to-end and end-to-side links, forming large meshworks that become insoluble ropy strands. These polymers are at first held together only by hydrogen bonding, but another clotting protein, Factor XIII, or fibrin stabilizing factor (itself activated by thrombin), introduces covalent bonds in the fibrin. Fibrin winds about the platelet aggregates at the site of vascular injury, converting the unstable platelet plug to a firm plug, providing definitive hemostasis.

Limiting Reactions   If unchecked, the generation of thrombin by the clotting cascade could lead to excessive vessel occlusion. Several types of limiting reactions confine the hemostatic plug to the site of vascular injury. The first of these is blood flow itself. As the vessel relaxes, returning blood flow dilutes activated clotting constituents and mechanically opposes continued hemostatic plug growth. Furthermore, both arterial and venous endothelial and smooth muscle cells can form a prostaglandin derivative, PGI_2, which is the most powerful inhibitor of platelet aggregation yet described. The importance of this compound as an endogenous limiting factor in hemostatic plug formation is not yet established. In addition, local inhibitors inactivate clotting intermediates. Of these, antithrombin may be the most significant. Hepatic clearance mechanisms remove circulating activated clotting factors.

One of the most important defense mechanisms is the fibrinolytic system. The active fibrinolytic enzyme, plasmin, digests both fibrin and fibrinogen. Plasmin is derived from its circulating zymogen, plasminogen. Vascular injury releases plasminogen activator from endothelial cells. Furthermore, activated factor XII itself leads to plasmin activation. Therefore the fibrinolytic system is triggered by the same stimuli that initiate clotting. Fibrinolysis and coagulation are both normal components of the hemostatic response to vascular injury. The digestion of fibrinogen by plasmin occurs at sites distinct from those susceptible to thrombin and proceeds through several stages. Early in the course of digestion plasmin cleaves small fragments from fibrinogen. The partly degraded fibrinogen can still react with thrombin, but it clots slowly, if at all. Therefore, the early plasmin digests of fibrinogen act as powerful anticoagulants, since they tie up thrombin with poorly functioning substrates. As plasmin reacts more extensively with fibrinogen, it produces smaller fibrinogen derivatives, which no longer bind thrombin. These fragments, however, do become incorporated into forming fibrin polymers, slowing the rate of polymerization, and weakening the resulting fibrin meshwork. Therefore the attack of plasmin on fibrinogen produces fragments that impede the thrombin-mediated formation of fibrin (Fig. 15). Interaction of the fibrinolytic system with the clotting cascade is essential in maintaining the patency of small blood vessels following injury.

Normal Platelet Physiology

Platelets are circulating cytoplasmic fragments derived from marrow precursors, megakaryocytes. In the marrow, primordial stem cells differentiate into three types of committed stem cells, each of which produces either red cells, white cells, or platelets. Committed stem cells, by definition, give rise either to new committed stem cells (thereby regenerating the precursor pool) or to cells that are destined to mature into the specific marrow cell line. Megakaryocytes mature from stem cells in a unique fashion, for they undergo nuclear division without cytoplasmic division. Therefore the earliest megakaryocyte (the "megakaryoblast") is diploid (2N), but on continued maturation nuclear components increase to 4N, 8N, 16N, and even to 32N. With each nuclear division the cytoplasmic mass increases. At any point in this process nuclear division may cease (it usually does so at 8N or 32N) and

Fig. 15 : Inter-
actions between
fibrinogen split pro-
ducts and thrombin-
mediated reactions.
Early split products
impair fibrin mono-
mer formation. Late
split products im-
pair fibrin monomer
polymerization.

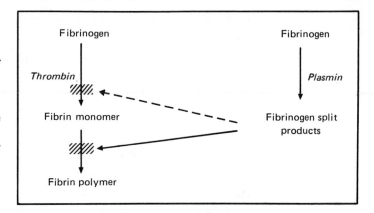

a second stage of maturation begin. Specific cytoplasmic or-
ganelles are formed, including the mitochondria and storage
granules that characterize the platelet. The megakaryocyte then
enters the third stage of maturation, as a network of demarcation
membranes invaginates from the plasma membrane, dividing the
cytoplasm into 50 or more compartments. Finally the cell rup-
tures, releasing the cytoplasmic segments, the platelets, into the
marrow sinusoid and thence into the bloodstream.

The process of megakaryocyte maturation and release is controlled by thrombopoietin, a regulatory hormone akin to erythropoietin. Thrombopoietin increases the number of committed
stem cells that enter into the maturation cycle; it increases the
number of nuclear divisions, thereby increasing cytoplasmic mass
and the ultimate number of platelets derived from each megakaryocyte; and it increases the rate of cytoplasmic maturation
and platelet release.

Once platelets are liberated into the circulation, they survive for
approximately 10 days. Of the total platelet mass, approximately
two-thirds circulates in the bloodstream. The remainder is sequestered in the spleen. In splenectomized patients the platelet count
rises sharply but transiently. By contrast, in patients with hypersplenism the platelet count is reduced because of splenic trapping
of the platelets.

Circulating platelets perform several functions. The first and
clearly the most important is the formation of the mechanical
hemostatic plug. In addition to ADP and thromboxane another
constituent is required for effective platelet plug formation. The
clotting protein Factor VIII is apparently made up of two components, one of which facilitates the interactions among clotting
Factor IX, calcium, phospholipid, and Factor X. The other component is required for the adherence of platelets to subendothelial
tissue. The mechanism by which Factor VIII protein participates

in the adherence of platelets to subendothelial tissue is unknown, since collagen will bind to platelets in its absence.

A second platelet function is to furnish the phospholipid surface necessary for the interactions of the clotting factors of the intrinsic pathway. A third platelet function is to furnish a cationic protein, called platelet factor 4, which neutralizes the action of heparin, a highly acidic anticoagulant. Platelets play an important role in restoring vascular integrity following injury. They secrete a factor or factors that stimulate(s) vascular smooth muscle cells to multiply, and thereby speed vascular repair.

Platelets also cause the phenomenon of clot retraction. When whole blood clots in a test tube, the clot slowly retracts, expressing serum from its interstices. The contraction is due to the platelet protein, thrombasthenin, which causes platelet pseudopods, to which fibrin adheres, to retract, compressing the clot. The role of retraction in hemostasis is not certain, but it may be important in plug stabilization.

Basic Tests of Hemostatic Function

In this book only those tests are described that are necessary for a preliminary assessment of hemostasis and its disorders. More detailed procedures can be found in more extended texts and in laboratory manuals.

History. The most important test of hemostasis is a thoughtful and complete history. Information to be sought includes family history of bleeding, age at onset of symptoms, location of bleeding, relation to trauma or surgery (description of response to dental extraction is helpful), diet, association with other illness, and ingestion of drugs. The pattern of inheritance of a bleeding disorder often points to a specific diagnosis: the two most common hereditary defects of the clotting system (Factor VIII and Factor IX deficiencies) are sex-linked recessive disorders. Certain defects are transmitted in an autosomal dominant pattern, while others are transmitted as autosomal recessives. Hereditary disorders are manifest soon after birth; acquired disorders may occur at any time. Disorders of the clotting system often produce bleeding into joints, while platelet abnormalities usually are associated with bleeding into the skin and mucus membranes. Bleeding that follows immediately after trauma usually reflects impaired primary hemostasis. By contrast, delayed onset of bleeding usually is due to a disorder of the clotting pathways. Diets depleted of vitamins may induce bleeding due to deficiencies of vitamin C or of vitamin K, particularly if broad spectrum antibiotics are also given. Ingestion of certain drugs, notably aspirin-containing compounds, may unmask mild bleeding disorders and produce frank hemorrhagic symptoms.

Platelet Counting. Enumeration of platelets is usually done either with an electronic counter or with a phase contrast microscope. An accurate estimate of the platelet count can be obtained from the standard blood film, however. A normal oil immersion field should contain about 15 to 30 platelets.

The bleeding time is a very useful assessment of primary hemostasis. In our laboratory we use only the Ivy bleeding time method and employ a template or a mechanical spring–driven blade to produce a standard incision on the forearm. The test is performed by inflating a blood pressure cuff on the arm to 40 mm of mercury and then making two incisions on the forearm. The time elapsed until bleeding ceases is recorded. The test should ordinarily not be performed if the platelet count is reduced below 80,000 per microliter. The bleeding time reflects vascular contraction, platelet function, and the participation of the non-clotting portion of the Factor VIII molecule, but it does not reflect the activity of the clotting pathways.

Prothrombin Time. The prothrombin time (PT) is a widely used test of coagulation. It measures the entire extrinsic pathway (its name is a misnomer). Whole blood is collected into an anticoagulant (usually citrate) that binds calcium and renders the blood incoagulable. The blood is centrifuged, and cell-free plasma is obtained. Tissue factor (usually a commercial preparation) is added, and the time to form a fibrin clot is recorded, usually by an automated device. The prothrombin time measures the activity of Factors VII, X, II, V, and I (fibrinogen). A deficiency of any of these factors prolongs the prothrombin time and so does an inhibitor directed against any of those factors. The test is unaffected by variations of Factors XII, XI, IX, and VIII or of platelets.

Partial Thromboplastin Time. The partial thromboplastin time (PTT) measures the intrinsic pathway of coagulation. Plasma is incubated with a finely powdered diatomaceous earth, usually kaolin, to provide maximal surface activation of Factor XII, and with phospholipids, to provide a platelet lipid substitute. Calcium is added, and the time to form a clot is measured. The test measures the activities of Factors XII, XI, IX, VIII, X, V, II (prothrombin) but is insensitive to VII or to platelets. The PTT is also prolonged by deficiencies of HMW kininogen or kallikrein.

Thrombin Time. The thrombin time is measured by adding a dilute solution of thrombin to plasma and recording the time to form a clot. The test measures the reactivity of plasma fibrinogen.

A normal prothrombin time establishes the integrity of the extrinsic pathway. A prolonged prothrombin time can reflect an isolated clotting factor abnormality or multiple defects. A normal partial thromboplastin time establishes the integrity of the intrinsic pathway. A normal prothrombin time, but prolonged partial thromboplastin time, suggests abnormalities of Factors XII, XI, IX, or VIII, singly or in combination. A prolonged prothrombin time but normal partial thromboplastin time suggests Factor VII deficiency. Prolongation of both tests suggests multiple deficiencies or an isolated depression of X, V, II, or I. The latter can be excluded by a normal thrombin time. More specific diagnoses require special coagulation assays of individual clotting factors. Circulating inhibitors may prolong all the routine clotting tests or may be directed at only a single clotting factor.

Disorders of Primary Hemostasis

The three major categories of abnormal primary hemostatic plug formation are vascular defects, quantitative disorders of platelets, and qualitative disorders of platelet function.

Vascular Defects

Vascular defects are of three types. Hereditary hemorrhagic telangiectasia (Osler-Weber-Rendu disease) is an autosomal dominant disorder characterized by the presence of small hemangiomas in the skin, gastrointestinal tract mucosa, nostrils, and occasionally in the lungs, liver, and spleen. Epistaxis and gastrointestinal bleeding are common. No specific therapy is available. Allergic purpura, or *vasculitis,* is caused by immune mechanisms that produce vascular necrosis, resulting in local bleeding into affected organs. Vasculitis may result from drug ingestion or it may follow certain viral infections. In many instances no etiology can be identified. When the vasculitis is manifested by skin lesions and joint and abdominal pain, it is termed *Henoch-Schönlein purpura.* This form of vasculitis occurs most often in children but may also be seen in adults. A third type of vascular defect reflects an intrinsic abnormality of the connective tissue supporting blood vessels. Vascular fragility may be due to inherited disorders of connective tissues, or it may reflect the consequences of prolonged steroid therapy or of vitamin C deficiency (scurvy).

Quantitative Platelet Disorders

Thrombocytopenia. Quantitative disorders of platelets are the most common cause of defects of primary hemostasis, and of these thrombocytopenia predominates. Thrombocytopenia may reflect decreased marrow production, increased peripheral destruction, increased sequestration of platelets in the spleen, or dilution by transfusion of blood products depleted of viable platelets. Decreased marrow production of platelets may occur in septic states, in uremia, following ionizing radiation, or as a result of replacement of the bone marrow by metastatic carcinoma, but the most common cause of marrow failure in clinical practice reflects the increasing use of drugs for chemotherapy of malignant disorders. Virtually all antitumor drugs suppress the marrow, and some agents, particularly cytosine arabinoside and alkylating drugs, cause severe thrombocytopenia. Folic acid deficiency, vitamin B_{12} deficiency, and excess alcohol ingestion may suppress platelet production as well. Hereditary disorders that cause thrombocytopenia are extremely rare but do occur.

Increased platelet destruction is most often due to immune mechanisms. Although many drugs cause thrombocytopenia, antibodies have been demonstrated to only a few. Quinidine induces the formation of an antiquinidine antibody. In the presence of quinidine the drug–antibody complex binds to the surface of the platelet. Complement is fixed, and the platelet is injured, resulting in its prompt removal by the spleen. Presumably, immune destruction of platelets caused by other drugs reflects a similar process. Idiopathic thrombocytopenic purpura (ITP) is an immune disorder that occurs in acute and chronic forms. Acute ITP is primarily a disease of children. Profound thrombocytopenia begins abruptly, usually several days to two weeks following a viral infection. Usually severe bleeding does not occur. The disease is often self-limited, lasting for a few weeks to a few months. In older children and adults ITP may run a more chronic course, beginning insidiously and remitting slowly. A circulating 7S gamma globulin, specific for platelets, is present and may be transmitted to the fetus if a pregnant woman develops ITP. Therapy with steroids often causes remission, but relapses may occur and may be an indication for splenectomy.

Posttransfusion purpura is a rare cause of thrombocytopenia. In addition to the common tissue-specific (HLA) antigens, platelets have specific antigens, among which the Pl^{A1} is the most important, present in over 98 percent of the population. Should a Pl^{A1}-negative donor receive Pl^{A1}-positive platelets, severe thrombocytopenia may develop, suggesting that antibodies directed against the donor's Pl^{A1}-positive platelets may form complexes that coat the recipient's Pl^{A1}-negative platelets, causing their destruction.

Nonimmune mechanisms also cause increased peripheral destruction of platelets. The *hemolytic-uremic syndrome* is a childhood disorder of unknown cause that results in vascular damage, most pronounced in the kidneys. Platelet-fibrin thrombi are deposited in the renal microcirculation. Red cells fragment as they are filtered through the fibrin beds, causing severe hemolysis. Platelet consumption by the thrombotic process is marked, and severe thrombocytopenia may occur. Renal failure is a direct consequence of the blocked renal vasculature. The severity of the disease is variable. Milder forms often remit spontaneously. In more severe cases, profound renal damage may cause death. Although steroids, antiplatelet agents, and anticoagulant drugs have been used to treat severe forms of the hemolytic-uremic syndrome, no clear evidence for their usefulness has been established.

Thrombotic thrombocytopenic purpura is a similar but more severe disorder that affects adults. The vascular damage is more widespread, usually involving the brain as well as the kidneys. The disorder is usually fatal, but recent attempts to treat it with corticosteroids, by splenectomy, or by exchange transfusion have been successful, for reasons not yet established. Other causes of increased peripheral destruction include localized increased consumption by coagulation within cavernous hemangiomas (the Kasabach-Merrit syndrome) and generalized increased consumption in the syndrome of *disseminated intravascular coagulation,* (see subsequent discussion under that heading).

Decreased platelet counts may also be caused by increased sequestration in enlarged spleens (*hypersplenism*) or may result from transfusion of banked blood or plasma that is devoid of viable platelets. The rapid transfusion of 8 or more units of these products usually causes moderate to marked thrombocytopenia, which can be prevented by the administration of fresh blood or of platelets as a routine measure during massive blood transfusion.

Bone marrow examination often helps distinguish among the causes of thrombocytopenia. When thrombocytopenia reflects decreased production, the marrow contains few megakaryocytes. Often other early cell precursors are also diminished. By contrast, when thrombocytopenia is due to increased peripheral destruction or increased splenic sequestration, the marrow contains numerous large megakaryocytes, reflecting thrombopoietin stimulation. The marrow is usually normal in acute dilutional thrombocytopenia.

Thrombocytosis. Thrombocytosis, an increase in the number of circulating platelets (usually above 1×10^6 per microliter), may be either *reactive* or *autonomous. Reactive thrombocytosis* denotes a condition in which the elevated platelet count is accompanied by increased numbers of megakaryocytes but in which the megakaryocyte size and ploidy are diminished. Therefore, although the marrow production of platelets is stimulated, the process is regulated. Reactive thrombocytosis occurs in conditions such as chronic infection, nonhematologic malignancies, and mild iron deficiency anemia. The stimulus to increased platelet formation is unknown. The platelets that circulate are normal in size and function. They cause neither bleeding nor thrombotic episodes. Therefore the elevated platelet count in reactive thrombocytosis is not an indication for therapy. By contrast *autonomous thrombocytosis* (idiopathic thrombocythemia) is a primary marrow disorder characterized by the presence of enlarged megakaryocytes with increased cytoplasmic mass and ploidy in the presence of an elevated peripheral platelet count. The platelets are abnormal and do not aggregate normally in response to epinephrine and ADP. Both bleeding and thrombotic episodes accompany this disorder and may respond to reduction of the total number of platelets through treatment with alkylating agents, although no firm guidelines for therapy have been established. Autonomous thrombocythemia often occurs in patients with polycythemia vera and may precede the appearance of increased numbers of red cells.

Qualitative Platelet Disorders

Disorders of platelet function can reflect impaired adhesion of platelets to subendothelial tissue, abnormal release of platelet constituents, or inability of platelets to respond to aggregating stimuli. Qualitative platelet disorders may be acquired or hereditary. Characteristically disorders of platelet function cause symptoms typical of impaired primary hemostasis: easy bruising, petechial hemorrhage, epistaxis, and bleeding from mucus membranes. In their milder forms they may escape detection until unmasked by severe trauma, surgical procedures, or the concomitant use of drugs such as aspirin, which impose additional defects on primary hemostatic mechanisms.

Acquired impairment of platelet adhesion to subendothelial connective tissue occurs in disorders that produce abnormal immunoglobulins (multiple myeloma) or macroglobulins (Waldenström's macroglobulinemia) that coat the platelets. Uremia is another major cause of acquired abnormal platelet adhesion. A circulating toxin or group of toxins, not yet clearly defined, prevents platelet adherence to connective tissue. Since many patients with uremia may also be thrombocytopenic, the combined defect of diminished platelet number and impaired function of the remaining platelets may cause severe bleeding into the gastrointestinal tract, pericardial sac, lungs, or brain. Hemodialysis may result in temporary removal of the circulating toxin, transiently restoring or improving platelet function.

Von Willebrand's disease is an inherited disorder of primary hemostasis characterized by diminished levels of Factor VIII protein. Both the coagulant properties of the protein and its platelet-adherence promoting activity are decreased. The nature of the defective platelet adherence in von Willebrand's disease is obscure, since platelets will adhere to collagen normally in vitro even in the absence of Factor VIII protein but fail to adhere normally to subendothelial tissue in patients with von Willebrand's disease. Other aspects of platelet function (response to aggregating agents, release of storage pool contents) are normal in von Willebrand's disease. When patients with von Willebrand's disease are given transfusions of blood products containing Factor VIII protein, they respond by synthesizing Factor VIII coagulant activity. The explanation for this phenomenon is not yet understood. Recently it has been shown that an antibiotic, ristocetin, will clump or agglutinate platelets and that the Factor VIII protein is required for this reaction. Plasma deficient in Factor VIII protein will not support ristocetin-induced platelet aggregation. Although ristocetin has no clinical usefulness, the antibiotic does serve as a useful reagent in the detection of von Willebrand's disease. In severely affected patients the Factor VIII protein is strikingly depressed (it may even be nondetectable), ristocetin-induced aggregation of platelets does not occur, the bleeding time is markedly prolonged, and bleeding is pronounced. In others less affected the bleeding time may be normal, ristocetin-induced aggregation may occur, and clinical symptoms may be mild. Factor VIII protein, however, is usually depressed below the normal range.

Von Willebrand's disease is transmitted with an autosomal dominant pattern of inheritance. The severity of the disease varies widely from generation to generation, and within families siblings may also have discrepant degrees of bleeding. Indeed, in a single patient the severity of symptoms may fluctuate, presumably reflecting changing degrees of Factor VIII synthesis. In females, pregnancy and ingestion of oral contraceptive agents raise the level of Factor VIII protein, often to normal values. The incidence of von Willebrand's disease is unknown. The introduction of relatively simple tests for Factor VIII protein and the awareness that the disorder may have only mild clinical symptoms have changed the previous concept that von Willebrand's disease is a rare disorder. It may in fact be one of the most frequent of all disorders of hemostasis.

Many drugs impair the release of platelet constituents. The most important are the anti-inflammatory agents that inhibit platelet cyclo-oxygenase, thereby blocking thromboxane A_2 formation. They also impair the release of ADP, serotonin, and Ca^{2+}. The relationship between the release reaction and thromboxane formation is not yet defined, but both are affected by similar agents. Aspirin has the most striking effect on platelets. It irreversibly acetylates certain platelet proteins. Its effect lasts for the entire life span of the platelet. Two hours after a normal subject ingests aspirin, his bleeding time is prolonged and stays elevated for days. Other anti-inflammatory drugs (indomethacin, phenylbutazone) also impair the release reaction, but the duration of their effect is limited to their biologic life span in the blood, usually only a few hours. In most normal subjects the prolongation of the bleeding time following aspirin is of minimal consequence, but in a few otherwise normal people the bleeding time response to aspirin is pronounced and may cause dangerous bleeding if trauma occurs during the peak response to aspirin. If a patient has any other disorder of hemostasis, ingestion may impose a major additional defect and may cause serious bleeding. *Aspirin should ordinarily not be given to patients with known abnormalities of hemostasis* except as a diagnostic challenge under controlled experimental conditions.

Hereditary disorders of the release reaction are of two types. The first is characterized by true impairment of release of the constituents of the storage granules. The concentration of the stored components (ADP, serotonin, Ca^{2+}, fibrinogen, cathepsins) is normal. Furthermore the platelet cytoarchitecture, as assessed by electron microscopy, is normal. However, in those patients in whom it has been measured, thromboxane formation is impaired. The nature of the defect is not understood. In severely affected patients the bleeding time is prolonged and clinical symptoms may be severe. In others the bleeding time may be normal or minimally prolonged. Bleeding may not occur unless an additional burden, such as aspirin ingestion, is incurred. The prevalence of this disorder is unknown, but it may be quite common. The pattern of inheritance is not established. The second form of inherited abnormalities of the release reaction is called *storage pool disease,* because the storage granules themselves are markedly reduced in number. Consequently the concentration of stored constituents is sharply lowered. In addition the morphology of the platelets is abnormal, reflecting the absence of the storage granules. Bleeding is usually severe. This disorder is rare, and its pattern of inheritance is not yet established.

Glanzmann's thrombasthenia is the only well-characterized hereditary disorder of platelet function in which the platelets fail to respond to ADP or other aggregating agents. This extremely rare disease is typified by low platelet-bound fibrinogen, abnormal platelet glycolytic activity, and impaired clot-retraction. It is transmitted as an autosomal recessive disorder.

Coagulation Disorders

Hereditary deficiencies are encountered for each of the clotting factors. Classic hemophilia (functional deficiency of Factor VIII) and Factor IX deficiency are transmitted as sex-linked recessive disorders; all the others are transmitted in an autosomal recessive pattern. Typically, hereditary clotting factor abnormalities are *single.* They are *stable* in their manifestations. They present early in childhood. Recurring bleeding into soft tissues, into the gastrointestinal and urinary tracts, and particularly into weight-bearing joints are characteristic.

Factor XII deficiency is exceedingly rare. Surprisingly, patients with this disorder suffer little or no bleeding. The defect, usually discovered accidentally, manifests itself in abnormal tests of the intrinsic pathway. Similarly, patients with hereditary deficiencies of prekallikrein or high molecular weight kininogen exhibit no untoward bleeding tendencies, although their blood clots abnormally slowly when assayed in vitro by the PTT. Factor XI deficiency, once thought to be rare, is now being diagnosed with increasing frequency. Therefore its incidence is not yet established. The disorder is found more frequently in Jews than in the general population. Spontaneous bleeding is unusual, but bleeding following trauma may be severe.

Factor IX deficiency is a sex-linked, recessive disorder. Therefore only males are clinically affected. Female carriers are usually asymptomatic. The offspring of a Factor IX–deficient male $(X^{-IX} \cdot Y)$ and a normal female $(X \cdot X)$ theoretically would be two normal sons $(X \cdot Y, \ X \cdot Y)$, and two carrier daughters $(X^{-IX} \cdot X)$ $(X^{-IX} \cdot X)$. The offspring of a carrier female $(X^{-IX} \cdot X)$ and a normal male $(X \cdot Y)$ would be a normal son $(X \cdot Y)$, one factor IX–deficient son $(X^{-IX} \cdot Y)$, one carrier daughter $(X^{-IX} \cdot X)$, and one normal daughter $(X \cdot X)$. Therefore all daughters of affected males are carriers, half the daughters of carriers are themselves carriers, and half the sons are affected. The incidence of the disorder is approximately 1 in 100,000. Bleeding is usually severe, resulting in crippling deformity of joints and repeated hemorrhage into soft tissues and viscera.

Classic hemophilia is a sex-linked recessive disease caused by a functional abnormality of the Factor VIII protein. For decades classic hemophilia was thought to be due to *absence* of Factor VIII, the antihemophilic globulin. We now recognize, however, that the Factor VIII protein contains at least two distinct components, or regions. One component is necessary for coagulation: it promotes the interaction of Factor IX and Factor X. A second region is required for normal adhesion of platelet aggregates. In hemophilia the clotting function of the Factor VIII protein is ablated, but the platelet-adhering component is normal. In von Willebrand's disease the concentration of the entire protein is diminished; therefore *both* the coagulant and platelet adherence-promoting activities are diminished. Classic hemophilia is the most frequently encountered hereditary disorder of the clotting proteins, occurring in 1 in 10,000-25,000 persons. One problem in establishing accurate estimates of its prevalence is the wide variation in Factor VIII levels in the normal population. The introduction of new methods for measuring the level of Factor VIII protein, as well as clotting activity, has made the diagnosis of hemophilia and the detection of the carrier state far more accurate.

Not all hemophiliacs are severe bleeders. Some, with less than 1 percent of the normal clotting activity, bleed spontaneously and have the typical disabling bleeding into the joints and other body cavities. Others, with 3 to 5 percent of normal clotting activity, rarely bleed spontaneously but experience hemorrhage after trauma. Those with levels between 5 and 15 percent of normal may escape detection until exposed to severe injury or surgical procedures. Often pronounced bleeding after dental extractions may be the first indication of mild hemophilia. The degree of abnormality is characteristic of the affected family, with little variation in severity from generation to generation. Replacement therapy with highly purified Factor VIII preparations has reduced sharply the incidence of lethal bleeding and has made surgery in hemophiliacs feasible. One of the most serious complications of hemophilia is the development of inhibitors directed against infused Factor VIII, rendering the patient refractory to further replacement therapy.

Deficiencies of Factors II, V, VII and X are each extremely rare. Patients with severe deficiencies have hemorrhagic complications similar to those of classic hemophilia.

Hereditary abnormalities affecting fibrinogen are of two types. In one form the plasma level of fibrinogen is very low, reflecting inadequate fibrinogen production. Surprisingly, bleeding symptoms are often minimal. Dysfibrinogenemia is another hereditary disorder of fibrinogen and is characterized by the production of abnormal fibrinogen molecules which react slowly with thrombin or which polymerize slowly after fibrinopeptides have been released. Again, bleeding symptoms are usually mild. One form of dysfibrinogenemia actually causes a thrombotic tendency. In distinction to other hereditary clotting factor deficiencies, abnormalities of fibrinogen cause prolongation of the thrombin time as well as the PTT and PT.

Hereditary deficiency of Factor XIII causes impaired wound healing, as well as faulty hemostasis. Factor XIII deficiency does not prolong the usual tests of clotting factors. It is detected by assays of the formation of covalent bonds in fibrin.

The principal mode of therapy in all inherited clotting factor deficiencies is replacement of the missing factor. A purified concentrate containing Factors II, VII, IX, and X is available for the treatment of Factor XI deficiency, and highly concentrated preparations of Factor VIII are available for the treatment of classic hemophilia. The most widely used preparation for the treatment of classic hemophilia is cryoprecipitate, a preparation made by freezing plasma and then allowing it to defrost at 4°C.

A precipitate, containing the bulk of the Factor VIII originally present in the plasma, forms. It can be resuspended in small amounts of plasma. Cryoprecipitate is the mainstay of treatment of routine bleeding in classic hemophilia. Because it contains only Factor VIII (and fibrinogen) in enriched amounts, cryoprecipitate is *not* useful for replacement therapy of disorders other than classic hemophilia. The remaining disorders are usually treated, when necessary, with transfusions of fresh frozen plasma, which contains all the clotting factors. Replacement therapy with plasma, however, may be limited by the large volume of fluid that may be required.

In contrast to hereditary clotting abnormalities acquired hemostatic defects are usually *multiple, acute* in onset, and *variable* in severity. One cause of an acquired hemostatic defect is the administration or surreptitious ingestion of warfarin, a drug that retards the synthesis of Factors II, VII, IX, and X. Vitamin K deficiency due to impaired fat absorption or to prolonged parenteral feeding in combination with administration of broad spectrum antibiotics, or arising in hemorrhagic disease of the newborn, also results in depressed synthesis of Factors II, VII, IX, and X. The liver makes virtually all the clotting factors except Factor VIII. Therefore depressed levels of clotting factors can occur in severe hepatic disease. Fibrinolysis may also be evident in advanced liver disease.

Dilution of clotting factors as well as of platelets may occur during massive transfusion therapy. Since Factors V and VIII and platelets do not survive in banked blood, rapid transfusion of many units may severely deplete these components.

Circulating inhibitors to clotting factors may arise following replacement therapy of hereditary deficiency states, but they may also accompany certain chronic illnesses, particularly lupus erythematosus, ulcerative colitis, and rheumatoid arthritis. Powerful inhibitors directed against Factor VIII sometimes occur postpartum or in otherwise healthy, elderly men. Occasionally certain drugs may induce circulating inhibitors as well. Many inhibitors cause little hemostatic difficulty, but some cause serious bleeding. Consumption or excess utilization of clotting factors can result from generalized activation of the hemostatic mechanism. This complex disorder, *disseminated intravascular coagulation,* will be described later.

APPROACH TO PATIENT WITH A SUSPECTED HEMORRHAGIC DISORDER

Evaluation of hemostasis is most commonly required in the preparation of a patient for a surgical procedure. The basic screening routine includes a careful history, complete physical examination, inspection of a blood smear for abnormalities of platelets or other formed elements, and an activated PTT. This routine will detect the vast majority of unsuspected bleeders. The whole blood clotting time and the prothrombin time are *not* adequate screening tests of hemostatic function. If a positive history of prior bleeding has been obtained, or if excess bleeding occurs during operation or in response to trauma, a more detailed examination is required. In addition to the previous procedures, additional tests, including the prothrombin time, thrombin time, and bleeding time (with aspirin challenge) should be done to determine which areas of the hemostatic sequence are involved. More specific tests can then be selected.

If a patient presents with an acute bleeding disorder, assessment must be rapid. If bleeding is confined to a single area, a local cause rather than a generalized hemostatic bleeding disorder should be suspected. Acute generalized bleeding may be caused by dilution of hemostatic constituents by massive transfusion; excess utilization of constituents by either disseminated coagulation or immune destruction; inhibition of clotting factors; failure of synthesis due to hepatic or marrow failure; ingestion of drugs (particularly coumarin anticoagulants or aspirin); dietary deficiency, especially of vitamin K; and generalized vascular injury. In contrast to the stable defect in inherited hemostatic disorders, many acquired causes of bleeding can operate at once. Often in acute bleeding states precise diagnosis and treatment may be impossible or may take too long. Fresh frozen plasma and platelet concentrates provide all the known clotting constituents and prove to be life-saving in emergency settings.

Thrombosis and Antithrombotic Therapy

Thrombosis is not a single pathologic entity. Three forms are separable by pathogenesis, by gross and ultrastructural morphology, by turnover of clotting constituents, and by response to antithrombotic therapy.

The White (Arterial) Thrombus

This lesion is initiated by vascular injury and endothelial denudation. The primary pathologic event is the reaction between platelets and exposed subendothelial tissue. In the forming arterial thrombus the platelet-fibrin mass grows along the wall of the injured vessel. As the thrombus becomes concentric, areas of red cells and fibrin are incorporated, reflecting local generation of thrombin. The continued disruption of the mural thrombus by axial blood flow and the redeposition of new platelet masses give the thrombus a laminar appearance, distinguishing it from the uniformly distributed red cell–fibrin meshwork of a clot that forms in vitro. The crucial features of the arterial thrombus are its genesis from an injured vessel wall and its growth by extension along the injured vessel wall. Only when the lumen becomes almost totally occluded does the coagulation mechanism become dominant.

The Red (Venous) Thrombus

In most venous thrombi there is no evidence for vascular injury in veins with recently formed thrombi, nor in the lining of valve pockets without thrombi. It is likely that turbulent flow in the proximity of valve cusps leads to selective deposition of platelets in such regions and that coagulation is initiated in these areas of turbulent platelet-rich blood. Whatever its cause, the venous thrombus grows by extension of the thrombus into the vein lumen, its propagation occurring primarily through coagulation. The resultant thrombus is composed primarily of red cells and fibrin, but because it grows in slowly flowing blood, platelets become enmeshed in it, giving it also a laminar appearance. The laminar structure of both the arterial and venous thrombus reflects their formation in flowing blood. Although both are distinct from a blood clot formed in vitro, their laminar similarity does not indicate that they share a common pathogenesis.

Disseminated Intravascular Coagulation (DIC)

The normal hemostatic response to vascular injury is a balanced concert of forces (1) that lead to the deposition of the hemostatic plug at the site of the injury and (2) that prevent the extension of the plug beyond the local site. A variety of diseases that lead to widespread vascular injury, such as endotoxinemia and heat stroke, or to the circulation of thromboplastic substances, such as amniotic fluid embolism and certain malignant mucin-secreting tumors, evoke a generalized rather than localized hemostatic response. Whether or not a bleeding diathesis or microvascular thrombosis or both occur depends on a balance of the generation of plasmin, thrombin, and fibrin degradation products. We recognize a spectrum in disseminated activation of the hemostatic mechanism. In disorders characterized by massive release into the circulation of particulate thromboplastin, or in instances in which tissue injury is particularly intense, fibrin deposition predominates, and the clinical consequences are primarily those of infarction. Rarely, certain tumors produce striking systemic fibrinolysis. Evidence of fibrin deposition may be absent, and bleeding predominates. More commonly, evidence is present for the elaboration of both thrombin and plasmin, but these come into balance, with little clinical evidence of bleeding or thrombosis although coagulation tests are grossly disturbed.

No generally available tests by themselves are diagnostic of disseminated intravascular coagulation. The most consistent findings are prolongation of the thrombin time, depression of fibrinogen, lowered platelet count, and the presence of fibrin-fibrinogen degradation products. In many cases, however, one or more of these abnormalities may not be present. It is difficult to make the diagnosis of disseminated intravascular coagulation in the presence of a normal thrombin time. Clotting factor levels are quite variable. They may be elevated, depressed, or unchanged. Red cell fragmentation is helpful when present but must be distinguished from other causes of abnormal red cell morphology.

The major challenge of this syndrome lies not in the diagnosis or therapy of the fulminant form of disseminated intravascular coagulation, but in the recognition of milder forms and in the selection for therapy of patients with laboratory evidence of disseminated intravascular coagulation but who are not yet in serious hemostatic difficulty. There is an astonishing lack of controlled clinical data to assist in this decision.

Antithrombotic Therapy

Four classes of drugs are presently employed to treat or prevent thrombosis. Each class of agents has a fundamentally different therapeutic premise and a different mode of action.

Antiplatelet Agents. The premise of antiplatelet drug therapy is that by interfering with the sequence initiated by adhesion of platelets to exposed subendothelial tissue and the subsequent buildup of platelet fibrin masses these drugs will aid in preventing the formation and in retarding the growth of the arterial thrombus. Agents now in use have been selected to interfere with the platelet sequence after adherence to collagen, to minimize the risk of hemorrhage.

Aspirin acts by inhibiting platelet cyclo-oxygenase, resulting in the blockage of production of cyclic endoperoxides and thromboxanes that participate in platelet aggregation. ADP release is also impaired by aspirin, but at this time the link between platelet prostaglandin formation and ADP release is not known. The effect of aspirin is permanent for all platelets exposed to aspirin. Aspirin is readily absorbed, and it is also rapidly hydrolyzed in plasma, with a biologic half-life of approximately twenty minutes. The salicylate moiety itself does not affect platelets. Therefore a single dose of aspirin is a *pulse,* exposed to the platelets for a short period, but with effects lasting for the ten-day life span of the platelet. The hemostatic effect is apparent within one hour of ingestion and is detectable for at least four days. The major toxic effect of aspirin is a tendency to induce gastrointestinal bleeding, a manifestation both of its direct local action on the gastric mucosa and its systemic antiplatelet action. In some patients with mild underlying disorders of hemostasis (which may have escaped prior detection) aspirin ingestion may produce severe hemorrhage following trauma or surgery. Large doses of aspirin may cause severe metabolic abnormalities and other forms of salicylate toxicity (vertigo, tinnitus, nausea, fever, confusion) and may exacerbate or provoke hepatitis or asthma. These toxic effects ordinarily are not seen at the usual daily doses (600–1,200 mg) of aspirin administered for its antiplatelet action. The rare urticarial reaction provoked by aspirin can occur at any dose.

Sulfinpyrazone is a drug that has mild anti-inflammatory and uricosuric actions. It impairs the second phase of platelet aggregation, the release reaction, but the mechanism of its action is not firmly established. The drug is rapidly absorbed and has a plasma half-life of approximately 3 hours. Unlike aspirin, sulfinpyrazone affects platelets only when the drug is present in the plasma. Toxic reactions are rare.

Dipyridamole is a vasodilator that impairs the responsiveness of platelets to ADP, although it does not itself block the release reaction. The metabolism of dipyridamole has not been fully studied. Toxic reactions include nausea, vomiting, and headaches.

Available data have produced a mixed and often contradictory assessment of the usefulness of antiplatelet agents. The different drugs appear to have limited effectiveness at best. They are not interchangeable in different clinical settings. Dipyridamole, given in addition to the oral anticoagulant warfarin, reduces the incidence of peripheral arterial embolization from artificial heart valves. Aspirin alone is not effective but allows reduction of the dose of dipyridamole. Sulfinpyrazone reduces the incidence of thrombi in arteriovenous shunts placed for chronic hemodialysis. Mass trials of aspirin in the prevention of *recurring* myocardial infarction are now underway, but given the uncertainty of the role of thrombosis as the cause of myocardial infarction and the many factors that can cause death once infarction has occurred, prevention of primary occurrence may be a truer test of the effectiveness of aspirin. Such trials involve massive investments and require a high degree of patient compliance. Another problem may be the increased incidence of bleeding in mass aspirin trials.

Fibrinolytic Agents. The premise of fibrinolytic therapy is that by activating endogenous plasminogen bound to fibrin within the interstices of a thrombus, fibrinolytic agents produce local digestion of a thrombus (thrombolysis) but do not cause systemic fibrinogenolysis. A corollary of this premise is that fibrinolytic therapy has no prophylactic value but is intended only to attack an existing thrombus.

Streptokinase, a bacterial enzyme, converts plasminogen to plasmin. In the general circulation both streptokinase and plasmin are inhibited, but at the surface of a thrombus, or within it, streptokinase activates plasminogen locally, and the plasmin is theoretically protected from the antiplasmin in the general circulation. The enzyme must be given by continuous infusion. Toxic reactions include pyrogenic reactions and bleeding. Urokinase is a human enzyme excreted by the kidney. It has been isolated and purified from urine. It is similar in action to streptokinase but does not cause pyrogenic reactions.

Although theoretically attractive, fibrinolytic therapy has limited clinical value in practice; generalized activation of plasminogen occurs, leading to a distinct bleeding tendency. To data, no convincing data have been collected that demonstrate that fibrinolytic therapy decreases mortality or morbidity from pulmonary embolism or coronary thrombosis. Fibrinolytic therapy may enhance dissolution of peripheral venous thrombi, but the value of this effect (compared to its distinct toxicity) remains to be proved.

Ancrod Therapy. The premise of Malayan pit viper venom (Ancrod) therapy is that by rendering the patient essentially afibrinogenemic, the treatment blocks the deposition or extension of a venous thrombus. Ancrod cleaves the α-chain of fibrinogen, releasing fibrinopeptide A, but it also partially degrades the remaining α-chain of fibrin monomer. The abnormal fibrin clots in the microcirculation. These clots contain non-cross-linked fibrin. Activation of plasminogen occurs by a mechanism not yet established, and the abnormal fibrin clots are rapidly dissolved. The venom must be given by continuous infusion. Occasional pyrogenic reactions and a mild bleeding tendency are the major toxic effects. Clinical trials of Ancrod have been limited but do show it to be effective in preventing extension of venous thrombi. To date the superiority of Ancrod over conventional anticoagulant therapy has not been shown.

Anticoagulant Therapy. The premise of anticoagulant therapy is that by retarding the synthesis of certain clotting factors or by accelerating the inactivation of clotting factors anticoagulants prevent the deposition or extension of stasis, venous-type thrombi. A corollary of this premise is that anticoagulants have no effect on established thrombi and that all anticoagulant therapy is prophylactic.

Heparin is a naturally occurring sulfated polysaccharide consisting of hexuronic acid, acetylated glucosamine, and many sulfuric acid ester groups. Its average molecular weight lies between 8 and 10,000. The molecule is extremely acidic because of its high sulfuric acid content. Heparin binds to a plasma α-globulin, variously known as the heparin cofactor or antithrombin III. It thereby strikingly potentiates the inhibitory action of this protein on thrombin and on activated factors X, IX, XI, and XII. The effect on Factor X outweighs the effect on thrombin. Heparin is an active anticoagulant in vitro and in vivo. Following an intravenous dose of heparin, 20 to 25 percent is recoverable unchanged in the urine. Most of the remainder is degraded in the liver. A small amount may be taken up by mast cells. The rate of clearance from plasma is variable, but the average half-time is approximately one hour. The major toxic effect of heparin is bleeding, usually from mucus membranes and open wounds. A specific antidote for heparin is protamine sulfate. Other toxic effects of heparin include thrombocytopenia, alopecia, and, on prolonged usage, metabolic bone disease.

There is no standard "dose" of heparin. When it is given by intermittent intravenous injection, the dosage is usually about 5,000 units every four hours. When given by continuous intravenous infusion, heparin therapy must be controlled by a clotting assay. After an initial loading dose the usual dosage is approximately 1,000 units per hour. Recent studies have shown continuous infusion to cause less bleeding than intermittent injection. In *low dose heparin therapy* the drug is given subcutaneously, 5,000 units every 8 to 12 hours, theoretically to provide preferential inhibition of activated Factor X, thereby affording antithrombotic protection but less risk of bleeding.

The coumarins are a class of water-soluble derivatives of coumaric acid. The most commonly used coumarin is warfarin. The coumarins impair the action of vitamin K on the hepatic synthesis of Factors II, VII, IX, and X. The precise mechanism of coumarin action is unknown. Vitamin K is essential for the γ-carboxylation of glutamic acid residues in Factors II, VII, IX and X, required for the binding of calcium by those clotting factors. Warfarin is completely absorbed from the gut. It is transported in plasma bound to albumin, from which it can be displaced by more tightly bound drugs. It is degraded in the liver by enzymes localized on the endoplasmic reticulum. The clearance of warfarin from the plasma varies widely from person to person, and therefore the dose must be individualized. The drug is effective only in vivo. It crosses the placenta and also appears in maternal milk. Therapy is monitored with the prothrombin time. If hemorrhage occurs, warfarin is discontinued, and plasma and vitamin K_1 are given. Drug–drug interactions are a major cause of hemorrhage in patients receiving warfarin. Although bleeding is the major toxic reaction, rare instances of hemorrhagic plate-like infarction of the skin occur in patients receiving warfarin.

Warfarin and full-dose heparin clearly prevent recurring pulmonary embolism. Their use is mandatory in patients with pulmonary embolism in the absence of contraindications to anticoagulant therapy. Warfarin also reduces the incidence of peripheral embolization in patients with valvular stenoses and atrial fibrillation and in patients with artificial heart valves. One recent large scale trial of low dose heparin has shown that it is effective in reducing fatal postoperative pulmonary embolism. The role of heparin in the treatment of disseminated intravascular coagulation remains controversial.

CASE DEVELOPMENT PROBLEMS: HEMOSTASIS

Patient History No. 1

A physician from an outlying community calls you, as a consultant, to help him with the following problem. A young boy of 6 was struck in the thigh by a baseball and subsequently developed an extensive hematoma. He was admitted to a local hospital, where the hematoma was drained. Following the operation the patient bled profusely, requiring 4 units of blood to control the bleeding. The physician was puzzled, because a prothrombin time determination done before operation (as required by the hospital) was normal. After the operation prothrombin times had been done on blood samples from the patient's mother and father. Again, both were normal.

1. What screening tests would you request? What further elements of the history would you explore? What factors are tested for in the prothrombin time? What factors are not measured?

Screening tests include a careful history and physical examination, examination of the peripheral smear, and partial thromboplastin time and prothrombin time tests. In this case further history revealed that the mother's nephew had bled following dental extraction. The patient was taking no medication at the time. You request that as many members of the family as possible come in for testing. The following data are obtained:

	Partial Thromboplastin Times (sec.)
Normal	35
Patient	52
Father	35
Mother	34
Mother's sister	35
Sister's son (patient's cousin)	58

2. Can you suggest a specific diagnosis?

The pattern of inheritance suggests a sex-linked recessive transmission, consistent with either Factor VIII or Factor IX deficiency. In this instance the patient was found to have a Factor VIII level of 5 percent, confirming the diagnosis of mild hemophilia.

3. Can you predict what the Factor VIII protein levels would be in this family?

Patient History No. 2

You are an intern on duty at Marvel Medical School University Hospital. One of the nurses on your ward tells you that she has developed a painful, swollen, discolored ankle following a relatively minor sprain. Anxious to display your diagnostic prowess, you agree to find the cause of her hemarthrosis.

1. How would you proceed? What tests would you order?

The history reveals that the patient has not had any prior episode as severe as this. On occasion her menstrual periods are heavy. She takes no medications other than intermittent Alka-Seltzer for indigestion. The laboratory data that you obtain are as follows:

CBC (including platelet count): normal
Prothrombin time: normal
Partial thromboplastin time: normal

Perplexed, you wonder if *anything* is wrong with the patient's hemostatic mechanism.

2. What tests would you do now?

A bleeding time should be done to determine the integrity of the primary hemostatic mechanism. Alerted by the history, you should do a bleeding time before and after the patient ingests aspirin. In this instance the Ivy template bleeding time before aspirin was 4½ minutes; after aspirin it was 22 minutes.

3. Have you established the diagnosis as von Willebrand's disease?

No, you have not established the diagnosis. Any mild disorder of primary hemostasis will be unmasked by aspirin. The patient could have either mild von Willebrand's disease, or a disorder of platelet function.

4. How would you establish the diagnosis of von Willebrand's disease?

Patient History No. 3

The following vignettes are examples of frequently encountered mishaps. Formulate your concept of the errors in clinical management.

1. A 75-year-old retired bartender was admitted with crushing substernal chest pain radiating to the left arm. Electrocardiograms revealed the presence of an acute myocardial infarction. Physical examination revealed gynecomastia, a slightly enlarged liver, and bilateral ankle edema. There was slight tenderness to palpation in the right calf. Laboratory findings included prothrombin time 15 seconds (control 13 seconds), total protein 4.8 gm/100 ml (globulin 3.0, albumin 1.8). Examination of the peripheral smear was normal. The patient was given an oral dose of warfarin of 30 mgs. Two days later the patient developed gross melena. The prothrombin time was 67 seconds.

2. A 58-year-old businessman was admitted with a classic myocardial infarction. During the hospitalization he was treated with phenobarbital and warfarin, which was controlled by frequent determinations of the prothrombin time. He was discharged on maintenance doses of warfarin and was to see his private physician in 3 weeks. Two weeks following discharge the patient developed hematuria. The prothrombin time was 52 seconds.

3. A 34-year-old housewife, a known epileptic whose seizures had been well controlled with diphenylhydantoin, was admitted with symptoms suggestive of pulmonary embolism. She was treated initially with heparin and then with warfarin. Although she was found to be markedly sensitive to warfarin, her dose was finally established at 2.5 mg every other day. She was discharged to her home, but called her private physician in 3 weeks complaining of a staggering gait and swollen gums.

4. A 32-year-old hemophiliac was admitted at 1 P.M. for treatment of bleeding into his left knee joint. After vigorous therapy his bleeding stopped. At two A.M. the patient complained of residual pain in the joint, and the house officer on call, aware of a potential problem with addiction, prescribed aspirin. The following day, there was evidence of recurrent bleeding into the joint.

SELECTED REFERENCES

Platelets and Primary Hemostasis

Deykin, D. Emerging concepts of platelet function. *N. Engl. J. Med.* 290: 144, 1974.

Hamberg, M., Svensson, J., and Samuelsson, B. Thromboxanes: A new group of biologically active compounds derived from prostaglandin endoperoxides. *Proc. Natl. Acad. Sci. U.S.A.* 72:2994, 1975.

Harker, L. A. and Finch, C. A.: Thrombokinetics in man. *J. Clin. Invest.* 48:963, 1969.

Harrington, W. J., Minnich, V., Hollingsworth, J. W., and Moore, C. V. Demonstration of a thrombocytopenic factor in the blood of patients with thrombocytopenic purpura. *J. Lab. Clin. Med.* 38:1, 1951.

418

Hoyer, L. W.   Von Willebrand's disease. *Prog. Hemostasis Thromb.* 3:231, 1976.

Mueller-Eckhardt, C.   Idiopathic thrombocytopenic purpura (ITP): Clinical and immunologic considerations. *Semin. Thromb. Hemostasis* 3:125, 1977.

Weiss, H. J.   Platelet physiology and abnormalities of platelet function. *N. Engl. J. Med.* 293:531, 1975.

Zimmerman, T. S., Ratnoff, O. D., and Powell, A. E.   Immunologic differentiation of classic hemophilia (factor VIII deficiency) and von Willebrand's disease, with observations on combined deficiencies of antihemophilic factor and proaccelerin (factor V) and an acquired circulating anticoagulant against antihemophilic factor. *J. Clin. Invest.* 50:244, 1971.

Coagulation Mechanism

Aledort, L. M. (ed.)   Recent advances in hemophilia. *Ann. N.Y. Acad. Sci.* 240:1975.

Bennett, B.   Coagulation pathways: Interrelationships and control mechanisms. *Semin. Hematol.* 14:301, 1977.

Esnof, M. P.   Biochemistry of blood coagulation. *Br. Med. Bull.* 33:213, 1977.

Feinstein, D. I. and Rapaport, S. I.   Acquired inhibitors of blood coagulation. *Prog. Hemostasis Thromb.* 1:75, 1972.

Kaplan, A. P., Meier, H. L., and Mandle, R., Jr.   The Hageman factor-dependent pathways of coagulation, fibrinolysis and kinin generation. *Semin. Thromb. Hemostasis* 3:1, 1976.

Mammen, E. F. (ed.)   Fibrinogen. *Semin. Throm. Hemostasis* 1:1, 2, 1974.

Suttie, J. W., and Jackson, C. M.   Prothrombin structure, activation and biosynthesis. *Physiol. Rev.* 57:1, 1977.

Thrombosis and Antithrombotic Therapy

Deykin, D.   Thrombogenesis. *N. Engl. J. Med.* 276:622, 1967.

Deykin, D.   The clinical challenge of disseminated intravascular coagulation. *N. Engl. J. Med.* 283:636, 1970.

Deykin, D.   Warfarin therapy. *N. Engl. J. Med.* 283:801, 1970.

Deykin, D.   Heparin therapy: Regimens and management. *Drugs* 13:46, 1977.

Harker, L. A.   Inhibitors of platelet function in the prevention of arterial thrombosis. *Ser. Haematologica* 8:105, 1976.

Stenflo, J.   Vitamin K, prothrombin and γ-carboxyglutamic acid. *N. Engl. J. Med.* 296:624, 1977.

Index